OXFORD MEDICAL PUBLICATIONS

Emergencies in Anaesthesia

T0177520

Published and forthcoming titles in the Emergencies series:

OXFORD MEDICAL PUBLICATIONS

Emergencies in Anaesthesia

THIRD EDITION

EDITED BY

Alastair Martin FRCA

Consultant Anaesthetist,
Royal Devon and Exeter NHS Foundation Trust, UK

Keith G. Allman MD FRCA

Consultant Anaesthetist,
Royal Devon and Exeter NHS Foundation Trust, UK

Andrew K. McIndoe FRCA

Consultant Anaesthetist and Senior Clinical Lecturer,
University Hospitals Bristol NHS Foundation Trust, UK

OXFORD
UNIVERSITY PRESS

OXFORD
UNIVERSITY PRESS

Great Clarendon Street, Oxford, OX2 6DP,
United Kingdom

Oxford University Press is a department of the University of Oxford.
It furthers the University's objective of excellence in research, scholarship,
and education by publishing worldwide. Oxford is a registered trade mark of
Oxford University Press in the UK and in certain other countries

© Oxford University Press 2020

The moral rights of the authors have been asserted

First Edition published in 2005
Second Edition published in 2009
Third Edition published in 2020

Published in the United States of America by Oxford University Press
198 Madison Avenue, New York, NY 10016, United States of America

British Library Cataloguing in Publication Data
Data available

Library of Congress Control Number: 2020935854

ISBN 978–0–19–875814–3

Printed and bound in Great Britain by
Ashford Colour Press Ltd.

Oxford University Press makes no representation, express or implied, that the
drug dosages in this book are correct. Readers must therefore always check
the product information and clinical procedures with the most up-to-date
published product information and data sheets provided by the manufacturers
and the most recent codes of conduct and safety regulations. The authors and
the publishers do not accept responsibility or legal liability for any errors in the
text or for the misuse or misapplication of material in this work. Except where
otherwise stated, drug dosages and recommendations are for the non-pregnant
adult who is not breast-feeding

Links to third party websites are provided by Oxford in good faith and
for information only. Oxford disclaims any responsibility for the materials
contained in any third party website referenced in this work.

Preface to the third edition

Welcome to this, the third edition of *Emergencies in Anaesthesia* and welcome also to our new Editor, Alastair Martin, who has taken on the onerous task of revamping this latest version.

Emergencies in Anaesthesia has been written to help anaesthetists anticipate different emergency situations that may arise in the various areas of anaesthetic practice. We have described topics that may need to be managed immediately or as soon as practicable and these include problems that may arise preoperatively, in theatre, or in recovery.

The successful management of any emergency arising during anaesthesia depends on the anaesthetist and their team reacting in a calm and logical way. Our ability to do this is much improved by experience, training, and preparation of both the individual and the team. Preparation for emergencies includes gaining the correct knowledge, skills, equipment and help, and protocols can provide a structure which helps us to focus and treat the likeliest causes, while remembering to exclude the rare.

We hope that *Emergencies in Anaesthesia* will stimulate readers to reflect on their knowledge and readiness to deal with any of the situations discussed. Additionally, since dealing with emergencies requires all members of the team to help, and for the theatres to be properly equipped, this book may serve to remind us what developments we need in our workplace. Dealing with the unexpected is always made easier by effective planning.

We would especially like to thank all our authors for their excellent work and, of course, our families for their continued support.

Alastair Martin
Keith G. Allman
Andrew K. McIndoe
February 2020

Contents

Contents

Abbreviations

P	primary
S	secondary
A–A	Alveolar–arterial
AAA	abdominal aortic aneurysm
AAGBI	Association of Anaesthetists of Great Britain and Ireland
ABC	Airway, Breathing, Circulation
ABGS	arterial blood gases
A&E	accident and emergency
ACE	angiotensin-converting enzyme
ACH	acetylcholine
ACHE	acetylcholinesterase
ACS	acute coronary syndrome
ACTH	adrenocorticotrophic hormone
ADH	antidiuretic hormone
ADP	accidental dural puncture
AEC	airway exchange catheter
AEDS	automated external defibrillators
AF	atrial fibrillation
AFE	amniotic fluid embolus
AHF	acute heart failure
AIDS	acquired immune deficiency syndrome
ALF	acute liver failure
ALI	acute lung injury
ALS	advanced life support
ALT	alanine aminotransferase
APL	automatic pressure limiting
APTR	activated partial thromboplastin ratio
APTT	activated partial thromboplastin time
ARDS	acute respiratory distress syndrome
ARF	acute renal failure
ASA	American Society of Anesthesiologists

ASAP	as soon as possible
AST	aspartate transaminase
ATLS	advanced trauma life support
ATN	acute tubular necrosis
AV	atrioventricular/arteriovenous
AVM	arteriovenous malformation
AXR	abdominal X-ray
BAL	bronchoalveolar lavage
BB	bronchial blockers
BCIS	bone cement implantation syndrome
BD	twice daily
BE	base excess
BIPAP	biphasic positive airway pressure
BLS	basic life support
BM	'blood sugar'
BMI	body mass index
BNP	b[rain]-natriuretic peptide
BP	blood pressure
BPF	bronchopleural fistula
BPM	beats per minute
BSA	body surface area
BTS	British Thoracic Society
BURP	Backwards, Upwards, Rightwards Pressure
CBF	cerebral blood flow
CCF	congestive cardiac failure
CCU	coronary care unit/critical care unit
CEA	carotid endarterectomy
CI	cardiac index
CICV	can't intubate ... can't ventilate
CK	creatine kinase
CK-MB	creatine kinase MB isoenzyme
CMV	cytomegalovirus
CNS	central nervous system

CO	cardiac output	ECM	external cardiac massage
COHB	carboxyhaemoglobin	ECMO	extracorporeal membrane oxygenation
COPD	chronic obstructive pulmonary disease	ECT	electroconvulsive therapy
CPAP	continuous positive airways pressure	ED	external diameter; emergency department
CPB	cardiopulmonary bypass	EDTA	ethylenediamine tetra-acetic acid
CPP	cerebral perfusion pressure	EEG	electroencephalogram
CPR	cardiopulmonary resuscitation	EMLA	eutectic mixture of local anaesthetics
CRP	C-reactive protein	ENT	ear, nose, throat
CS	Caesarean section	ERPC	evacuation of retained products of conception
CSE	combined spinal/epidural	ET	endotracheal
CSF	cerebrospinal fluid	$ETCO_2$	end-tidal CO_2
CSM	Committee on Safety of Medicines	ETT	endotracheal tube
CSW	cerebral salt-wasting	EU	European Union
CSWS	cerebral salt-wasting syndrome	EUA	examination under anaesthetic
CT	computed tomography	FAST	Focused Assessment with Sonography for Trauma
CTPA	computed tomography pulmonary angiogram	FB	foreign body
CV	central venous	FBAO	foreign body airway obstruction
CVC	central venous catheter	FBC	full blood count
CVE	cerebrovascular episode	FEV_1	forced expiratory volume in 1 second
CVP	central venous pressure	FFP	fresh frozen plasma
CVS	cardiovascular system	FGF	fresh gas flow
CXR	chest X-ray	F_IAA	inspired fraction of anaesthetic agent
DAS	Difficult Airway Society	F_IO_2	inspired fraction of O_2
DBS	double-burst stimulation	FOB	fibreoptic bronchoscope
DC	direct current	FOI	fibreoptic intubation
DDAVP	1-deamino-8-D-arginine vasopressin	FONA	front of neck access
DHI	dynamic hyperinflation	FRC	functional residual capacity
DI	diabetes insipidus	FT_c	corrected flow time
DIC	disseminated intravascular coagulation	GA	general anaesthesia
DKA	diabetic ketoacidosis	G&S	group and save
DLT	double-lumen tube	GCS	Glasgow coma scale
DMV	difficult mask ventilation	GFR	glomular filtration rate
DNAR	do not attempt resuscitation	GI	gastrointestinal
DVT	deep vein thrombosis	GIT	gastrointestinal tract
ECG	electrocardiogram		

G-6-PD	glucose-6-phosphate dehydrogenase		IVRA	intravenous regional anaesthesia
GTN	glyceryl trinitrate		JVP	jugular venous pressure
GU	genitourinary		KCL	potassium chloride
HB	haemoglobin		LA	local anaesthetic/left atrium
HBV	hepatitis B virus		LBBB	left bundle branch block
HCV	hepatitis C virus		LFT	liver function test
HDU	high dependency unit		LMA	laryngeal mask airway
HIB	*Haemophilus influenzae b* (vaccine)		LMWH	low molecular weight heparin
			LOC	loss of consciousness
HIV	human immunodeficiency virus		LSCS	lower segment Caesarean section
HME	heat and moisture exchanger		LV	left ventricle
HR	heart rate		LVAD	left ventricular assist device
IA	intra-arterial		LVF	left ventricular failure
IAP	intra-abdominal pressure		LVH	left ventricular hypertrophy
IBP	invasive blood pressure monitoring		LVSWI	left ventricular stroke work index
ICD	implantable cardioverter defibrillator		MA	mean acceleration
			MAC	minimum alveolar concentration
ICH	intracerebral haemorrhage		MAOIS	monoamine oxidase inhibitors
ICP	intracranial pressure		MAP	mean arterial pressure
ICS	Intensive Care Society		MC&S	microscopy, culture and sensitivity
ICU	intensive care unit			
ID	internal diameter		MDI	metered dose inhaler
IGE	immunoglobulin E		MEN	multiple endocrine neoplasia
ILCOR	International Liaison Committee on Resuscitation		METHB	methaemoglobin
			MH	malignant hyperthermia
I:E RATIO	inspiratory:expiratory ratio		MHRA	Medicines and Healthcare products Regulatory Agency
IHD	ischaemic heart disease			
ILMA	intubating laryngeal mask airway		MI	myocardial infarction
			MRI	magnetic resonance imaging
IM	intramuscular(ly)		MSU	midstream urine
INR	international normalized ratio		NAI	non-accidental injury
IO	intraosseous		NG	nasogastric
IPPV	intermittent positive pressure ventilation		NHS	National Health Service
			NIBP	non-invasive blood pressure
ITU	intensive therapy unit		NICE	National Institute for Health and Care Excellence
IU	international units			
IV	intravenous		NIDDM	non-insulin-dependent diabetes mellitus
IVC	inferior vena cava			
IVCT	*in vitro* contracture testing			
IVI	intravenous infusion			

NRLS	National Reporting and Learning System	PEP	postexposure prophylaxis
NSAIDS	non-steroidal anti-inflammatory drugs	PICC	peripherally inserted central catheter
NSTEACS	non-ST segment elevation acute coronary syndromes	PICCO	pulse contour cardiac output
NSTEMI	non-ST elevation myocardial infarction	PICU	paediatric intensive care unit
OD	once daily	PIH	pregnancy-induced hypertension
ODP	operating department practitioner	PLMA	ProSeal LMA
		PO	by mouth
OGD	oesophago-gastroduodenoscopy	PO_2	partial pressure O_2
OLV	one-lung ventilation	PONV	postoperative nausea and vomiting
OMV	Oxford Miniature Vaporizer	PPI	proton pump inhibitor
PA	pulmonary artery	PR	per rectum
PABA	para-aminobenzoic acid	PRN	when required
PAC	pulmonary artery catheter	PT	prothrombin
$PACO_2$	partial pressure arterial CO_2	PTH	parathyroid hormone
PACU	post-anaesthetic care unit	PTT	partial thromboplastin time
PAFC	pulmonary artery flotation catheter	PUD	peptic ulcer disease
		PV	peak velocity
PALS	paediatric advanced life support	PVR	pulmonary vascular resistance
		QDS	four times daily
PAO_2	partial pressure arterial O_2	QSOFA	quick sepsis-related organ failure assessment
PAP	positive airways pressure/pulmonary artery pressure	RA	right atrium
P_{aw}	airway pressure	RAE	Ring–Adair–Elwyn
PAWP/PAOP	pulmonary artery wedge pressure/pulmonary artery occlusion pressure	RBBB	right bundle branch block
		RBC	red blood cell(s)
		RF	recombinant factor
PBLS	paediatric basic life support	ROSC	return of spontaneous circulation
PCA	patient-controlled analgesia		
PCI	percutaneous coronary intervention	RS	respiratory system
		RSI	rapid sequence induction
PCV	pressure-controlled ventilation	RTA	road traffic accident/motor vehicle accident
PCWP	pulmonary capillary wedge pressure		
		RUL	right upper lobe
PDPH	postdural puncture headache	RV	right ventricle
PE	pulmonary embolism/phenytoin equivalents	SAD	supraglottic airway device
		SAG-M	saline adenine glucose–mannitol
PEA	pulseless electrical activity	SAH	subarachnoid haemorrhage
PEEP	positive end-expiratory pressure	SAO_2	arterial oxygen saturation
PEFR	peak expiratory flow rate	SBCU	special baby care unit

SC	subcutaneous(ly)
SCD	sickle cell disease
SCI	spinal cord injury
ScvO$_2$	central venous O$_2$ saturation
SD	stroke distance
SHOT	Serious Hazards of Transfusion
SIADH	syndrome of inappropriate antidiuretic hormone secretion
SIRS	systemic inflammatory response syndrome
SL	sublingual
SLE	systemic lupus erythematosus
SLT	single-lumen endotracheal tube
SNP	sodium nitroprusside
SOFA	sepsis-related organ failure assessment
SPO$_2$	peripheral oxygen saturation
SSRI	selective serotonin-reuptake inhibitor
STEMI	ST elevation myocardial infarction
SV	stroke volume
SVC	superior vena cava
SVI	stroke volume index
SVR	systemic vascular resistance
SVRI	systemic vascular resistance index
SVT	supraventricular tachycardia
T$_3$	tri-iodothyronine
T$_4$	thyroxine
TAVI	transcatheter aortic valve implantation
TB	tuberculosis
TBW	total body water
TCA	tricyclic antidepressants
TCI	target controlled infusion
TC/XE	technetium/xenon
TDS	three times daily

TEDS	thromboembolism deterrent stockings
TEG	thromboelastography
TFTS	thyroid function tests
TIA	transient ischaemic attack
TIVA	total intravenous anaesthesia
TMJ	temporomandibular joint
TOE	transoesophageal echocardiography
TOF	train-of-four
T-PA	tissue plasminogen activator
TPN	total parenteral nutrition
TRALI	transfusion-related acute lung injury
TSH	thyroid stimulating hormone
TT	tracheal tube
TURP	transurethral resection of the prostate
U	unit
U&ES	urea and electrolytes
URTI	urinary tract infection
US	ultrasound
USS	ultrasound scan
UTI	urinary tract infection
UV	ultraviolet
VATS	video-assisted thoracoscopy
VES	ventricular ectopics
VF	ventricular fibrillation
VOO	ventricular asynchronous
VP	ventriculoperitoneal (shunt)
VSD	ventricular septal defect
VT	tidal volume
VT	ventricular tachycardia
VTE	venous thromboembolism
WFNS	World Federation of Neurological Surgeons
WHO	World Health Organization
WPW	Wolff–Parkinson–White (syndrome)
YAG	yttrium–aluminium–garnet (laser)

Note on drug dosages

Some of the drugs and dosages are suggested outside of those stated in the British National Formulary (BNF) because the book describes the use of drugs in specialist situations. Always refer to the BNF and product literature before using any drug with which you are unfamiliar.

Contributors to the third edition

James Bennett
Consultant Anaesthetist,
Conquest Hospital, East Sussex
Healthcare NHS Trust, Hastings,
United Kingdom

Jim Blackburn
Anaesthesia, North Bristol NHS
Trust, Honorary Associate
Lecturer, University of Bristol,
United Kingdom

Hannah Blanshard
Consultant in Anaesthesia,
University Hospitals Bristol NHS
Foundation Trust, Bristol, United
Kingdom

Tim Cook
Consultant in Anaesthesia and
Intensive Care Medicine, Royal
United Hospital, Bath, United
Kingdom

Louise Cossey
Anaesthetic Registrar, University
Hospitals Plymouth NHS Trust,
Plymouth, United Kingdom

Jules Cranshaw
Consultant in Anaesthesia
and Intensive Care Medicine,
Royal Bournemouth Hospital,
Bournemouth, United Kingdom

Owen Davies
Consultant Anaesthetist,
Christchurch Public Hospital,
Christchurch, New Zealand

Craig Dunlop
Consultant in Cardiothoracic
Anaesthesia and Intensive Care
Medicine, University Hospitals
Plymouth NHS Trust, Plymouth,
United Kingdom

Charles Gibson
Consultant in Anaesthesia
and Intensive Care Medicine,
Royal Devon and Exeter NHS
Foundation Trust, Exeter, United
Kingdom

Gerard Gould
Consultant Anaesthetist,
Conquest Hospital, East Sussex
NHS Trust, Hastings, United
Kingdom

Kim J. Gupta
Consultant in Anaesthesia
and Intensive Care Medicine,
Royal United Hospital NHS
Trust, Bath, United Kingdom

Katharine Hunt
Consultant Neuroanaesthetist,
National Hospital for Neurology
and Neurosurgery, University
College London Hospitals,
London, United Kingdom

John Isaac
Consultant Anaesthetist,
University Hospitals Birmingham
NHS Foundation Trust,
Birmingham, United Kingdom

Michael Kinsella
Consultant Obstetric
Anaesthetist, St. Michael's
Hospital, University Hospitals
Bristol NHS Foundation Trust,
Bristol, United Kingdom

Daniel Lutman
Chief of Heart and Lung,
Children's Acute Transport
Consultant, Great Ormond
Street Children's Hospital,
London, United Kingdom

Bruce McCormick
Consultant Anaesthetist,
Royal Devon and Exeter NHS
Foundation Trust, Exeter, United
Kingdom

Simon Mercer
Director of Medical Education,
Liverpool University Hospitals
NHS Foundation Trust, Aintree
University Hospital, Liverpool,
United Kingdom

Jerry Nolan
Consultant in Anaesthesia and
Intensive Care Medicine, Royal
United Hospital, Bath; Professor
of Resuscitation Medicine,
University of Warwick,
Warwick, United Kingdom

Neil Rasburn
Consultant Anaesthetist,
University Hospitals Bristol NHS
Foundation Trust, Bristol, United
Kingdom

Mark Scrutton
Consultant Obstetric
Anaesthetist, St. Michael's
Hospital University Hospitals
Bristol NHS Foundation Trust,
Bristol, United Kingdom

Mark Stoneham
Consultant Anaesthetist and
Honorary Clinical Senior
Lecturer, Nuffield Department
of Anaesthetics, Oxford, United
Kingdom

Kath Sutherland
Specialty Registrar in
Anaesthesia, Bristol Royal
Children's Hospital, University
Hospitals Bristol NHS
Foundation Trust, Bristol, United
Kingdom

Benjamin Walton
Consultant in ICM and
Anaesthesia, North Bristol NHS
Trust, Bristol, United Kingdom

Manni Waraich
Consultant in Neurointensive
Care & Neuroanaesthetics,
National Hospital for Neurology
and Neurosurgery, University
College London Hospitals,
London, United Kingdom

Nerida Williams
Intensive Care Registrar,
National Capital Private
Hospital, Canberra, Australia

Contributors to the first edition

Ciara Ambrose
Specialist Registrar in Anaesthesia, Southmead Hospital, Bristol, United Kingdom

Davinia Bennett
Fellow in Liver Transplant, Anaesthesia and Intensive Care, Queen Elizabeth Hospital, University of Birmingham NHS Trust, Birmingham, United Kingdom

Colin Berry
Consultant Anaesthetist, Royal Devon and Exeter NHS Trust, Exeter, United Kingdom

Hannah Blanshard
Specialist Registrar in Anaesthesia, Bristol Royal Infirmary, Bristol, United Kingdom

Elaine Boyle
Specialist Registrar, Neonatal Unit, Royal Infirmary of Edinburgh, Edinburgh, United Kingdom

Tim Cook
Consultant Anaesthetist, Royal United Hospital, Bath, United Kingdom

Jules Cranshaw
Specialist Registrar in Anaesthesia, Bristol Royal Infirmary, Bristol, United Kingdom

R.D. Evans
Reader, University of Oxford, Nuffield Department of Anaesthetics, Radcliffe Infirmary, Oxford, United Kingdom

Gerard Gould
Fellow in Thoracic Anaesthesia, Guy's and St Thomas' Hospital, London, United Kingdom

Kim J. Gupta
Consultant Anaesthetist, Bath, United Kingdom

Katharine Hunt
Consultant Neuroanaesthetist, National Hospital for Neurology and Neurosurgery, London, United Kingdom

John Isaac
Consultant Anaesthetist, University Hospital, Birmingham, United Kingdom

Michael Kinsella
Consultant Obstetric Anaesthetist, United Bristol Healthcare NHS Trust, Bristol, United Kingdom

Chris Langrish
Specialist Registrar in Anaesthesia, Bristol, United Kingdom

Stephen J. Mather
Consultant in Anaesthesia and Perioperative Medicine, United Bristol Healthcare NHS Trust, Bristol, United Kingdom

Bruce McCormick
Senior Lecturer, Queen Elizabeth Hospital, Balantyre, Malawi, Africa; Specialist Registrar in Anaesthesia and Intensive Care Medicine, Frenchay Hospital, Bristol, United Kingdom

Jerry Nolan
Consultant in Anaesthesia and Intensive Care Medicine, Bath, United Kingdom

Aidan O'Donnell
Specialist Registrar in Anaesthesia, Royal Infirmary of Edinburgh, Edinburgh, United Kingdom

Adrian Pearce
Consultant Anaesthetist, Guy's and St Thomas' Hospital, London, United Kingdom

Richard H. Riley
Clinical Associate Professor of Anaesthesia, University of Western Australia, Australia

Mark Scrutton
Consultant Obstetric Anaesthetist, United Bristol Healthcare NHS Trust, Bristol, United Kingdom

Martin Smith
Consultant Neuroanaesthetist and Honorary Lecturer in Anaesthesia, National Hospital for Neurology and Neurosurgery, London, United Kingdom

Ben Stenson
Consultant Neonatologist, Royal Infirmary of Edinburgh, Edinburgh, United Kingdom

Mark Stoneham
Consultant Anaesthetist and Honorary Clinical Senior Lecturer, Nuffield Department of Anaesthetics, Oxford, United Kingdom

Ranjit Verma
Consultant Anaesthetist, Derby City General Hospital, Derby, United Kingdom

Benjamin Walton
Specialist Registrar in Anaesthesia, Bristol, United Kingdom

David Wilkinson
Anaesthetic Practitioner, Royal Devon and Exeter NHS Trust, Exeter, United Kingdom

Chapter 1

Crisis management and human factors

Simon Mercer

⑦ Human factors

Introduction

The roles human factors play in the management of emergencies and crisis situations are becoming increasingly recognized in healthcare. They have gained political momentum following a concordat from the National Quality Board in 2013.

Human factors are described as 'the cognitive, social, and personal resource skills that complement technical skills and contribute to safe and efficient task performance'.

The terms human factors, crisis resource management, and non-technical skills are often interchangeable. They are in a sense the study of how interactions between organizations, tasks, and the individual worker impact on human behaviour and affect systems performance. Many patient safety incidents are related to a lack of attention to human factors and the way that our systems are designed.

In 2011, the 4th National Audit Project of the Royal College of Anaesthetists and the Difficult Airway Society reported on major complications of airway management in the United Kingdom. Specific human factor failures were identified as contributory and these included failures of communication, decision-making, and leadership. A further analysis revealed that there may have been problems with up to four human factors in each reportable case. In another high-profile case, human factors were implicated in the death of a patient attributable to how the anaesthetic was conducted and the behaviours of those in the anaesthetic room.

A change in culture is required to ensure that human factors are adopted throughout healthcare organizations and that systems are designed to avoid 'latent organizational failures'.

Further reading

Bromiley, M. (2008). Have you ever made a mistake? *Bulletin of the Royal College of Anaesthetists*, **48**, 2442–5.

Carayon, P., Xie, A., Kianfar S. (2014). Human factors and ergonomics as a patient safety practice. *BMJ Quality & Safety*, **23**, 196–205.

Department of Health (2000). *An Organisation with a Memory*. London, UK: Department of Health.

Fletcher, G., McGeorge, P., Flin, R.H., Glavin, R.J., Maran, N.J. (2002). The role of non-technical skills in anaesthesia: a review of current literature. *British Journal of Anaesthesia*, **88**, 418–29.

Flin, R.H., O'Connor, P., Crichton, M. (2008). *Safety at the Sharp End: A Guide to Non-Technical Skills*. Farnham, UK: Ashgate Publishing, Ltd.

NHS England. *Human Factors in Healthcare—A Concordat from the National Quality Board*. Available at: http://www.england.nhs.uk/wp-content/uploads/2013/11/nqb-hum-fact-concord.pdf

① Preparation prior to an emergency

It is vital to involve the whole team in crisis management simulation and training. Regular 'in situ' drills allow for the practice of many common emergencies.

Although many emergencies cannot be planned for, if there is time then the following should be considered:

Preparation for an on-call event will include confirming

☑ Where am I supposed to go (where is the emergency dept?)
☑ Who is assisting me on this shift? Who is my consultant on call?
☑ Who else is available to help me?
☑ What bleep number is the operating department practitioner (ODP) available on?
☑ What are the other key numbers required?
  • Transfusion
  • Critical care
  • Emergency theatre coordinator
☑ Are there any specific standard operating procedures I need to be aware of?
☑ Is there any equipment I need to be familiar with?
  • Rapid infuser
  • Anaesthetic machine
  • Infusion pumps
  • Ventilators

Standard operating procedures

Standard operating procedures (SOPs), protocols, and checklists are very useful as aide-mémoires in a crisis situation and can reduce errors, particularly drug errors. Anaesthesia as a specialty has several national peer-reviewed SOPs for emergencies that individuals should be familiar with. These include:
• Anaphylaxis
• Malignant hyperthermia
• Can't Intubate, Can't Ventilate
• Local Anaesthetic Toxicity
• Resuscitation Council Guidelines
• Massive Haemorrhage

WHO checklist

This is a specific checklist that should be completed prior to surgery starting (the **sign in**), before the surgical incision (the **timeout**) and at the end of surgery (the **sign out**). This three-part checklist has been reported to cut deaths by more than 40% and complications by more than one-third.

It allows the whole team to be aware of the patient, the operation, and any special circumstances, ensuring the same mental model is followed by the whole team. It provides an opportunity to raise concerns and mitigates 'Never Events'.

Among other things, The WHO checklist ensures:
- All members of the team know who everyone is.
- The correct patient is receiving the correct operation.
- Relevant investigations are available (imaging, group & save).
- Patient allergy status is confirmed.
- Antibiotic prophylaxis has been considered.
- Any equipment concerns.
- Any specific concerns about the surgery that the surgeon wishes to make the team aware of.
- Any recovery issues.

Preparing to receive a trauma patient or standby patient

- ☑ Determine the team leader.
- ☑ Designate roles and responsibilities.
- ☑ Call for additional help if required (senior help might be away from the hospital out of hours).
- ☑ Conduct a team brief based on the pre-hospital alert—this will outline the likely mental model (or the likely course of events).
- ☑ Consider drawing up a 'wet pack' of drugs (this will include induction agent, muscle relaxants, opiates, and others anticipated drugs such as antibiotics and tranexamic acid).
- ☑ Consider setting up additional equipment such as a rapid infuser.
- ☑ Contacting other agencies in the hospital such as theatres, intensive care, radiology, and transfusion.
- ☑ In some hospitals the CT scanner might need to be turned on.
- ☑ Transfusion might need to plan for additional blood products from the regional network.
- ☑ The theatre coordinator might be required to prepare an operating theatre.

Further reading

Arbous, M.S., Meursing, A.E., van Kleef, J.W., et al. (2005). Impact of anesthesia management characteristics on severe morbidity and mortality. *Anesthesiology*, **102**, 257–68.

Gaba, D.M. (2010). Crisis resource management and teamwork training in anaesthesia. *British Journal of Anaesthesia*, **105**, 3–6.

Haynes, A.B., Weiser, T.G., Berry, W.R., et al. (2009). A surgical safety checklist to reduce morbidity and mortality in a global population. *New England Journal of Medicine*, **360**, 491–9.

NHS England (2018). *Never Events Policy and Framework*. Available at: https://improvement.nhs.uk/documents/2265/Revised_Never_Events_policy_and_framework_FINAL.pdf

⚙ During the incident

Key human factors are important to ensure that an anaesthetist can function during an emergency or critical incident. Seek help at the earliest opportunity.

Situational awareness

This is a dynamic state and it is vital that the lead anaesthetist maintains situational awareness at all times to avoid being 'caught out'.

Three elements have been described:
1. Perception of elements in the environment.
2. Comprehension of the current situation.
3. Projection of the future status.

or more simply:
1. **Gathering information**—from the pre-hospital alert, the patient handover, the monitors, patient history (and previous case notes), blood tests (ABGs), imaging (X-rays, scans, and ultrasound).
2. **Making sense of the information according to a mental model.** (For example, a patient with a Glasgow coma scale (GCS) of 3/15 follow a head injury will require intubation, ventilation, and then a CT scan).
3. **Anticipating and planning for the future.** (For example, following a CT scan a patient with a head injury might need transferring for neurosurgery).

Situational awareness can be lost at any of these stages:
- Errors in gathering information.
- Misinterpretation of the information.
- Failure to act on the information received.
- Failure to plan ahead.

In addition to these, situational awareness can be lost due to:
- Poor leadership (lack of guidance, conflict in the team).
- Distractions (noisy environment, interruptions, overloading from numerous alarms).
- Ambiguity in the information gathered (e.g. a historical normal blood pressure reading being assumed to be current in conjunction with an extreme tachycardia in trauma).
- Fixation on one particular task (e.g. intubation or arterial cannulation).
- Involuntary automaticity (seeing what you expect to see and not looking further).

It is important that thoughts are verbalized so that the team know what the leader is thinking. Maintain situational awareness by:

☑ Stepping back and maintaining 'an all-round look'.
☑ Not being drawn into performing a technical task.
☑ Handing over the leadership with a formal handover if the leader is the only person able to fulfil a technical task (e.g. intubation). The leadership can be returned once the task is completed.
☑ Verbalizing thoughts and reviewing actions.
☑ Updating the team at regular intervals.

Leadership

It is important that the team know who the leader is, and this must be announced if there is any ambiguity. The leader is responsible for:

☑ Task allocation and prioritization.
☑ Coordination of tasks.
☑ Planning ahead.
☑ Motivating, encouraging.
☑ Maintaining situational awareness by standing back and not being drawn into performing a technical role.

Communication

During an emergency or critical incident, good communication is vital. When under stress, individuals can become quiet and this can hinder communication. Communication can be improved by:

☑ Limiting the noise in the area (this requires discipline).
☑ Ensuring that communication flows from the leader to the followers and vice-versa.
☑ Allocating tasks to people by their name or pointing to them instead of just asking generalized questions.
☑ Ensuring that instructions are understood by using feedback loops (i.e. a team member receiving a task repeats the instruction back to the leader and then informs the leader once the task is completed).
☑ Using 'sit reps' (short updates) to ensure that team members involved in technical tasks maintain situational awareness.

When requesting help, use a structured system such as SBAR:

● S Situation
● B Background
● A Assessment
● R Recommendation

The UK Defence Medical Services have developed the mnemonic **TBCS** to conduct a brief 'sit-rep' (or update) during damage control resuscitation every 10–30 min:

● T—Time since the start of surgery.
● B—**B**lood (units given & rate of transfusion) and **B**lood gas results.
● C—**C**lotting (from the RoTEM™) & **C**old (current temperature).
● S—Surgical progress or discussions on new surgical plan.

Teamwork

Emergency teams often have the following characteristics
- They are multidisciplinary with individuals having different roles.
- They have a common goal (e.g. stabilizing a critically ill patient).
- They have a limited lifespan (i.e. members have other roles to return to once the team goal is achieved).

They are also obliged to ensure that
- They support each other.
- Work through any conflicts that arise during the crisis situation.
- Exchange information effectively.
- Coordinate activities that are required to perform the task.

Decision-making

Decision-making can utilize the following:
- Recognition-primed (e.g. based on previous experiences).
- Rule-based (e.g. use preprepared guidelines and protocols).
- Option appraisal.
- Solution generation or creative decision-making.

Further reading

Endsley, M.R. (1995). Toward a theory of situation awareness in dynamic systems. *Human Factors: The Journal of the Human Factors and Ergonomics Society*, **37**, 32–64.

Fortune, P.-M., Davis, M., Hanson, J., Phillips, B. (2012). *Human Factors in the Health Care Setting: A Pocket Guide for Clinical Instructors*. New York, NY: John Wiley & Sons, Ch. 7, p. 59.

Pierre, M.S., Hofinger, G., Buerschaper, C., Simon, R. (2011). *Crisis Management in Acute Care Settings*, 2nd edition. Cham, Switzerland: Springer.

Rall, M., Glavin, R.J., Flin, R. (2008). The '10-seconds-for-10-minutes principle'. Why things go wrong and stopping them get worse. *Bulletin of the Royal College of Anaesthetists*, **51**, 2614–16.

Toft, B., Mascie-Taylor, H. (2005). Involuntary automaticity: a work-system induced risk to safe health care. *Health Services Management Research*, **18**, 211–16.

⑦ After the incident

Debriefing

Debriefing is very important after the event has taken place. Experiential learning allows individuals the opportunity to review what has happened and then focus on what their actions will be in the future. The Association of Anaesthetists of Great Britain and Ireland have produced guidelines on dealing with the aftermath of a catastrophe and the tasks that must take place.

The person conducting the debrief should try to:

- ☑ Arrange the debrief as soon as possible after the event.
- ☑ Hold the debrief in a quiet and private room away from the clinical environment.
- ☑ Conduct the debrief in a calm atmosphere (this might be difficult after a stressful event).
- ☑ Ensure all involved have a chance to speak and if necessary 'air their grievances'.
- ☑ Ensure what is said is constructive.
- ☑ Ensure the debrief covers all the issues that people wish to discuss.
- ☑ Ensure the debrief is done in a manner that is not confrontational and that people don't feel they are being singled out.
- ☑ Draw everything together at the end of the debrief and summarize the key points.

It might be necessary to arrange for a further debrief to take place at a later date.

Further reading

Association of Anaesthetists. *Catastrophes in Anaesthetic Practice*. Available at: http://www.aagbi. org/sites/default/files/catastrophes05.pdf

Cardiovascular

Jerry Nolan and Craig Dunlop

☠: Asystole and pulseless electrical activity (PEA)

Definition
Asystole: Cardiac arrest associated with the absence of cardiac electrical activity.
PEA: Cardiac arrest associated with organized cardiac electrical activity.

Presentation
- **Asystole:** No electrical activity on the ECG—the baseline usually undulates slowly on the monitor. No palpable central pulses (carotid or femoral). Occasionally, atrial electrical activity continues in the absence of ventricular electrical activity. This 'P-wave asystole' may respond to electrical pacing.
- **PEA:** Organized electrical ECG activity which would normally be consistent with a pulse. No palpable central pulses (carotid or femoral).

Immediate management
(➲ See Figures 2.1 and 2.2 (adult in-hospital resuscitation and ALS algorithms, respectively), pp. 12, 13.)
- ☑ Stop any surgical activity likely to be causing excessive vagal stimulation (e.g. traction on peritoneum).
- ☑ Establish clear airway and ventilate with 100% oxygen.
- ☑ Give chest compressions at 100–120 per min—if a tracheal tube or supraglottic airway is in situ, do not interrupt compressions for ventilation.
- ☑ The end-tidal CO_2 can indicate the effectiveness of chest compressions—aim to achieve an $ETCO_2$ value ≥20 mmHg during CPR.
- ☑ If asystole has been caused by surgical stimulation of the vagus, give IV atropine in increments of 0.5 mg.
- ☑ Give adrenaline 1 mg IV if PEA, or if asystole is not immediately resolved by stopping surgical activity or injecting atropine. Repeat this dose of adrenaline every 3–5 min until spontaneous circulation is restored.

Subsequent management
- ☑ Treat reversible causes of asystole (➲ see 'Exclusions/Causes', p. 11).
- ☑ Rapid infusion of fluid (including blood if severe haemorrhage).
- ☑ Consider pacing if complete heart block (third-degree) or Möbitz Type II AV block. This can be achieved using a transcutaneous pacer while awaiting someone skilled in transvenous pacing. Alternatively start an isoprenaline infusion (starting dose 5.0 μg/min).
- ☑ If resuscitation is successful, life-saving surgery (e.g. to control haemorrhage) should be completed.

☑ Unless the period of CPR has been very brief (perhaps less than 3 min), the patient should remain intubated and be transferred to the critical care unit.

☑ Following prolonged cardiac arrest, if there is a possibility of neurological injury, consider targeted temperature management.

☑ Obtain a CXR, 12-lead ECG, arterial blood gases, and plasma electrolyte analysis.

☑ ⊃ See 'Post-resuscitation care', p. 373.

Investigations
U&Es, ABGs, ECG, CXR.

Risk factors
- Procedures associated with excessive vagal activity (e.g. gynaecological/eye surgery).
- Pre-existing complete heart block, second-degree heart block, or trifascicular heart block.

Exclusions/Causes
- Disconnected ECG lead—this appears on the monitor as a completely straight line.
- Hypoxia—obstructed airway, oesophageal intubation, bronchial intubation, oxygen failure.
- Hypovolaemia—haemorrhagic shock (particularly with induction of anaesthesia), anaphylaxis.
- Hypo/hyperkalaemia and metabolic disorders—renal failure, suxamethonium-induced hyperkalaemia after burns.
- Hypothermia—unlikely.
- Tension pneumothorax—especially in the trauma patient or after central venous catheter insertion.
- Tamponade—after penetrating trauma.
- Toxic/therapeutic disorders—after drug overdose (self-inflicted or iatrogenic).
- Thromboembolism—massive pulmonary embolus.

Paediatric implications
- The same principles apply to the treatment of asystole in children.
- Hypoxia is more likely as primary cause.
- Refer to 'Paediatric ALS' for drug doses (⊃ pp. 130–3).

Special considerations
- Asystole associated with excessive vagal stimulation or injection of suxamethonium will usually resolve spontaneously on stopping the cause. Give atropine (0.5–1 mg IV) or glycopyrronium (200–600 µg IV); occasionally, a brief period of chest compressions is required.
- Under these conditions, follow-up investigations are usually unnecessary.
- In other circumstances asystole is associated with a poor prognosis unless there is a potentially reversible cause that can be treated immediately.

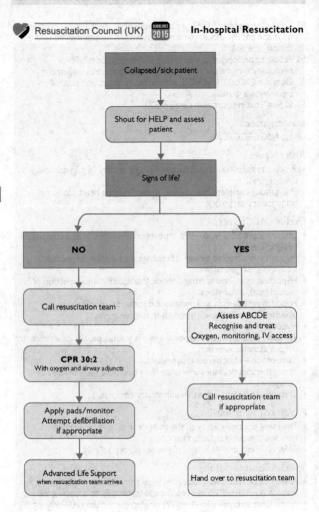

Figure 2.1 Adult in-hospital resuscitation.
Reproduced with the kind permission of the Resuscitation Council (UK).

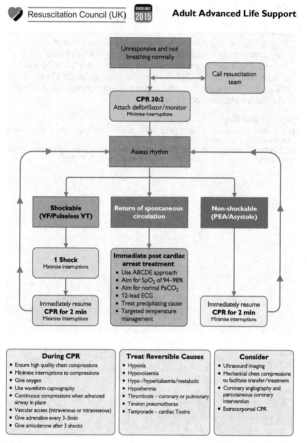

Figure 2.2 Advanced life support (adults).

Reproduced with the kind permission of the Resuscitation Council (UK).

- If the patient has an arterial line at the time of cardiac arrest it can be used in addition to the $ETCO_2$ to optimize the quality of chest compressions.
- Targeted temperature management should be considered after resuscitation from in-hospital cardiac arrest regardless of initial rhythm. The recommended target temperature is in the range 32–36°C and is maintained for at least 24 h; aim for the target defined by local protocols. Cooling can be initiated in the operating room using cold IV fluid and/or external cooling (e.g. ice).

Further reading

Nolan, J., Soar, J., Hampshire, S., et al. (eds) (2016). *Advanced Life Support*, 7th edition. London, UK: Resuscitation Council UK.

Soar, J., Nolan, J.P., Bottiger, B.W., et al. (2015). European Resuscitation Council guidelines for resuscitation 2015 section 3 adult advanced life support. *Resuscitation*, **95**, 99–146.

:☠: Ventricular fibrillation

Definition

Cardiac arrest is associated with an irregular, chaotic, broad-complex, fast rhythm on the ECG.

Presentation

- Characteristic appearance of VF on ECG.
- No palpable central pulses (carotid or femoral).

Immediate management

(See Figure 2.2, ALS (adults) algorithm, ➔ p. 13.)

1. Confirm cardiac arrest – check for signs of life or if trained to do so, breathing and pulse simultaneously.
2. Call resuscitation team.
3. Perform uninterrupted chest compressions while applying self-adhesive defibrillation/monitoring pads—one below the right clavicle and the other in the V_6 position in the mid-axillary line.
4. Plan actions before pausing CPR for rhythm analysis and communicate these to the team.
5. Stop chest compressions; confirm VF/pVT from the ECG. This pause in chest compressions should be brief and no longer than 5 s.
6. Resume chest compressions immediately; warn all rescuers **other than the individual performing the chest compressions** to 'stand clear' and remove any oxygen delivery device as appropriate.
7. The designated person selects the appropriate energy on the defibrillator and presses the charge button. Choose an energy setting of at least 150 J for the first shock, the same or a higher energy for subsequent shocks, or follow the manufacturer's guidance for the particular defibrillator. If unsure of the correct energy level for a defibrillator, choose the highest available energy.
8. Ensure that the rescuer giving the compressions is the only person touching the patient.
9. Once the defibrillator is charged and the safety check is complete, tell the rescuer doing the chest compressions to 'stand clear'; when clear, give the shock.
10. After shock delivery immediately restart CPR using a ratio of 30:2, starting with chest compressions. If an advanced airway is in situ give continuous chest compressions while ventilating the lungs at ten breaths per minute. Do not pause to reassess the rhythm or feel for a pulse. The total pause in chest compressions should be brief and no longer than 5 s.
11. Continue CPR for 2 min; the team leader prepares the team for the next pause in CPR.
12. Pause briefly to check the monitor.
13. If VF/pVT, repeat steps 6–12 and deliver a second shock.
14. If VF/pVT persists, repeat steps 6–8 and deliver a third shock. Resume chest compressions immediately. Give adrenaline 1 mg IV and amiodarone 300 mg IV while performing a further 2 min CPR.

Withhold adrenaline if there are signs of return of spontaneous circulation (ROSC) during CPR.

15. Repeat this 2 min CPR—rhythm/pulse check—defibrillation sequence if VF/pVT persists.
16. Give further adrenaline 1 mg IV after alternate shocks (i.e. approximately every 3–5 min).
17. If organized electrical activity compatible with a cardiac output is seen during a rhythm check, seek evidence of ROSC (check for signs of life, a central pulse, and end-tidal CO_2 if available).
    a. If there is ROSC, start post-resuscitation care.
    b. If there are no signs of ROSC, continue CPR and switch to the non-shockable algorithm.
18. If asystole is seen, continue CPR and switch to the non-shockable algorithm.

Witnessed VF/pVT while connected to a defibrillator
☑ If the patient is already connected to a defibrillator at the onset of VF/pVT, give up to three quick successive (stacked) shocks.
☑ Rapidly check for a rhythm change and, if appropriate, ROSC after each defibrillation attempt.
☑ Start chest compressions and continue CPR for 2 min if the third shock is unsuccessful.

Subsequent management
☑ Exclude potentially reversible causes if VF persists.
☑ If resuscitation is successful, life-saving surgery (e.g. to control haemorrhage) should be completed.
☑ Unless the period of CPR has been very brief (perhaps less than 3 min), the patient should remain intubated and be transferred to the critical care unit.
☑ Consider targeted temperature management (➲ see 'Post-resuscitation care', p. 389).

Investigations
U&Es, ABGs, ECG, CXR.

Risk factors
- Recent myocardial infarction.
- Ischaemic heart disease.
- Excessive endogenous or exogenous catecholamines.
- Hypokalaemia.
- Irritation of myocardium by guidewire during insertion of central venous catheter.

Exclusions
- Artefact on the ECG—interference from diathermy or patient movement.

- Polymorphic ventricular tachycardia—in the absence of a pulse, treatment is still defibrillation.
- Atrial fibrillation in the presence of atrioventricular accessory pathway—often capable of conducting very rapidly.

Paediatric implications

- VF cardiac arrest is unusual in children.
- The same principles apply to the treatment of VF in children.
- Refer to paediatric ALS for appropriate shock energies and drug doses (➔ see p. 130).

Special considerations

- Electrical defibrillation can be accomplished using self-adhesive patches or, less commonly, manual paddles and gel pads. One electrode is applied just below the right clavicle and the other in the left mid-axillary line in approximately the fifth intercostal space (lead V_6). Self-adhesive patches can be applied prophylactically to those patients deemed to be at very high risk of VF intraoperatively.
- The treatment of pulseless ventricular tachycardia is the same as for VF.
- AEDs or shock-advisory defibrillators (with a manual override function) are deployed commonly outside of critical care areas. The need to stop chest compressions while these devices analyse the rhythm is a significant disadvantage and anyone capable of rhythm interpretation should operate these devices in manual mode.

Further reading

Nolan, J., Soar, J., Hampshire, S., et al. (eds) (2016). *Advanced Life Support*, 7th edition. London, UK: Resuscitation Council UK.

Soar, J., Nolan, J.P., Bottiger, B.W., et al. (2015). European Resuscitation Council guidelines for resuscitation 2015 section 3 adult advanced life support. *Resuscitation*, **95**, 99–146.

☼ Intraoperative arrhythmias: bradycardia

Definition

Ventricular rate <60 bpm. Absolute bradycardia (<40 bpm); relative bradycardia (heart rate inappropriate for haemodynamic state of patient). May be sinus or associated with AV block/sick sinus syndrome.

Presentation

- Ventricular rate <60 bpm.
- 12-lead ECG to define rhythm.

Immediate management

(🢂 See Figure 2.3, 'Adult bradycardia algorithm', p. 19.)
☑ Urgent correction of any hypoxaemia.
☑ Check for a pulse—if there is no pulse (pulseless electrical activity—PEA) start CPR and treat as for asystole (🢂 p. 10).
☑ May not need any action in absence of cardiovascular compromise (blood pressure is acceptable and peripheral perfusion is adequate).
☑ Correct other underlying causes—stop surgical stimulation, which is likely to increase vagal activity.
☑ Atropine (500 µg increments up to 3 mg IV), glycopyrronium (200–600 µg IV) or ephedrine (6–9 mg IV).
☑ Consider isoprenaline (starting at 5.0 µg/min) or adrenaline (2–10 µg/min) if persistent.
☑ External transcutaneous pacing if fails to respond to drug treatment—this is used until a transvenous pacing wire or permanent pacing system can be inserted. When initiating external transcutaneous pacing, the typical current required to achieve electrical capture is 50–100 mA.

Subsequent management

☑ Treat precipitating reversible causes (electrolyte abnormalities).
☑ Stop drugs that prolong QT interval (e.g. amiodarone, sotalol, erythromycin, disopyramide, procainamide, quinidine, haloperidol, chlorpromazine).
☑ In patients with persisting bradycardia, a 12-lead ECG will enable assessment of heart block.

Investigations

ECG, U&Es, ABGs.

Risk factors/causes

Sinus bradycardia may be caused by:
- Vagal stimulation during surgery.
- Drugs (β-blockers, digoxin, amiodarone, anticholinesterases, suxamethonium).

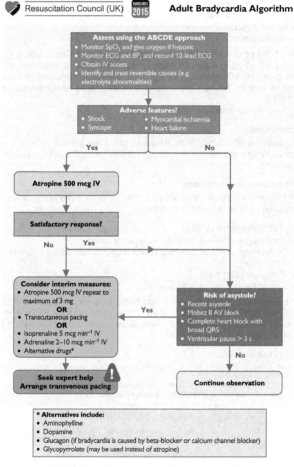

Figure 2.3 Adult bradycardia algorithm (includes rates inappropriately slow for haemodynamic state).

Reproduced with the kind permission of the Resuscitation Council (UK).

- Sick sinus syndrome.
- Myocardial infarction.
- Raised intracranial pressure.
- Hypothermia.

Third-degree atrioventricular block and second-degree Möbitz type II AV block will result in significant bradycardia, haemodynamic instability, and the possibility of asystole. Other significant risk factors associated with the risk of asystole include a recent episode of asystole or ventricular pauses of >3 s.

Severe hypoxaemia will cause bradycardia.

Exclusions

Appropriate sinus bradycardia associated with adequate cardiac output—check history and current medication (patient taking β-blockers, athletic patients).

Paediatric implications

In children, bradycardia is usually secondary to hypoxia and adequate oxygenation must be restored immediately.

Special considerations

Indications for referral for preoperative pacing include:
- Second-degree AV block—Möbitz type II or 2:1 (intermittent failure of conduction).
- Complete heart block.
- Symptomatic sinus node disease.

Asymptomatic bundle branch block, bifascicular, trifascicular, and first-degree heart block are not indications for preoperative pacing. Pacing is not usually required for Möbitz type I second-degree AV block (Wenckebach) unless the patient is symptomatic.

Further reading

Nolan, J., Soar, J., Hampshire, S., et al. (eds) (2016). *Advanced Life Support*, 7th edition. London, UK: Resuscitation Council UK.

Soar, J., Nolan, J.P., Bottiger, B.W., et al. (2015). European Resuscitation Council guidelines for resuscitation 2015 section 3 adult advanced life support. *Resuscitation*, **95**, 99–146.

⚠ Intraoperative arrhythmias: atrial fibrillation

Definition
Chaotic and uncoordinated atrial depolarization and an **irregularly irregular** ventricular rate.

Presentation
- An irregularly irregular QRS complex on the ECG associated with rapid chaotic atrial activity with deflections in size and rate but without visible P waves. A 12-lead ECG provides the best opportunity to confirm atrial fibrillation (AF).
- The refractory period of the AV node determines the ventricular rate. In the absence of drug treatment or disease the ventricular rate will be 120–200 bpm.

Immediate management
(➲ See Figure 2.4, 'Adult tachycardia algorithm', p.24.)
- ☑ Treatment of AF depends on whether it is paroxysmal or persistent. If the onset of AF is recent (within 48 h) and is associated with significant cardiovascular compromise (hypotension, rate >150 bpm, cardiac failure, associated valve disease), treatment should include:
  - attempted restoration of sinus rhythm by electrical synchronized cardioversion starting with 120–150 J. If the first shock does not terminate the arrhythmia, give up to two more shocks of increasing energy up to the maximum setting of the defibrillator.
  - immediate correction of precipitating causes, such as electrolyte abnormalities.
- ☑ If electrical cardioversion fails, attempt chemical cardioversion with amiodarone 300 mg IV over 1 h followed by 900 mg IV over 23 h. Amiodarone will slow the ventricular rate even if it fails to restore sinus rhythm.
- ☑ In patients with a life-threatening deterioration in haemodynamic stability following the onset of AF, emergency electrical cardioversion should be performed, irrespective of the duration of the AF. In these cases, give a therapeutic dose of heparin.
- ☑ In patients with non-life-threatening haemodynamic instability, if the AF has been present for more than 48 h, anticoagulation is required before attempting cardioversion (risk of embolizing any blood clot in the atrium):
  - rate control can be achieved with an intravenous β-blocker, such as esmolol, atenolol, or metoprolol.
  - a rate-controlling calcium antagonist is a good option but the best of these drugs, diltiazem, is not available for IV use in the UK.
  - in the presence of heart failure, rate control can be achieved with digoxin 500 µg IV, repeated after 2–4 h.

Subsequent management

☑ Treat precipitating reversible causes (electrolyte abnormalities, hypovolaemia, sepsis). If digoxin is used, ensure therapeutic levels (1–2 ng/mL). Anticoagulate unless contraindicated.

☑ Patients remaining in AF require 3 weeks of full anticoagulation before attempting cardioversion. In patients with persistent AF, a rate-control strategy is the preferred initial option except in people:
  - whose atrial fibrillation has a reversible cause.
  - who have heart failure thought to be primarily caused by atrial fibrillation.
  - with new-onset atrial fibrillation.
  - with atrial flutter whose condition is considered suitable for an ablation strategy to restore sinus rhythm.
  - for whom a rhythm control strategy would be more suitable based on clinical judgement.

☑ Patients in AF started on amiodarone to control rate must be converted to an alternative drug (e.g. β-blocker or diltiazem) for rate control (long-term complications associated with amiodarone).

☑ The goals for rate control are to produce a resting heart rate of 60–90 bpm and not >110 bpm after slight exercise.

Investigations
ECG, U&Es, ABGs, TFTs, Mg^{++}.

Risk factors
Common causes of AF include:
- Myocardial ischaemia.
- Sepsis.
- Rheumatic heart disease.
- Electrolyte abnormalities (especially hypokalaemia or hypomagnesaemia).
- Hypertension.
- Thoracic and cardiac surgery.

Exclusions
- Frequent atrial ectopic beats can give the appearance of AF.
- Other supraventricular tachycardias are regular—but at very fast rates it can be difficult to distinguish these from AF.
- Atrial flutter is characterized by rapid and regular atrial activity with a rate of 250–350 bpm. This creates characteristic saw-tooth flutter waves on the ECG best seen in leads II and V1. There is usually AV block of between 2:1 and 8:1. Thus, atrial flutter at 300 bpm and a 2:1 block will result in a ventricular rate of 150 bpm.

Special considerations
Long-term anticoagulation is normally recommended for men with a CHA_2DS_2VASc score of 1 and women with a CHA_2DS_2VASc score of 2 (Table 2.1). Anticoagulation may be with apixaban, dabigatran, rivaroxaban, or warfarin.

Table 2.1 Components of the CHA_2DS_2VASc score

Risk factor	Score
Congestive heart failure	1
Hypertension	1
Age ≥ 75	2
Age 65–74	1
Diabetes mellitus	1
Stroke/TIA/thromboembolism	2
Vascular disease	1
Sex female	1

Further reading

National Institute for Clinical Health and Excellence (2014). *NICE Clinical Guideline 180. Atrial Fibrillation: The Management of Atrial Fibrillation*. Available at: http://www.nice.org.uk/guidance/cg180

Nolan, J., Soar, J., Hampshire, S., et al. (eds) (2016). *Advanced Life Support*, 7th edition. London, UK: Resuscitation Council UK.

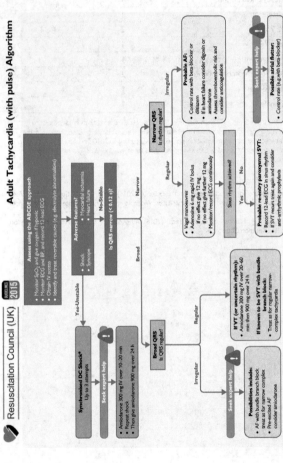

Figure 2.4 Adult tachycardia algorithm.

:⚙: Intraoperative arrhythmias: narrow-complex tachycardia

Definition
Regular, narrow-complex (QRS <0.12 s duration) tachycardia arising from above the ventricles. Includes sinus tachycardia, atrial tachycardia, junctional tachycardia, and atrial flutter.

Presentation
- ECG demonstrating narrow-complex tachycardia (QRS <0.12 s) with rate 100–300 bpm.
- Presence of normal P wave implies sinus tachycardia.
- Flutter waves (typically 300 bpm) present in atrial flutter. A 2:1 block is common and results in a ventricular rate of 150 bpm.
- During a junctional tachycardia the P waves may be hidden behind the QRS complexes or, if they are visible, they are often inverted or of abnormal morphology.
- A 12-lead ECG taken during sinus rhythm may reveal evidence of an accessory pathway:
  - short PR interval.
  - slurred upstroke on the R wave (the delta wave).

Immediate management
(⊕ See Figure 2.4, 'Adult tachycardia algorithm', p. 24.)
- ☑ If sinus tachycardia, treat underlying causes (⊕ see 'Risk factors', p. 26).
- ☑ Having excluded sinus tachycardia, attempt vagal manoeuvres such as carotid sinus massage.
- ☑ Give adenosine 6 mg IV by rapid bolus, followed if necessary by up to two doses of 12 mg. Adenosine may terminate the arrhythmia or will temporarily slow the ventricular rate, enabling the diagnosis of the underlying rhythm (e.g. flutter waves may become more visible). Side effects of adenosine include flushing, dyspnoea, and headache.
- ☑ If cardiovascular compromise (systolic blood pressure <90 mmHg, heart failure, reduced conscious level, evidence of myocardial ischaemia), attempt electrical synchronized cardioversion using 70–120 J. If the first shock does not terminate the arrhythmia, give up to two more shocks of increasing energy up to the maximum setting of the defibrillator.
- ☑ If cardioversion is not achieved, give amiodarone 300 mg IV over 10–20 min, then repeat shock. Follow this with amiodarone 900 mg IV over 23 h.
- ☑ In the absence of cardiovascular compromise, there are several options for drug treatment that will control ventricular rate and may produce cardioversion to sinus rhythm (e.g. amiodarone 300 mg IV over 20–60 min followed by 900 mg IV over 23 h, esmolol 50–200 µg/kg/min, or verapamil 2.5–5 mg IV).

Subsequent management

☑ Treat precipitating reversible causes (electrolyte abnormalities, hypovolaemia, sepsis).
☑ Look for evidence of an accessory pathway.
☑ Patients with evidence of an accessory pathway will need referral to a cardiologist.

Investigations
ECG, U&Es, ABGs, TFTs.

Risk factors
Common causes of sinus tachycardia include:
• Inadequate anaesthesia and/or analgesia
• Hypovolaemia
• Hypoxaemia
• Hypercapnia
• Sepsis

Supraventricular tachycardias may be caused by an atrioventricular accessory pathway causing a pre-excitation antidromic (re-entry) arrhythmia (e.g. Wolff–Parkinson–White (WPW) syndrome).

Exclusions
• Awareness/light anaesthesia—check delivery of inhalational/ intravenous agent to the patient.
• Ventricular tachycardia will cause broad QRS complexes (>0.12 s).
• Fast atrial fibrillation can appear regular, but close inspection of a 12-lead ECG should enable the correct diagnosis.

Special considerations
Supraventricular tachycardias associated with aberrant conduction pathways will produce wide-complex tachycardias resembling **ventricular** tachycardia. If the patient is severely compromised, the appropriate treatment is as for ventricular tachycardia (➲ see 'Broad-complex tachycardias', p. 27).

Further reading

Nolan, J., Soar, J., Hampshire, S., et al. (eds) (2016). *Advanced Life Support*, 7th edition. London, UK: Resuscitation Council UK.

Page, R.L., Joglar, J.A., Caldwell, M.A., et al. (2015). ACC/AHA/HRS guideline for the management of adult patients with supraventricular tachycardia: a report of the American College of Cardiology/American Heart Association Task Force on Clinical Practice Guidelines and the Heart Rhythm Society. *Journal of American College of Cardiology*, **133**, E506–74.

✸ Intraoperative arrhythmias: broad-complex tachycardia

Definition

Tachycardia arising from the ventricles (ventricular tachycardia, VT) or a supraventricular tachycardia (SVT) associated with aberrant conduction. QRS >0.12 s. duration. Torsade de pointes is a specific polymorphic form of VT.

Presentation

- Broad-complex tachycardia with rate >100 bpm.
- History of ischaemic heart disease, visible independent P waves, fusion, or capture beats imply VT rather than SVT.
- In the patient without haemodynamic compromise, adenosine (6 mg by rapid IV bolus followed if necessary by up to two doses of 12 mg) can be used to differentiate VT from SVT with aberrant conduction.
- Causes of an irregular broad-complex tachycardia include torsade de pointes, pre-excited AF, and AF with bundle branch block. Torsade de pointes is a polymorphic form of VT characterized by beat-to-beat variation, a constantly changing axis, and a prolonged QT interval.

Immediate management

(➲ See Figure 2.4, 'Adult tachycardia algorithm', p. 24.)

☑ Feel for pulse—if pulseless VT, treat as for VF with immediate attempted defibrillation. Give unsynchronized shocks—see 'Ventricular fibrillation', p. 15.

☑ In the presence of cardiovascular compromise (systolic blood pressure <90 mmHg, heart failure, reduced conscious level, evidence of myocardial ischaemia), attempt electrical **synchronized** cardioversion using 120–150 J. If the first shock does not terminate the arrhythmia, give up to two more shocks of increasing energy up to the maximum setting of the defibrillator.

☑ Correct any electrolyte abnormalities such as hypokalaemia or hypomagnesaemia. If the patient is taking a regular diuretic, assume the presence of hypomagnesaemia and give magnesium 2 g IV.

☑ If attempted electrical cardioversion fails, give amiodarone 300 mg over 10–20 min IV and repeat attempted electrical cardioversion.

☑ In the absence of haemodynamic compromise, correct any electrolyte abnormalities and attempt chemical cardioversion with amiodarone 300 mg IV over 20–60 min—followed by 900 mg IV over 23 h, with electrical cardioversion if necessary.

☑ If torsade de pointes is present, give magnesium 2 g IV over 10 min and correct any electrolyte abnormalities such as hypokalaemia.

Subsequent management

☑ Treat precipitating reversible causes (e.g. electrolyte abnormalities in the presence of a prolonged QT interval).

☑ Stop drugs that prolong the QT interval.

☑ Persistent or recurrence of a broad-complex tachycardia will necessitate urgent referral to a cardiologist—may use alternative antiarrhythmic drugs or overdrive pacing.

Investigations

ECG, U&Es, ABGs, Mg^{++}.

Risk factors

Causes of VT include:

- Ischaemic heart disease.
- Ventricular scarring after myocardial infarction or previous cardiac surgery.
- Right ventricular failure.
- Electrolyte abnormalities in patients with prolonged QT interval (tricyclic antidepressants, antihistamines, phenothiazines; or Brugada syndrome). These conditions may also precipitate torsade de pointes.
- Supraventricular tachycardias caused by an atrioventricular accessory pathway causing a pre-excitation antidromic (re-entry) arrhythmia (e.g. Wolff–Parkinson–White (WPW) syndrome), may cause a broad-complex tachycardia.

Exclusions

- Supraventricular tachycardia with aberrant conduction—in an emergency the treatment is as for ventricular tachycardia.
- Sinus tachycardia with bundle branch block—P waves will precede each QRS complex.

Special considerations

- Intravenous lidocaine (50 mg IV over 2 min repeated every 5 min to a maximum of 200 mg) may be considered for recurrent sustained VT or VF not responding to β-blockers or amiodarone or in the case of contraindications to amiodarone.

Further reading

Nolan, J., Soar, J., Hampshire, S., et al. (eds) (2016). *Advanced Life Support*, 7th edition. London, UK: Resuscitation Council UK.

Priori, S.G., Blomstrom-Lundqvist, C. (co-chairs) (2015). The Task Force for the Management of Patients with Ventricular Arrhythmias and the Prevention of Sudden Cardiac Death of the European Society of Cardiology (ESC). 2015 ESC Guidelines for the management of patients with ventricular arrhythmias and the prevention of sudden cardiac death. *European Heart Journal*, **36**, 2793–867.

☼ Intraoperative hypotension

Definition
Systolic arterial blood pressure <20% preoperative value.

Presentation
- Hypotension detected by non-invasive or invasive blood pressure monitoring.
- Assess peripheral circulation:
  - **warm peripheries** imply vasodilation—consider overdose of anaesthetic (check end-tidal volatile or intravenous anaesthesia pump settings) or high regional block, sepsis (fever, tachycardia, precipitating cause), histamine releasing drugs, anaphylaxis.
  - **cold peripheries** imply hypovolaemia or pump failure.
- A tachycardia will accompany most causes of hypotension (hypovolaemia, sepsis, cardiogenic shock). A bradycardia may be the primary cause—it will also accompany a high neuraxial block. Spinal cord injury is a rare cause of hypotension accompanied by bradycardia.

Immediate management
- ☑ ABC—ensure adequate oxygenation and ventilation and increase F_iO_2 if required.
- ☑ Check for blood loss and ensure that venous return is not being impaired inadvertently by surgeons (e.g. direct compression of the inferior vena cava, excessive intra-abdominal pressure during laparoscopic surgery).
- ☑ Consider excessive losses from redistribution and quickly assess peripheral perfusion.
- ☑ Give fluid bolus of 10 mL/kg crystalloid to optimize filling pressure and assess response (heart rate, blood pressure, CVP if available). A head-down or legs-up position will rapidly increase venous return while fluid is being given.
- ☑ Reduce general anaesthetic if appropriate.
- ☑ Insert an arterial cannula for continuous blood pressure monitoring.
- ☑ Consider vasoconstrictor or inotrope:
  - if peripherally vasodilated and response to fluid challenge is poor, give a bolus of vasoconstrictor, for example, metaraminol (0.5–1.0 mg IV) or phenylephrine (0.25–0.5 mg IV).
  - after an appropriate fluid challenge, if peripheral perfusion is poor and the cardiac output is likely to be low, give ephedrine 6 mg IV and consider starting an infusion of an inotrope such as dobutamine (2–5 µg/kg/min) or adrenaline (0.1–0.2 µg/kg/min).

Subsequent management
If hypotension persists, further management may include:
☑ Use of a cardiac output system (e.g. PiCCO, LiDCO, oesophageal Doppler) to enable formal assessment of fluid responsiveness and cardiac output.
☑ Check urine output to assess renal perfusion.
☑ Infusion of noradrenaline ($0.1–0.2$ µg/kg/min or more as required) if hypotension persists and the patient remains vasodilated (e.g. septic shock).
☑ Infusion of dobutamine ($2–5$ µg/kg/min) if poor cardiac output and hypotensive despite adequate fluid volume. A persistent metabolic acidosis and rising serum lactate may also imply inadequate cardiac output and oxygen delivery.
☑ Patients with persistent hypotension, oliguria, and significant acidaemia will need admission to a critical care unit postoperatively.

Investigations
ECG, CXR, ABGs, haemoglobin, cardiac enzymes.

Risk factors/causes
Causes of intraoperative hypotension include:
- Hypovolaemia
- Haemorrhage
- Capillary leak (septic shock, anaphylaxis)
- Dehydration (diarrhoea and/or vomiting)
- Obstructed venous return (tension pneumothorax, compression of IVC)
- Vasodilation
- High spinal or epidural block
- Excessive anaesthetic or other vasodilating drugs
- Anaphylactic or anaphylactoid reaction, or septic shock
- Addisonian crisis
- Obstructive shock
- Pulmonary embolism
- Air embolism
- Amniotic fluid embolism
- Pump failure
  - left and/or right ventricular failure
- Arrhythmia

Exclusions
- Measurement errors:
  - damped arterial line measurement errors.
  - interference with non-invasive blood pressure cuff.
- Hypovolaemia—will usually be accompanied by tachycardia, cool peripheries, collapsed veins (low CVP), and an arterial trace with a marked respiratory swing or stroke volume variation >10%.
- Suspect dehydration—if the patient has been thirsty, has a dry tongue and sunken eyes, and has elevated urea and creatinine.

- Pulmonary/gas embolism—suspect if the patient had a pre-existing low CVP and open venous bed. Signs include a decrease in end-tidal CO_2, decrease in S_aO_2, and increase in CVP.
- Suspect microembolism—from intramedullary cavity in the presence of long-bone fractures or intramedullary surgery.
- Cardiac failure—suspect if the patient has distended neck veins (high CVP), tachycardia, cool peripheries, pulmonary oedema (hypoxaemia, fine crackles on auscultation of the lungs), and ischaemic changes on the ECG.
- Anaphylaxis—will be accompanied, variably, by tachycardia, erythema, rash, urticaria, wheeze, and angioedema.

Paediatric implications
- The same principles apply to the treatment of hypotension in children.
- Fluid boluses of 10 mL/kg should be used and repeated as necessary.

Special considerations
- Patients on β-blockers may not mount an appropriate tachycardia.
- In young, healthy patients a short period of hypotension is unlikely to be harmful as long as cardiac output is well maintained. Patients with ischaemic heart disease and/or chronic hypertension will require a higher blood pressure to maintain vital organ perfusion.

☼ Intraoperative hypertension

Definition

Blood pressure >15% above baseline.
Systolic >160 mmHg or diastolic >100 mmHg.
Severe hypertension: systolic >180 mmHg or diastolic >110 mmHg.

Presentation

- Hypertension detected by non-invasive or invasive blood pressure monitoring.

Immediate management

- ☑ ABC
- ☑ Stop surgery until controlled. Increase F_iO_2 if required. Increase ventilation if hypercapnic. Confirm readings. Increase depth of anaesthesia. Give analgesia. Give vasodilator and/or β-blocker and/ or α-blocker.

Consider and treat potential causes:

- ☑ Hypoxia/hypercapnia—ABC; also check S_pO_2 and end-tidal CO_2.
- ☑ Inadequate depth of anaesthesia—check end-tidal volatile anaesthetic concentration, check TIVA pump and IV cannula, check depth of anaesthesia monitor (e.g. BIS).
- ☑ Inadequate analgesia—if in doubt, give alfentanil 10–20 µg/kg IV or remifentanil 0.5 µg/kg IV and observe effect.
- ☑ Measurement error—repeat non-invasive BP while palpating distal pulse (return of pulse approximates systolic pressure); check transducer height if using invasive blood pressure monitoring.
- ☑ Iatrogenic drug response—recheck ampoules (e.g. cocaine or ephedrine given instead of morphine) and confirm dilution of vasopressors or inotropes.
- ☑ Pre-eclampsia—if the patient is over 20 weeks' pregnant, check for proteinuria, platelet count, clotting studies, and liver function tests (➲ see 'Pre-eclampsia', p. 166).
- ☑ Intracranial hypertension—check for Cushing response (hypertension and bradycardia) and dilated pupil (➲ see 'Raised intracranial pressure', p. 190).
- ☑ Assuming this is not a physiological response to a correctable cause, the aim of symptomatic management is to prevent myocardial ischaemia/infarction or hypertensive stroke. In addition to increasing the depth of anaesthesia and giving more analgesia, treatment options include:
  - vasodilators:
    - hydralazine 5 mg slow IV every 15 min.
    - GTN (50 mg/50 mL starting at 3 mL/h IV and titrate to effect).
    - sodium nitroprusside for resistant hypertension (0.5–1.5 µg/kg/ min).

- β-blockade, particularly if hypertension is accompanied by tachycardia:
  - IV metoprolol 1–2 mg increments.
  - IV labetalol 5–10 mg increments (β:α block ratio 7:1).
  - IV esmolol 0.5 mg/kg loading dose followed by an infusion of 50–200 μg/kg/min.

Subsequent management

☑ Remifentanil 0.25–0.5 μg/kg/min will provide intense analgesia and will help if surgical stimulation is difficult to overcome by other means.
☑ Check 12-lead ECG postoperatively and cardiac troponin after 12 h if there is thought to have been severe myocardial ischaemia or infarction.
☑ Close monitoring of blood pressure. Treat any underlying chronic cause (essential hypertension, hyperthyroidism, phaeochromocytoma).

Investigations

ECG, troponin, thyroid function tests, 24 h urinary catecholamine excretion.

Risk factors/causes

- Inadequate depth of anaesthesia/analgesia.
- Tracheal intubation/extubation.
- Untreated essential hypertension or 'white coat' hypertension preoperatively (increased lability).
- Aortic surgery—cross-clamping, particularly above the renal arteries, greatly increases systemic vascular resistance.
- Hypercapnia.
- Hypoxia.
- Pregnancy-induced hypertension.
- Drugs—MAOIs (+ pethidine), ketamine, ergometrine, systemic absorption of adrenaline-containing solutions, phenylephrine eyedrops, cocaine.
- Family history of multiple endocrine neoplasia (type 2) syndrome, medullary thyroid carcinoma, Conn's syndrome.
- Acute head injury/Raised intracranial pressure.
- Thyroid storm causing elevated T_4 and T_3 levels.
- Phaeochromocytoma causing elevated plasma noradrenaline levels.
- Malignant hyperthermia.

Exclusions

- Measurement errors:
  - blood pressure cuff too small.
  - interference with non-invasive blood pressure cuff.
  - transducer for non-invasive blood pressure too low in relation to the patient's heart or incorrectly zeroed.

Special considerations
If hypertension is thought to reflect intracranial hypertension, undertake a CT scan of the brain to exclude pathology amenable to neurosurgical intervention. Ensure that MAP is maintained >80 mmHg, head-up tilt, unobstructed SVC drainage, and normocapnia. Consider mannitol and temporary period of hyperventilation.

⚙ Intraoperative myocardial ischaemia

(➔ See also 'Acute coronary syndromes', pp. 335–7.)

Definition

Inadequate myocardial oxygen supply in relation to demand.

Presentation

- ECG displays ST segment depression (ischaemia) or ST segment elevation (evolving acute myocardial infarction). These changes can be analysed properly only by looking at more than one lead. Ideally, obtain a 12-lead ECG immediately, especially if there is suspicion of ST elevation.
- Impaired myocardial function may cause hypotension and/or pulmonary oedema—assess peripheral perfusion, auscultate for fine crackles that signify left ventricular failure and pulmonary oedema.
- Ischaemia of the cardiac conduction system may cause severe ventricular arrhythmias—these will exacerbate myocardial ischaemia.
- Echocardiography may show a non-contracting ischaemic region of the myocardium bulging outward during systole (dyskinesis).
- Myocardial infarction will be accompanied by an increase in cardiac troponin— a significant increase in this cardiac marker in the absence of ST segment elevation implies non-ST elevation myocardial infarction (NSTEMI). A reliable value for troponin can be achieved only after 12 h.

Immediate management

☑ ABC—restore oxygen delivery to the myocardium:
- increase F_iO_2 if required.
- give fluid if hypovolaemic, and blood if severely anaemic— myocardial oxygen extraction is normally very high, a combination of coronary artery disease and severe acute anaemia will quickly cause myocardial ischaemia which can be reversed by restoring an adequate haemoglobin concentration (70–90 g/L).
- cardiac output system may indicate fluid responsiveness and guide fluid replacement.
- if ischaemic changes persist despite restoration of adequate volume, consider vasopressor (e.g. noradrenaline) if hypotensive or an inodilator (e.g. dobutamine) if blood pressure adequate but cardiac output is poor.

☑ Reduce myocardial oxygen demand:
- if tachycardia is present, reduce heart rate with β-blocker and/or analgesia (metoprolol 1–2 mg IV increments, esmolol 0.5 mg/kg IV loading dose followed by an infusion of 50–200 µg/kg/min).
- treat tachyarrhythmias as appropriate (see treatment of supraventricular and ventricular arrhythmias, ➔ pp. 25, 27).

- if hypertensive, treat underlying cause and consider GTN infusion to reduce afterload (50 mg/50 mL starting at 3 mL/h IV and titrate to effect). In the first instance, to hasten delivery, 400 µg GTN can be sprayed under the patient's tongue.
☑ If ST segment elevation is present, immediately record a 12-lead ECG—if acute myocardial infarction confirmed, consider urgent transfer for percutaneous coronary intervention—give aspirin (300 mg chewed/NG) and ticagrelor (180 mg) or prasugrel (60 mg).

Subsequent management
☑ Postoperatively—repeat 12-lead ECG, titrate inspired oxygen concentration to a target S_pO_2 of 94–98% and maintain adequate mean arterial blood pressure.
☑ If myocardial ischaemia persists, continue intravenous nitrate.
☑ Request urgent cardiac echo to assess myocardial function.
☑ Persistent myocardial ischaemia despite optimizing preload, afterload, and myocardial contractility will necessitate full anticoagulation with heparin (unless absolutely contraindicated) and referral to a cardiologist for further investigation.
☑ Measurement of cardiac troponin will enable risk assessment (which will direct further treatment) and exclusion or confirmation of myocardial infarction.
☑ In the presence of an evolving ST elevation myocardial infarction (STEMI), every effort should be made to undertake coronary angiography and percutaneous coronary intervention (PCI) as rapidly as possible.

Investigations
ECG, FBC, troponin (12 h after the event).

Risk factors
- Pre-existing coronary artery disease:
  - in the presence of coronary artery disease, hypotension, hypovolaemia, or anaemia is more likely to cause myocardial ischaemia.
  - spontaneous plaque rupture with partial or total occlusion of a coronary artery may also be the primary cause of myocardial ischaemia or infarction.

Exclusions
- Conduction abnormalities, such as bundle branch block, may be confused with ST segment changes that accompany myocardial ischaemia or infarction.
- Incorrectly placed ECG electrodes during surgery—always place in a standard position before induction and assess the normal trace. Changes are more likely to be seen and be significant.

Special considerations
If the patient is conscious, myocardial ischaemia and/or infarction is likely to be accompanied by angina.

Further reading
Timmis, A. (2015). Acute coronary syndromes. *British Medical Journal*, **351**, h5253.

☼ Cardiac tamponade

Definition
Low cardiac output state from mechanical compression of the heart.

Presentation
- Typically, after penetrating chest trauma or cardiac surgery.
- Systemic hypotension with elevated and equalized ventricular filling pressures (RA (CVP) and LA (PCWP)); decreased pulse pressure; raised JVP; pulsus paradoxus; no prominent 'y' descent on central venous pulse wave.
- Oliguria.
- Poor peripheral perfusion, cyanosis, metabolic acidosis, hypoxaemia.
- Dyspnoea.
- Sudden decrease/cessation of chest drainage in patient previously bleeding heavily after cardiac surgery.
- Cardiac arrest.

Immediate management
- ☑ ABC—100% O_2.
- ☑ Assess vital signs.
- ☑ Establish adequate IV access; give IV fluids, inotropic support.
- ☑ Post-cardiac surgery—cautiously 'milk' chest drains; attempt to clear clots from drains by sucking inside them with soft-tip suction catheter. Call for surgical help; alert theatres; prepare to open chest (on cardiac recovery area if necessary).
- ☑ Do NOT remove penetrating foreign body if present.
- ☑ Unless in cardiac arrest, anaesthetize before chest opening: choose technique which minimizes vasodilatation; intubation and ventilation will be required as chest will be opened; be prepared to open chest (wire cutters) immediately after induction.
- ☑ Open chest immediately if haemodynamics cannot be controlled.
- ☑ If in cardiac arrest caused by cardiac tamponade following penetrating thoracic trauma, immediate resuscitative thoracotomy is required.
- ☑ Pericardiocentesis may gain time and lessen the haemodynamic insult of anaesthesia (rarely used in acute situation).
- ☑ Request blood, and clotting factors as necessary.

Subsequent management
- ☑ Maintain filling pressures and sympathetic tone; avoid bradycardia.
- ☑ Anticipate blood pressure overshoot immediately on chest opening and relief of tamponade; usually rapid recovery of haemodynamic stability following mediastinal evacuation.
- ☑ Ensure surgeon identifies bleeding point and clears drains of clots.
- ☑ Correct metabolic acidosis.

☑ Positive pressure ventilation will worsen tamponade and hypotension.
☑ Repeat antibiotics if chest is reopened.

Investigations

Chest X-ray (widened mediastinum), ECG (low voltage, electrical alternans, T-wave abnormalities), echocardiogram/TOE (pericardial fluid collection, small non-filling ventricles).

Risk factors

- Chest trauma (particularly penetrating)
- Recent cardiac surgery, especially if:
  - heavy bleeding through chest drains postoperatively
  - pleurae NOT opened perioperatively
  - reoperations
- Coagulopathy (both hyper- and hypocoagulable)
- Hypothermia

Exclusions

- Tension pneumothorax
- Cardiogenic shock/myocardial failure/MI
- Pulmonary embolus
- Overtransfusion, fluid overload
- Anaphylaxis

Paediatric implications

- Cardiac tamponade can occur with very low volumes of blood in the mediastinum.
- Can be very sudden and present as cardiac arrest.
- Increased risk with cyanotic conditions, complex reoperations, and impaired coagulation associated with hepatic congestion.

Special considerations

- Electrical alternans—beat-to-beat shift in QRS axis associated with mechanical swinging of the heart in a large accumulation of fluid. Virtually pathognomonic of cardiac tamponade, though not always seen.
- High index of suspicion for cardiac tamponade after cardiac surgery.
- Only **definitive** diagnosis is made by opening chest—even small pericardial collections on echocardiography can have large haemodynamic consequences if pressing on the right atrium.
- Diagnosis can be very difficult, especially if possible failure/overload.
- If severe, impaired coronary flow may cause myocardial ischaemia, further complicating diagnosis.
- Presentation can be slow or very rapid.
- Hypocoagulable patients are more likely to bleed into the pericardium.
- Hypercoagulable patients are more likely to clot off chest drains.

- Patients with cardiac tamponade caused by penetrating trauma, including stabbed hearts and gunshot wounds, should be taken to theatre immediately and a pericardial exploration performed. Patients in cardiac arrest following penetrating thoracic trauma require immediate resuscitative thoracotomy (usually in the emergency department). Percutaneous pericardial drainage (pericardiocentesis) is usually ineffective and should not be performed unless surgery is unavailable.

:☼: Pulmonary embolus

Definition
Obstruction of pulmonary circulation by thromboembolus.

Presentation
- Chest pain (typically pleuritic). Dyspnoea, tachypnoea, haemoptysis.
- Hypoxaemia or increased A–a P_{O_2} gradient.
- Hypotension, tachycardia, dysrhythmia, cyanosis, poor peripheral perfusion, raised JVP/CVP, decreased end-tidal CO_2.
- Oliguria.
- Cardiovascular collapse, cardiac arrest.

Immediate management
☑ ABC—100% O_2, intubation/ventilation if arrested/in extremis.
☑ Define severity:
- non-massive PE—no RV dysfunction.
- submassive PE—right ventricular dilation and hypokinesis without systemic hypotension. Symptoms of chest pain and dyspnoea.
- massive PE—severe haemodynamic and ventilatory impairment with increased RV afterload.

Medical treatment
Non-massive and submassive PE
☑ Anticoagulation—therapeutic dose of low molecular weight heparin (e.g. enoxaparin 1.5 mg/kg every 24 h is first choice). Unfractionated heparin (10 000 units load, then 1500–2000 units/h aiming for APTT 1.5–2.5 × normal) is preferred if severe renal impairment, for those at high risk of bleeding, older people, or those extremely under- or overweight.

Massive PE
☑ Wide-bore IV access, fluid resuscitation, central access.
☑ Monitor vital signs (including invasive arterial and central venous pressure).
☑ Inotropic support as required.
☑ Thrombolysis (alteplase, rt-PA 10 mg over 1–2 min then 90 mg over 2 h; tenecteplase, t-PA 30–50 mg bolus). Surgery within the previous 1–2 weeks is a relative contraindication to thrombolysis. Thrombolysis is also considered in some cases of submassive PE.
☑ Consider surgical embolectomy if thrombolytic therapy is contraindicated.

Subsequent management

☑ Consider insertion of inferior vena cava filter if anticoagulation is contraindicated.
☑ Surgical embolectomy—if severe, deteriorating state, failed medical treatment, collapse, arrest, and in a centre that has this facility.
☑ Transvenous embolectomy (in a centre with this facility).

Investigations

- Arterial blood gases (hypoxaemia, hypercapnia or respiratory alkalosis, metabolic acidosis).
- Immediate transthoracic echocardiography.
- Chest X-ray (oligaemic lung fields, prominent PA).
- ECG:
  - Sinus tachycardia.
  - '$S_I Q_{III} T_{III}$' 20–50%.
  - T-wave inversion anteriorly 85%.
  - right heart strain 75%.
- CTPA.
- Troponin—an elevated value may identify those with submassive PE who may benefit from thrombolysis.

Risk factors

- Prolonged stasis/immobility, paralysis, recent air travel.
- Postoperative patients (classically 10 days), especially following prolonged and extensive pelvic/abdominal dissections; vascular damage.
- Previous history of DVT/thromboembolism.
- Hypercoagulability, obesity, oral contraceptives, malignancy, elderly.
- Heart failure.

Exclusions

- Myocardial infarction
- Respiratory tract infection, pneumonia
- Pneumothorax
- Cardiac tamponade
- Bronchial neoplasm; acute airway obstruction
- Sepsis

Special considerations

Anaesthetic management for emergency surgical embolectomy

☑ Avoid hypotension on induction ('fixed cardiac output'— decreased ventricular loading can lead to arrest).
☑ Have wide-bore intravenous, central venous, invasive arterial access established, and surgical team scrubbed before induction.
☑ Consider femoral vessel cannulation under LA.
☑ General aim is to maintain low pulmonary vascular resistance to offload right ventricle (but NOT cause excessive systemic vasodilatation), maintain cardiac output, and maintain coronary flow.
☑ If inotropes required, adrenaline may be the best compromise.

☑ Aggressive fluid therapy to maintain circulating blood volume (increased central blood volume causes pulmonary dilatation; little risk of pulmonary oedema but further RV failure possible).

☑ Avoid hypoxaemia and hypercapnia (more important than the increase in intrathoracic pressure during IPPV) as this will reduce PVR.

☑ Gentle hand ventilation during pulmonary arteriotomy on bypass to massage clots back out of PA.

☑ Manage pulmonary haemorrhage (may be copious bleeding from tracheal tube):
  • crossmatch blood, order clotting factors—especially if prior use of thrombolysis.
  • frequent ETT suction.
  • PEEP.
  • consider double lumen endobronchial tube if side known.
  • may require pneumonectomy.

Further reading

Konstantinides, S.V., Torbicki, A., Agnelli, G., et al. (2014). 2014 ESC Guidelines on the diagnosis and management of acute pulmonary embolism. *European Heart Journal*, **35**, 3033–80.

☼ Cardiac trauma

Definition
Blunt or penetrating injury to heart or great vessels.

Presentation
- Chest bruising, shock, hypotension, hypovolaemia, hypoxaemia.
- Poor peripheral perfusion, unequal/absent peripheral pulses, dysrhythmia, cardiac tamponade. Haemothorax—dull chest percussion, decreased breath sounds.
- May be coexisting injuries of other thoracic structures:
  - chest wall trauma (rib fracture, sternal fracture, sucking wound, flail segment).
  - pulmonary contusion (haemoptysis, haemothorax, hypoxaemia).
  - tracheobronchial rupture (stridor, dyspnoea, pneumothorax, hypoxaemia).
  - diaphragmatic rupture (dyspnoea, hypoxaemia, chest 'bowel' sounds).
  - oesophageal rupture (pain, dysphagia, mediastinal air on CXR).

Immediate management
- ☑ General management strategy as for all trauma cases. Neck immobilization.
- ☑ ABC—100% O_2.
- ☑ Wide-bore intravenous access, fluid resuscitation.
- ☑ Intubate/ventilate if necessary.
- ☑ Rapidly establish nature and extent of injuries—cardiac contusion is notoriously difficult to diagnose, rarely an isolated injury, sternal/rib fractures are a common though not essential association.
- ☑ Have high index of suspicion in all cases of blunt chest injury. Critical factor is adequacy of cardiac function.
- ☑ If penetrating implement in place, do not remove.
- ☑ Haemodynamic instability/inadequacy may be hypovolaemia, cardiac tamponade, blunt thoracic aortic injury, or primary myocardial dysfunction.
- ☑ Central venous access, invasive arterial monitoring (right arm).
- ☑ Chest drain if haemothorax/pneumothorax; observe rate of bleeding/air leak (theatre if excessive).
- ☑ Order blood and clotting factors, organize theatres.
- ☑ Analgesia.
- ☑ If blunt aortic injury is suspected, in the absence of head injury, aim for a systolic blood pressure of 80–90 mmHg until definitive repair/stenting is achieved.

Subsequent management
- ☑ Anaesthetic considerations. Assume full stomach; obtain control of airway and ventilation; if airway cannot be controlled (e.g. lower tracheal rupture) urgent bypass may be the only option.
- ☑ Antibiotics, tetanus.

Cardiac contusion:
- ☑ monitor haemodynamics and ECG.
- ☑ inotropes and antidysrhythmics as required.
- ☑ remember to treat other injuries.
- ☑ coronary artery injury very rare but may require coronary grafting.

Cardiac or great vessel rupture/perforation:
- ☑ ongoing resuscitation.
- ☑ theatre for urgent surgical repair.
- ☑ order blood and clotting factors.
- ☑ like aortic dissection, blunt thoracic aortic injury can present with proximal hypertension.
- ☑ typically median sternotomy.
- ☑ cardiorrhaphy may be performed on beating heart without bypass; if intracardiac damage, bypass will be required. Remember to give heparin (300 units/kg) before aortic/femoral cannulation. Bleeding may be brisk when chest is opened, requiring chest sucker-to-femoral artery bypass.
- ☑ blunt thoracic aortic injuries now increasingly managed with endovascular stent grafts.
  - Cardiac tamponade— see p. 38.
  - Aortic dissection— see p. 46.

Investigations

Chest X-ray (rib/sternal fractures, widened mediastinum, haemothorax), ECG (dysrhythmia, non-specific or ST segment changes), echocardiogram, CT scan (contrast, spiral), aortogram, troponin.

Risk factors
- Travel, notably road traffic accident (RTA)
- Use of seatbelts an important factor in car accidents
- Velocity of impact

Exclusions
- Haemorrhage from other sites
- Cardiac tamponade
- Aortic dissection
- Primary myocardial dysfunction
- May be coexisting injuries besides thorax (neck, head, abdomen, limbs)

Classification
- Blunt (non-penetrating):
  - blunt cardiac injury ('cardiac contusion')
  - cardiac rupture
  - aortic dissection
  - great vessel tear/rupture
- Penetrating—implement may or may not be in place
  - cardiac perforation
  - great vessel perforation

☀ Thoracic aortic dissection

Definition
Intimal tear creating a false lumen in the wall of the aorta.

Presentation
- Sudden-onset 'tearing' chest pain radiating to back.
- Severe hypertension; differential blood pressure in different limbs (some may be hypotensive/pulseless).
- Signs of acute aortic regurgitation (wide pulse pressure, collapsing pulse).
- Areas of poor peripheral perfusion. Oliguria.
- May present in cardiovascular collapse/cardiac arrest as:
  - cardiac tamponade (if ruptured into pericardium)
  - haemothorax (if ruptured into pleural space).
- When on cardiopulmonary bypass, presents as sudden decreased venous return and mean arterial pressure, with increased arterial 'line pressure' (i.e. pressure measured by perfusionist in arterial tubing returning blood from pump).

Immediate management
- ☑ ABC—100% O_2.
- ☑ Wide-bore peripheral IV access.
- ☑ Invasive arterial monitoring, central intravenous access, urinary catheter.
- ☑ Control BP—decrease myocardial contractility (essential) ± vasodilatation (helpful). Aim for systolic arterial pressure ≤110 mmHg.
- ☑ α_1/β_1-blockade (e.g. labetalol 5 mg boluses or infusion 2 mg/min until satisfactory response; max dose 200 mg).
- ☑ Sodium nitroprusside infusion (initially 0.3 µg/kg/min, increasing to max of 1.5 µg/kg/min until satisfactory response).
- ☑ Analgesia (e.g. IV morphine).
- ☑ Monitor all pulses; neurological examination (cerebral and spinal cord perfusion).
- ☑ Arrange theatres or transfer.

Subsequent management
Type 'A' dissection
- ☑ Surgical procedure is interposition of a tubular graft of the ascending aorta and resuspension of aortic valve; occasionally, the valve/aortic root must be replaced and coronaries reimplanted (same anaesthetic management) **or** surgery involves arch (requires deep hypothermic circulatory arrest for cerebral protection). Usually no coronary angiogram is available and therefore the state of the coronary arteries is unknown in these patients.
- ☑ Use the right radial/brachial artery for monitoring; if dissection involves this limb, it will be pulseless, therefore use the left arm.

Classification

- Type 'A'—involving ascending aorta (i.e. proximal, regardless of possible distal extension):
  - urgent surgical management.
  - median sternotomy approach.
  - often associated with aortic valve regurgitation (disrupted aortic annulus).
- Type 'B'—involving descending thoracic aorta only (i.e. distal, not involving ascending aorta):
  - usually initial conservative medical management but may proceed urgently to theatre for thoracotomy if complicated (rupture, uncontrollable BP, distal vascular compromise).
  - increasingly managed by endovascular stenting.
  - often associated with spinal cord ischaemia.

☑ Wide-bore IV access/central venous access/PAFC introducer preinduction. Nasopharyngeal, rectal, and peripheral temperature probes. PA flotation catheter useful but don't delay surgery for placement.

☑ Control BP (aim for systolic arterial pressure of 80–90 mmHg):
  - particularly avoid BP rise (may cause aortic rupture) on intubation, induction, and sternotomy (fentanyl, esmolol).
  - use volatile anaesthetic/labetalol/vasodilator infusion to maintain pressure reduction.

☑ Manage aortic regurgitation—avoid bradycardias (isoprenaline, atropine), decrease afterload (isoprenaline, vasodilators), avoid severe diastolic hypotension (reduction in coronary perfusion).

☑ Femoral artery cannulation for bypass, usually before sternotomy.

☑ Remember to give heparin before cannulation (300 units/kg). Anticipate major blood loss and coagulopathy—crossmatch blood (6 units), order clotting factors, tranexamic acid.

☑ Anticipate myocardial dysfunction (myocardial hypertrophy, prolonged bypass and cross-clamp times, dissection involving coronaries).

☑ Be aware that false lumen may have been cannulated—attempt to verify correct location by monitoring nasopharyngeal ('brain') and rectal ('core') temperatures during start of hypothermia on bypass—head temperature MUST cool with rectal temperature; check pupils; urine output.

☑ If surgery involves arch, deep hypothermic circulatory arrest will be required (consider cerebral and renal protection, e.g. thiopental 10 mg/kg; methylprednisolone 30 mg/kg).

☑ Anticipate hypotension on decannulation of femoral artery (lactate release)—sodium bicarbonate 50–100 mmol.

Type 'B' dissection

☑ Increasingly endovascular if surgical repair required.

☑ If open, then left lateral thoracotomy; double lumen endobronchial tube.

☑ Not performed on bypass but:

- one-lung ventilation.
- aorta cross-clamped with severe proximal hypertension (BP control) and haemodynamic upset on unclamping (NaHCO₃, inotropes).
- use right radial/brachial artery for invasive BP monitoring in case left subclavian artery is clamped.
- consider renal protection before aortic cross-clamp applied.
- risk of spinal cord ischaemia (consider steroid, barbiturate, spinal drain for spinal cord protection).
☑ Severe bleeding common—crossmatch blood (6 units), clotting factors, tranexamic acid, use cell saver if available.

Investigations

Chest X-ray (widened mediastinum; loss of aortic knuckle; displacement of intimal calcification), ECG (hypertrophy, strain, myocardial ischaemia if coronary involvement), CT aortogram (intimal flap, true and false lumen), MRI scan (intimal flap, true and false lumen), echocardiogram, ABGs (metabolic acidosis, mesenteric ischaemia).

Risk factors

- Hypertension
- Marfan's syndrome, connective tissue disease, cystic medial necrosis
- Chest trauma
- Atherosclerosis
- Cardiac surgery (intraoperative complication)

Exclusions

- Myocardial infarction
- Pulmonary embolus
- Acutely extending thoracic aortic aneurysm

Transferring thoracic aortic rupture patient to a cardiac centre

☑ Stabilize patient, wide-bore intravenous access, oxygen.
☑ Analgesia (morphine, fentanyl).
☑ Monitor cardiorespiratory status (BP, ECG, SₚO₂).
☑ Intubate and ventilate if necessary (cardiostable induction).
☑ Maintain haemodynamic stability—control systolic arterial pressure between 80 and 90 mmHg (e.g. labetalol infusion). Avoid overtransfusion with intravenous fluids.
☑ Ensure receiving hospital is fully notified. Transfer rapidly.
☑ Take blood with patient; maintain monitoring, BP control, and analgesia/sedation.

☼ Aortic stenosis

Definition

Obstruction of outflow through the aortic valve during systole, resulting in pressure loading of left ventricle. Severe when aortic valve area less than 1 cm^2 (normal 2.5–3.5 cm^2). (➲ See 'Classification of aortic stenosis', Table 2.2.)

Presentation

- Most commonly progressive exertional dyspnoea, angina, and syncope.
- Symptoms may not correlate well with disease severity.
- Classical examination finding is an ejection systolic murmur at the second right intercostal space, radiating to the neck.
- May be a slow rising pulse, carotid and precordial thrills.
- Left ventricular hypertrophy leads to diastolic heart dysfunction, with signs of failure in advanced decompensated disease.

Investigations

ECG—LV hypertrophy, secondary ST segment and T-wave changes, conduction defects.

CXR—often unremarkable. Occasionally valvular calcification or poststenotic dilatation of aorta. Pulmonary congestion suggests advanced disease or combined pathology.

Echocardiography—assess anatomy and grade severity, exclude other pathology, define ventricular function.

Cardiac catheterization or CT angiography to exclude coexisting coronary artery disease.

Risk factors

- Most commonly degenerative calcific disease.
- Congenital bicuspid valves tend to present at an earlier age.

Exclusions

- Coexisting coronary artery disease
- Combined valvular lesions

Table 2.2 Classification of aortic stenosis

	Peak velocity (m/s)	Mean pressure gradient (mmHg)	Aortic valve Area (cm^2)
Mild	<3.0	<20	>1.5
Moderate	3.0–4.0	20–40	1.0–1.5
Severe	>4.0	>40	<1.0

Perioperative management

Symptomatic patients and those with severe disease are at risk of sudden perioperative death and should be deferred where possible for consideration of valve replacement. If urgent, then:

☑ Establish adequate IV access and preinduction arterial BP monitoring.
☑ CVC may aid vasopressor administration.
☑ Haemodynamic goals are aimed at maintaining myocardial oxygen delivery.
☑ An opiate based technique is generally favoured to achieve this (fentanyl, remifentanil).
☑ Low normal heart rate (50–70).
☑ Maintain SVR with α-agonists (metaraminol/phenylephrine/noradrenaline) titrated to achieve BP at preinduction levels.
☑ Normovolaemia, avoid excessive fluid boluses.
☑ Treat arrhythmias aggressively.
☑ Neuraxial blockade should be used with extreme caution.
☑ Regional techniques may provide ideal analgesia and aid achieving haemodynamic goals.
☑ Postoperative care should continue in a critical care setting for all but the most minor procedures.
☑ Appropriate antibiotic prophylaxis as per local guidelines.

Special considerations

- Balloon aortic valvuloplasty may be considered as a temporizing measure, though is not without its own risks and benefit is not sustained.
- High risk patients are increasingly referred for TAVI; however, open valve replacement remains the gold standard.
- CPR is relatively ineffective.
- Beware the symptomatic patient with low reported gradient—may herald failing ventricle with severe disease.
- Carefully titrated neuraxial blockade has been used successfully for the management of obstetric patients but remains high risk.

☼ Aortic regurgitation

Definition

Abnormal retrograde flow through aortic valve during diastole with resulting volume loading of left ventricle. Severe when regurgitant fraction greater than 50%.

Presentation

- Chronic regurgitation develops over several years and is well tolerated.
- Increasing dyspnoea once compensatory mechanisms overcome.
- Palpitations if atrial fibrillation present (LA dilatation).
- Early diastolic murmur heard at second right intercostal space.
- Widened pulse pressure ('waterhammer' pulse, Corrigan's sign).
- Acutely presents with pulmonary oedema as left ventricle unable to compensate for sudden increased volume load.

Investigations

ECG—left ventricular hypertrophy, atrial fibrillation.
CXR—cardiomegaly, pulmonary congestion.
Echocardiography—assess aetiology and grade severity, exclude other pathology, define ventricular function.
CT aortogram—aortic root and/or ascending aortic dilatation, dissection in acute presentation.

Perioperative management

- ☑ Chronic regurgitant lesions generally tolerate anaesthesia well.
- ☑ Adequate IV access, arterial line for major surgery.
- ☑ Aim for high normal heart rate (80–100) to minimize regurgitant time.
- ☑ Low normal SVR augments forward flow and increases stroke volume.
- ☑ Maintain normovolaemia.
- ☑ Treat new arrhythmias, although tachycardia may be better tolerated than with stenotic lesions.
- ☑ Neuraxial blockade is generally well tolerated.
- ☑ Appropriate antibiotic prophylaxis as per local guidelines.

Risk factors

- Aetiology of chronic regurgitation may be degenerative, annular dilatation secondary to connective tissue disorders, longstanding hypertension, inflammatory disease, congenital abnormalities, rheumatic heart disease.
- Acute presentations secondary to aortic dissection or endocarditis.

Exclusions

- Aortic dissection
- Endocarditis

Special considerations
- Acute presentations require referral for urgent valve replacement.
- Severe regurgitation may be associated with low diastolic pressures and compromise coronary filling—vasopressors may be required despite the adverse effect on regurgitant fraction and cardiac output.
- In chronic presentations refer for consideration of replacement when severe and symptomatic or evidence of ventricular dysfunction.
- Intra-aortic balloon pumps worsen regurgitation and are contraindicated.

☼ Mitral stenosis

Definition

Obstruction of flow through the mitral valve during diastole resulting in pressure loading of left atrium. Severe when valve area less than 1 cm² (normal 4–6 cm²). (➲ See 'Classification of mitral stenosis', Table 2.3.)

Presentation

- Often asymptomatic until advanced disease as a result of compensatory mechanisms.
- As these are overcome then dyspnoea, fatigue, and frequent lower respiratory tract infections and haemoptysis.
- Progression to pulmonary oedema and pulmonary hypertension.
- AF is common, but new onset may result in acute decompensation.
- Mid-diastolic murmur heard best at apex.
- May progress to signs of right heart failure (elevated JVP, hepatomegaly, peripheral oedema).

Investigations

ECG—commonly AF, but broad/notched P waves (p-mitrale) if SR.
CXR—enlarged left atrium, valvular calcification, pulmonary congestion.
Echocardiography—assess anatomy and grade severity, exclude other pathology, define ventricular function.

Perioperative management

- ☑ Establish adequate IV access and preinduction arterial BP monitoring.
- ☑ CVC may aid vasopressor administration.
- ☑ Management of anticoagulation may be required.
- ☑ Aim for a low/normal heart rate (50–70) to allow LV filling.
- ☑ An opiate based technique is generally favoured to achieve this.
- ☑ Fixed output state in common with aortic stenosis—maintain SVR with α-agonists (metaraminol/phenylephrine/noradrenaline).
- ☑ Aim for normovolaemia—fluid overload may be poorly tolerated.
- ☑ Neuraxial blockade should be used with extreme caution.
- ☑ Regional techniques may provide ideal analgesia and aid achieving haemodynamic goals.
- ☑ Treat arrhythmias aggressively, although cardioversion of established AF unlikely to be successful. Rate control with cautious short acting β-blockade (i.e. esmolol) may be helpful.
- ☑ Avoid hypoxia, hypercapnia, acidosis, N₂O—may exacerbate pulmonary hypertension.
- ☑ Postoperative care should continue in a critical care setting for all but the most minor procedures.
- ☑ Appropriate antibiotic prophylaxis as per local guidelines.

Table 2.3 Classification of mitral stenosis

	Mean pressure gradient (mmHg)	Mitral valve Area (cm²)
Mild	<5	>1.5
Moderate	5–10	1.0–1.5
Severe	>10	<1.0

Risk factors

- Rheumatic heart disease remains leading cause worldwide.
- In developed world usually degenerative calcification or endocarditis, more rarely infiltrative disorders or congenital abnormalities.

Exclusions

- Coexisting coronary artery disease
- Combined valvular lesions

Special considerations

- Select cases may benefit from percutaneous mitral valvuloplasty.
- Valve replacement is the preferred treatment for those with symptomatic disease.
- Pregnancy is poorly tolerated (increased circulating volume, tachycardia) and may be first presentation.
- Early cautious neuraxial analgesia facilitates delivery.
- Oxytocin causes tachycardia and vasodilatation—administer cautiously.

☼ Mitral regurgitation

Definition

Abnormal retrograde flow through mitral valve during systole with resulting volume loading of left atrium and ventricle. Severe when regurgitant fraction greater than 50%.

Presentation

- Fatigue, dyspnoea.
- Severe disease with pulmonary oedema and pulmonary hypertension.
- Right sided heart failure (elevated JVP, hepatomegaly, peripheral oedema).
- Acute presentations with pulmonary oedema and circulatory collapse as the left atrium is unable to compensate for the sudden volume load.
- Look for features of ischaemia and endocarditis.
- Pansystolic murmur at apex.

Investigations

ECG—commonly atrial fibrillation, LA enlargement if sinus rhythm, ischaemic changes.

CXR—cardiomegaly, valvular calcification.

Echocardiography—assess aetiology, grade severity, define ventricular function (including right side) and regional wall motion abnormalities, exclude LA thrombus (if atrial fibrillation). Ejection fraction is falsely high as large volume may be retrograde.

Perioperative management

- ☑ Chronic regurgitant lesions without symptoms generally tolerate anaesthesia well.
- ☑ Adequate IV access, arterial line for major surgery.
- ☑ Management of anticoagulation may be required.
- ☑ Aim for high normal heart rate (80–100) to minimize regurgitant time.
- ☑ Low normal SVR augments forward flow and increases stroke volume.
- ☑ Maintain normovolaemia—may be difficult to estimate, but aim to keep well filled.
- ☑ Treat new arrhythmias, although tachycardia may be better tolerated than with stenotic lesions.
- ☑ Avoid hypoxia, hypercapnia, acidosis, N_2O—may exacerbate pulmonary hypertension.
- ☑ Neuraxial blockade is generally well tolerated.
- ☑ Appropriate antibiotic prophylaxis as per local guidelines.

Risk factors

- Valve dysfunction may be primary or secondary.
- Primary causes may be related to:
  - leaflet pathology: degenerative (myxomatous) disease, prolapse, endocarditis, rheumatic heart disease.
  - chordal/papillary muscle rupture: ischaemia, endocarditis.
- Secondary causes ('functional' MR) related to ventricular dysfunction, either as a result of annular dilatation or regional wall motion abnormalities.

Exclusions

- Myocardial ischaemia
- Endocarditis

Special considerations

- Acute presentations require referral for urgent valve repair or replacement.
- Ventilation, vasodilator therapy, and diuresis may be required acutely.
- Hypotension may limit vasodilator use and require vasopressor support despite its adverse effects on regurgitant fraction.
- Intra-aortic balloon pump insertion provides useful bridging therapy by reducing afterload and augmenting coronary perfusion.
- Chronic primary regurgitation should be referred for consideration of surgery when severe and symptomatic or with declining ventricular function.
- The surgical management of chronic regurgitation of secondary aetiology is less clear and requires multidisciplinary input into the decision-making process.
- Percutaneous techniques are relatively new with long-term outcomes unclear, but may be considered for high-risk patients unsuitable for conventional surgical approaches.

Further reading

Holmes, K., Gibbison, B., Vohra, H. (2017). Mitral valve and mitral valve disease. *British Journal of Anaesthesia Education*, **17**(**1**), 1–9.

Nishimura, R.A., Otto, C.M., Bonow, R.O., et al. (2014). 2014 AHA/ACC guideline for the management of patients with valvular heart disease. *Circulation*, **129**, e521–e643.

Respiratory

Tim Cook and Benjamin Walton

☼ Hypercapnia

Definition
P_aCO_2 >6.3 kPa (50 mmHg).

Presentation
Raised end-tidal CO_2 or P_aCO_2.

Immediate management
- ☑ Increase inspired O_2 to maintain S_pO_2 >95%.
- ☑ Check/increase minute ventilation. If patient is breathing spontaneously, then exclude excessive depth of anaesthesia and consider starting assisted ventilation.
- ☑ Compare measured inspired/expired tidal volumes for evidence of circuit leaks leading to reduced tidal volume. Check TT or SGA cuff pressure.
- ☑ Examine the capnograph trace to exclude rebreathing of CO_2. If detected, increase fresh gas flow or change CO_2 absorbent in circle system.
- ☑ Check for disconnections within the breathing system that increase dead space (e.g. internal limb of a Bain circuit).
- ☑ Ensure expiratory valves of circle system are not sticking.
- ☑ If safe functioning of the circuit is in doubt, change to alternative means of assisted ventilation. Remember to maintain adequate anaesthesia.

Subsequent management
- ☑ If P_aCO_2 or $ETCO_2$ continues to rise, exclude malignant hyperthermia, thyroid storm and other hyperthermic states.

Investigations
ABGs to confirm elevated P_aCO_2, and check for elevated base deficit suggestive of metabolic problem. Temperature, K^+ and creatine kinase if malignant hyperthermia suspected.

Risk factors/causes
- Increased CO_2 production—including pyrexia, sepsis, malignant hyperthermia, neuroleptic malignant syndrome, serotonin syndrome, reperfusion injury, thyroid storm.
- Decreased CO_2 clearance—respiratory depression, bronchospasm, inadequate minute volume during IPPV, inappropriate or faulty breathing system, partial airway obstruction, ineffective breathing during SV, excessive dead space.
- Increased CO_2 delivery to the lungs—abdominal insufflation with CO_2, capnothorax.
- Rebreathed CO_2—exhausted soda lime, inadequate FGF in partial rebreathing system, circuit valve fault, CO_2 in the fresh gas mixture.

Exclusions
- Malignant hyperthermia (➔ p. 280).
- A degree of hypoventilation is common during anaesthesia with SV.

Paediatric implications
Small increases in equipment dead space may significantly compromise the elimination of expired carbon dioxide. When using a T-piece breathing circuit, a FGF >5 L/min is required to prevent rebreathing.

Special considerations
- In the vast majority of cases, intraoperative hypercapnia is not clinically significant. In the absence of dysrhythmias or raised intracranial pressure specific treatment is not needed.
- The toxic child/adolescent with sepsis may have a very high metabolic rate and raised CO_2.

☼ Hypocapnia

Definition
P_aCO_2 <4.5 kPa (35 mmHg).

Presentation
Reduced end-tidal CO_2 or P_aCO_2.

Immediate management

No $ETCO_2$

☑ Check patient, monitors, connections, and ventilator at the same time as switching to 100% O_2 and confirming presence of a pulse. Is capnograph correctly attached? Is ventilator on?

☑ If cardiac arrest confirmed, perform advanced life support (➜ see p. 13). But note, capnography is low but not flat during CPR (or cardiac arrest) if the lungs are being ventilated.

☑ Try to distinguish between disconnection, airway misplacement, and obstruction. Hand ventilate with 100% O_2 looking for chest movement (remove drapes if necessary). Observe for chest movement.

☑ If disconnection—reconnect.

☑ If airway misplaced (including oesophageal intubation)—replace.

☑ If obstruction—urgently try to identify whether obstruction is (i) patient and airway or (ii) anaesthetic circuit.

☑ To exclude patient and airway obstruction (➜ see p. 75):
  • check position of TT/SGA.
  • Consider passing suction catheter down TT/SGA to confirm patency.
  • Exclude complete laryngospasm, foreign body, or displacement. If in doubt, remove airway device and replace.

☑ To exclude/manage circuit obstruction: change to self-inflating bag with 100% O_2 if circuit obstruction suspected and not remedied immediately. Keep $ETCO_2$ monitoring if possible. Ensure **new** HME filter.

Low $ETCO_2$

☑ Check patient's vital signs (pulse, S_pO_2, BP, temperature) and monitors.

☑ Look for causes of low cardiac output (e.g. reduction in venous return due to caval compression, concealed blood loss, pulmonary embolus, myocardial ischaemia), ➜ see also 'Intraoperative hypotension', p. 29.

☑ Is the patient being overventilated—is the respiratory rate or tidal volume high?

☑ Consider possibility of air/gas embolism (➜ p. 77). If likely, ask the surgeon to compress any bleeding points or irrigate wound.

☑ Check ABGs. Does the P_aCO_2 correlate with the $ETCO_2$? If not, does $ETCO_2$ monitor need replacing/recalibrating?

Subsequent management

- ☑ If equipment problem detected, ensure this is corrected for subsequent cases.
- ☑ Compromised elderly patients may have low metabolic rates. Adjust ventilation to produce normal $ETCO_2$ as this may cause excessive cerebral vasoconstriction.
- ☑ Consider hypothyroidism—a rare underlying cause (⊕ see p. 353).

Investigations

- ABGs

Risk factors

Elderly patients undergoing major surgery (hypovolaemia, hypothermia, metabolic rate).

Exclusions/Causes

- **No $ETCO_2$**—implies no ventilation or analyser disconnected/faulty.
  - Check pulse/S_pO_2, airway, and circuit, CO_2 analyser, and connection.
  - Is the ventilator on?
  - Remember oesophageal intubation and accidental extubation.
- **Low $ETCO_2$**—consider rate of fall.
  - patient—reduced cardiac output or cardiac arrest or reduced CO_2 production (hypothermia/hypotension/anaphylaxis/embolism). Impaired gas exchange or compensated metabolic acidosis. Obstructing airway.
  - anaesthetic—hyperventilation, anaesthesia too deep.
  - equipment—monitor, sampling.

Special considerations

It is important to note that during cardiac arrest, both with CPR and without it, if there lungs are being ventilated there will be an attenuated (low value) trace but it will nto be flat. If there is no trace, oesophageal Intubation should be excluded.

Beware the elderly, hypotensive, hypovolaemic patient. A low P_aCO_2 will further compromise cerebral circulation. Reduce ventilation and resuscitate.

Futher reading

No trace = wrong place https://www.youtube.com/watch?reload=9&v=t97G65bignQ

Cook TM, Harrop-Griffiths W. Capnography prevents avoidable deaths BMJ 2019; 364 doi: https://doi.org/10.1136/bmj.l439

☼: Hypoxaemia during anaesthesia

Definition
Inadequate arterial oxygen content.

Presentation
- S_aO_2 <90% with good perfusion. Cyanosis.
- Bradycardia in children.

Immediate management
- ☑ Change to 100% oxygen—confirm with oxygen analyser. Change oxygen source if doubt.
- ☑ Ventilate manually with large tidal volumes—check chest movement.
- ☑ If there is possible circuit leak or obstruction, switch to a self-inflating bag or remove and replace airway components until problem disappears. Change HME filter.
- ☑ If circuit is patent but ventilation is obstructed, suction or flexible bronchoscopy down TT/SGA to clear—replace and use facemask if necessary.
- ☑ If chest movement or auscultation is asymmetrical, consider possibility of pneumothorax (especially tension) or bronchial intubation.
- ☑ Listen for added sounds suggesting bronchospasm, oedema, or aspiration.
- ☑ Check pulse and blood pressure—exclude hypovolaemia/heart failure.
- ☑ If atelectasis is suspected (elderly, smokers, obese, supine), alveolar recruitment may be achieved by CPAP of 30 cmH_2O for 30 s followed by IPPV with PEEP.

Subsequent management
- ☑ CXR postoperatively (or on table).
- ☑ Consider and correct anaemia, hypovolaemia, carbon monoxide poisoning, sickle cell disease which will all worsen the impact of hypoxaemia.
- ☑ Consider severe right to left shunt (may present as hypoxia).

Investigations
ABGs, CXR, bronchoscopy.

Risk factors/causes
- Reduced F_IO_2—anaesthetic gas failure (➲ see p. 408).
- Reduced alveolar ventilation—depressed respiration, airway/circuit disconnection, airway obstruction, circuit obstruction, oesophageal intubation, accidental extubation, or bronchial intubation, bronchospasm/asthma, residual neuromuscular blockade.

- Increased ventilation/perfusion mismatch—chronic lung disease, interstitial lung problem (oedema, infection), PE, aspiration, airway collapse, atelectasis, obesity.

Exclusions

- Faulty S_pO_2 probe or poor position, surgical diathermy, or excessive patient movement (e.g. shivering or seizure activity). Check trace as well as the saturation number, reposition the probe to obtain a better trace—if in doubt, check ABGs. Oximeters also may misread during poor perfusion: check blood pressure.
- Anaphylaxis may present as hypoxia—hypotension will usually be a feature.
- Methaemoglobinaemia. Pulse oximetry readings falsely low due to the misinterpretation of methaemoglobin for deoxyhaemoglobin by pulse oximeter (typically reads approximately 85%).
Methylene blue (methylthioninium chloride) injection (e.g. for parathyroid/renal surgery) and patent blue (for sentinel node identification in breast surgery) have similar effects. As hypoxaemia may co-exist, do not assume a low S_pO_2 is due to these causes.
- Carboxyhaemoglobin produces a falsely high pulse oximeter reading. Exclude by bench oximetry readings from ABGs.

Paediatric implications

- Due to higher oxygen consumption and smaller FRC, rapid desaturation is more likely.
- Severe hypoxia may cause (or present as) bradycardia progressing to asystolic cardiac arrest.
- The infant lung is more susceptible to both mucus obstruction and atelectasis, so intubation, frequent tracheal suctioning, and administration of PEEP may be beneficial.
- Congenital heart disease. Treat aggressively with 100% oxygen to reduce PVR. Adrenaline and IV fluid to increase SVR, thus diminishing right to left shunt. Seek expert advice.

Special considerations

Cyanosis is only **clinically** detectable when the amount of deoxygenated haemoglobin is greater than 50 g/L. An anaemic patient may therefore be extremely hypoxic, yet not appear cyanosed.

☼ Non-tension pneumothorax

(➔ See also 'Pneumothorax during one-lung ventilation', p. 232)

Definition

Air in the pleural space.

Presentation

- Dyspnoea, cough, pleuritic chest pain, hypoxia.
- Asymmetric chest expansion with reduced air entry and hyper-resonance on percussion (signsoften absent/vague). Increased airway pressures during IPPV.
- Erect CXR—absent lung markings lateral to lung edge. Diagnosis more difficult with supine CXR. Anterior pneumothorax may occur in trauma/ICU—needs CT for diagnosis.
- Loss of lung sliding on lung ultrasound

Immediate management

☑ Increase oxygen delivery to achieve normoxia. IV access.
☑ Exclude tension pneumothorax (hypotension, significant respiratory distress). Tracheal deviation and jugular venous distension are late signs and often absent—➔ see p. 66 and 475.
☑ If tension pneumothorax is suspected, perform needle decompression (second intercostal space mid-clavicular line or thoracostomy, 66) followed by intercostal drain insertion (➔ p. 472–475).
☑ Nitrous oxide will worsen pneumothorax and should not be used.
☑ IPPV may worsen pneumothorax. Convert to spontaneous ventilation if possible. Reduce ventilation volumes/pressures until definitive drain inserted.

Subsequent management

- Pneumothorax can be classified as 1° (i.e. in a healthy patient) or 2° (i.e. in a patient with underlying chest disease). Prognosis is worse in 2° pneumothorax.
- The size of a pneumothorax can be estimated on CXR by measurement at the level of the hilum.
- Guidelines are designed for non-anaesthetic settings and earlier drainage may be indicated during anaesthesia.
    ☑ Patients on IPPV should have an intercostal drain inserted unless immediate weaning from IPPV is possible.
    ☑ 1° pneumothorax if symptomatic and/or >2 cm: needle aspiration. If unsuccessful, try one repeat aspiration, then insert intercostal drain. If asymptomatic and <2 cm—observe.
    ☑ 2° pneumothorax—if symptomatic, >2 cm, or patient >50 years old: intercostal drain, otherwise try aspiration. If <1 cm can observe.

☑ Persistent air leak—consider applying suction after 48 h (high volume/low pressure, 10–20 cmH$_2$O). Refer to thoracic surgery for further treatment (e.g. pleurodesis or pleurectomy).

Investigations

CXR, CT for complex cases.

Risk factors

- Secondary pneumothorax—associated with medical conditions: emphysema, Marfan's and Ehlers–Danlos syndromes.
- High-speed trauma—exclude pneumothorax before anaesthesia or IPPV. Prophylactic chest drain advised.
- Procedures— internal jugular or subclavian line, percutaneous tracheostomy, regional anaesthesia, post-CPR. May present some hours after procedure.
- IPPV-related—COPD, asthma, ARDS.
- Surgery-related—laparoscopic surgery, thoracic surgery, nephrectomy, percutaneous nephrolithotomy.

Exclusions

- Tension pneumothorax, lung bulla, major PE, lung collapse (opposite side). Diaphragm rupture (stomach in chest).
- During IPPV—bronchial intubation, pulmonary collapse.
- Bronchopleural fistula (post-thoracic surgery/severe trauma).

Special considerations

- Rapid re-expansion of the collapsed lung may be associated with pulmonary oedema. Monitor closely.
- Chest drain insertion (⊃ p. 472–5).
- Clamping chest tubes before removal: contentious. No evidence that clamping the drain improves re-expansion rates after drain removal. May detect small air leaks.
- Clamping for transfer is rarely, if ever, indicated. Clamping creates the risk of re-accumulation of a simple pneumothorax and converting a simple pneumothorax into a tension pneumothorax.
- Morbidity due to pain associated with intercostal drains is underestimated. Injection of interpleural local anaesthetic through the chest drain (e.g. 20 mL 0.25% bupivacaine 8 hourly prn) reduces pain without significant morbidity.

Further reading

MacDuff, A., Arnold, A., Harvey, J., BTS Pleural Disease Guideline Group Thorax (2010). Management of spontaneous pneumothorax: British Thoracic Society Pleural Disease Guideline 2010. *Thorax*, **65** Suppl 2, ii18–31.

☠ **Tension pneumothorax**

(➔ See also 'Pneumothorax during one-lung ventilation', p. 232.)

Definition
Accumulation of air under pressure in the pleural space.

Presentation
- Dyspnoea, cough, chest pain, hypoxia/cyanosis. Asymmetric chest expansion with reduced air entry and hyperresonance on percussion. Tracheal deviation away from the affected side (late sign).
- Hypotension and tachycardia, neck vein distension. Airway pressures increased on IPPV. Cardiovascular collapse.
- CXR—pneumothorax with deviation of mediastinal structures. Occasionally bilateral tension pneumothoraces occur—difficult to diagnose. Clinically resembles severe asthma.
- Loss of lung sliding on lung ultrasound

Immediate management
- ☑ High flow 100% oxygen. IV access.
- ☑ Needle decompression in the second intercostal space, mid-clavicular line of the affected side. Seeker needle to confirm, then a large-bore cannula of sufficient length to reach the pleural space (e.g. 16 G or larger in adults).
- ☑ Listen for audible hiss of air under pressure. The cannula should remain in place and open to atmospheric pressure until an intercostal drain is inserted.
- ☑ Thoracostomy, in the ventilated patient, is an alternative and increasingly recommended.

Subsequent management
- ☑ Intercostal drain insertion on the side of the needle decompression, ➔ see p. 472–5.
- ☑ If decompression did not confirm tension pneumothorax, an intercostal drain may still be required, as a pneumothorax may develop after needle decompression.

Investigations
Clinical diagnosis. Treatment should not await CXR. However, CXR is diagnostic.

Risk factors
- Trauma (blunt or penetrating)—often associated with rib fractures. CPR.
- Prolonged or high-pressure IPPV particularly in ARDS.
- CVC placement, regional anaesthesia (may occur some hours after insertion).

- Simple pneumothorax may become tension pneumothorax—IPPV, N_2O, or inappropriate clamping of intercostal drains.
- Surgery-related—laparoscopic surgery, thoracic surgery, nephrectomy, percutaneous nephrolithotomy.

Exclusions

- Airway obstruction.
- Bronchial intubation.
- Asthma, bronchospasm, and anaphylaxis may present with both respiratory and cardiovascular collapse, but respiratory signs are likely to be bilateral.

Paediatric implications

Small children are particularly at risk, especially with meconium aspiration or IPPV. Tension pneumothorax may present as hypoxia, hypotension, or bradycardia.

Special considerations

- Bronchopleural fistula (Ⓔ see p. 225).
- The development of tension in a pneumothorax is not dependent on the size of the pneumothorax.
- Avoid N_2O in patients at risk.

Further reading

MacDuff, A., Arnold, A., Harvey, J., BTS Pleural Disease Guideline Group Thorax (2010). Management of spontaneous pneumothorax: British Thoracic Society Pleural Disease Guideline 2010. *Thorax*, **65** Suppl 2, ii18–31.

☼ Pulmonary oedema

Definition
Increased extracellular pulmonary fluid.

Presentation
- Dyspnoea, hypoxia, sweating, tachycardia, pink frothy sputum, elevated JVP, gallop rhythm. Lung auscultation—fine inspiratory crepitations and quiet bases.
- Decreasing compliance on IPPV .
- CXR—pulmonary oedema (classical bat's wing, Kerley B lines, fluid in horizontal fissure), cardiomegaly if due to cardiac cause.

Immediate management
- ☑ 100% O_2 and sit patient up if practical. IV access.
- ☑ Furosemide 50 mg IV and diamorphine 1.5–5 mg IV.
- ☑ If BP >100 mmHg systolic—GTN (50 mg in 50 mL at 0–10 mL/h).
- ☑ Consider CPAP (5–10 cmH$_2$O) or PEEP.

Subsequent management
- ☑ Intubation and IPPV if not responding.
- ☑ If hypotension (<100 mmHg systolic) consider inotropic support (commonly dobutamine 1–15 µg/kg/min).
- ☑ Repeat furosemide, urinary catheter.
- ☑ If acute MI, refer for emergency angiography/PCI or consider thrombolysis as appropriate.
- ☑ Intra-aortic balloon counter pulsation.

Investigations
- ECG (tachycardia, ischaemia, myocardial infarction, LVH), CXR, ABGs.
- Echocardiography will detail valve function and contractility.

Risk factors/causes
- Fluid overload
- Heart failure
- Neurogenic
- Increased capillary permeability (sepsis/ALI)
- Following airway obstruction (post-obstructive pressure pulmonary oedema)
- Pulmonary aspiration

Exclusions
- Chest infection, severe asthma, anaphylaxis, pulmonary embolus, aspiration.
- Distinguish between high venous pressure (heart failure) and capillary leak (e.g. ALI).

Paediatric implication

In children non-cardiac causes (e.g. obstructive airway problems) are more common than in adults.

Special considerations

- LVF is commonest cause of pulmonary oedema.
- Opioids and furosemide also act as vasodilators.
- Differentiating between ALI and cardiogenic pulmonary oedema is difficult. ALI is likely with trigger events causing systemic inflammation (e.g. sepsis/major trauma/pancreatitis, and others). ALI: usually normal ECG and CXR showing diffuse bilateral shadowing without cardiomegaly or upper lobe pulmonary venous distension.
- LVF in extremis—venesection (250–500 mL) can buy time.

☢: Severe bronchospasm

(➔ See also 'Acute severe asthma in children', p. 136.)

Definition
- Life-threatening bronchospasm. This is an inflammatory condition, associated with mucus plugging and bronchial mucosal oedema.

Presentation
- Tachypnoea, hypoxia, tachycardia, cyanosis, hyperexpanded lung fields, wheeze or silent chest, reduced conscious level, exhaustion, hypotension.
- IPPV—increased airway pressure, up-sloping expiratory capnograph trace, slow expiratory phase, air trapping, wheeze may be audible or absent.

Immediate management
- ☑ 100% O_2, IV access.
- ☑ Nebulized salbutamol 5 mg. Repeat as indicated, if necessarily back-to-back.
- ☑ Nebulized ipratropium bromide 0.5 mg (4–6 hourly).
- ☑ IV salbutamol if not responding (250 µg slow bolus then 5–20 µg/min).
- ☑ Hydrocortisone 100 mg IV 6 hourly or prednisolone orally 40–50 mg/day.
- ☑ In extremis (decreasing conscious level) adrenaline may be used:
  - nebulizer 5 mg (5 mL of 1 in 1000).
  - IV 10 µg (0.1 mL 1:10 000) increasing to 100 µg (1 mL 1:10 000) depending on response.
  - beware arrhythmias in the presence of hypoxia and hypercapnia.
  - if intravenous access is not available, intramuscular administration 0.5–1 mg (0.5–1 mL 1:1000) may be used.
- ☑ Magnesium 1.2–2 g IV over 20 min.
- ☑ If bronchospasm follows induction of anaesthesia, stop all potential anaesthetic precipitants (including desflurane), maintain with isoflurane, sevoflurane, or TIVA. Try salbutamol inhaler 6–8 puffs through adaptor (➔ see p. 453). Consider anaphylaxis as cause (➔ p. 271). Exclude circuit/airway obstruction (➔ p. 413).

Subsequent management
- ☑ CXR—exclude pneumothorax (uncommon but may be fatal).
- ☑ If no response to initial management consider:
  - aminophylline (5 mg/kg over 20 min then infusion 0.5–0.7 mg/kg/h with ECG monitoring). Omit loading dose if already on maintenance.
- ☑ Consider ICU and IPPV.
- ☑ Volatile anaesthetics (isoflurane/sevoflurane) and ketamine sometimes help bronchodilatation.

Investigations

- ABGs—rising CO_2 ominous as suggests exhaustion.
- CXR—exclude pneumothorax.
- FBC, U&Es (check K^+ which can fall with β_2 agonist therapy).

Risk factors

- History of asthma (especially poor control/ICU/IPPV).
- Non-compliance with treatment or monitoring. Psychosocial factors.
- May be precipitated by induction of anaesthesia, tracheal intubation, or light anaesthesia. Most bronchospasm in this situation will settle rapidly.
- Administration of inappropriate drug. Use of NSAIDs, atracurium, D-tubocurarine, mivacurium, barbiturates, neostigmine, morphine, and oxytocin in susceptible individuals (only a few asthmatics are sensitive to NSAIDs and they can usually be identified from the preoperative history, but cross-sensitivity does occur within this group).

Exclusions

- Anaphylaxis, laryngospasm, glottis or subglottic airway obstruction, foreign body, aspiration, pneumothorax, pulmonary oedema.
- Circuit or airway obstruction including malpositioned SGA.

Paediatric implications

- Same basic principles as in adults, but more frightening!
- ⊃ See p. 136.

Special considerations

- Optimize asthma before anaesthesia.
- Routine prescription of antibiotics is not indicated in acute asthma.
- No single drug is predictably effective in any one patient—treatment is with maximal therapy and then reduce.
- Beware of hypokalaemia and lactic acidaemia caused by repeated β-agonist therapy.
- Heliox has the theoretical advantage of increasing flow in the airways. However, the reduced F_IO_2 (20–30%) is usually too significant for it to have a place in the management of life-threatening asthma. It is not recommended in BTS guidelines.
- During IPPV severe gas trapping may raise intrathoracic pressure, reduce venous return, and impair cardiac output necessitating intermittent disconnection of the circuit from the patient.
- Dehydration is common with severe asthma and, coupled with high airway pressures during IPPV, may lead to marked hypotension.
- The report of the UK-wide National Review of Asthma Deaths in 2014 reported >200 asthma deaths per annum. Most deaths occurred before admission. Previous admissions and psychosocial factors are associated with subsequent mortality. Inadequate treatment with steroids, inadequate objective monitoring, and underuse of written management plans were factors in fatalities.

Initiation of ventilation and ventilation strategy

☑ Indications for ventilation include exhaustion, worsening hypoxia, rising CO_2 (even when still in the normal range), reduced conscious level, and respiratory arrest.

☑ Whenever possible, induction should take place in ICU with senior staff. Be careful when moving critically ill asthmatics. Asthma is frequently underestimated, and brittle asthmatics may deteriorate dramatically in a matter of minutes.

☑ Use intravenous induction (propofol or ketamine) combined with an opioid and relaxant (vecuronium or rocuronium). RSI only if indicated. Sedate with opioids and propofol or ketamine infusion. Inhalational agents (sevoflurane or isoflurane) can be used. Muscle relaxants will facilitate IPPV, but are not bronchodilators.

☑ High airway pressures are inevitable to overcome airways resistance.

☑ Patients may have high levels of intrinsic PEEP and marked air trapping due to failure of expiration. Alveolar distension can impair venous return and cardiac filling.

• Long expiratory phases should be used to ensure adequate expiration.
• If hypotension is a feature, try disconnecting the patient from the ventilator, ventilate manually at 4–5 bpm on 100% oxygen, and observe for lung deflation.
• Manual chest compression has also been used (to augment lung deflation) but is controversial.
• If necessary, low-pressure PEEP may be tried to open airways and aid expiration. Some ventilators have an intrinsic PEEP function (PEEPi) to assess treatment.

☑ Permissive hypercapnia is indicated to avoid iatrogenic complications of ventilation.

Further reading

British Thoracic Society; Scottish Intercollegiate Guidelines Network (2014). British guideline on the management of asthma. *Thorax,* **69** Suppl 1, 1–192.

Royal College of Physicians (2014). *Why Asthma Still Kills: The National Review of Asthma Deaths (NRAD); Confidential Enquiry Report 2014.* London, UK: Royal College of Physicians. Available at: http://www.rcplondon.ac.uk/sites/default/files/why-asthma-still-kills-full-report.pdf

☠ Massive haemoptysis

Definition

Lower airway bleeding causing significant morbidity and/or mortality.

Presentation

- Extensive blood from airway, visible blood in TT, or on tracheal suction.
- Deteriorating gas exchange or pulmonary compliance.
- Cardiovascular instability (unlikely to precede significant disruption of gas exchange).

Immediate management

☑ ABC ... 100% O_2. IV access. Call for help.
☑ Intubation and IPPV may be required urgently or immediately.
☑ High airway pressures may be required if bleeding is extensive.
☑ Position patient appropriately—lateral (with bleeding lung dependent).
☑ Ensure efficient suction is available.
☑ Lung isolation if soiling of other lung is significant problem. (➲ See 'Pneumothorax during one-lung ventilation', p. 232.)
☑ Volume replacement.
☑ Crossmatch blood and blood products.
☑ Early bronchoscopy to identify cause.

Subsequent management

☑ Dependent on cause— sources of advice include thoracic or respiratory teams or radiology.
☑ Correct any coagulopathy.
☑ Intubation technique will depend on the clinical situation and the experience of the anaesthetist. If the source of bleeding is known, then lung isolation (using intentional endobronchial intubation, a double lumen tube or a bronchial blocker) will prevent soiling.
☑ Rigid bronchoscopy may be needed for surgical treatment.
☑ Radiological bronchial artery embolization has a high chance of controlling bleeding. Rebleeding is common and requires expectant postprocedural care.
☑ Emergency surgery carries a high mortality and should be reserved for patients in whom other measures have failed and those with adequate lung function.

Investigations

FBC, U&Es, coagulation, radiology imaging, bronchoscopy.

Risk factors

- Coagulopathy, acute invasion of blood vessel (e.g. trauma, neoplasm, abscess), bronchiectasis, pre-existing vascular abnormality

(e.g. AVM), pulmonary vasculitis (e.g. granulomatosis with with polyangiitis: previously known as Wegener's granulomatosis).
• Complication of tracheostomy, or pulmonary artery rupture caused by Swann-Ganz catheter.
• Malposition of chest drain.

Exclusions
Gastrointestinal haemorrhage, upper airway bleeding.

Special considerations
• Endobronchial isolation may be life-saving.

☼ Difficult controlled ventilation

Definition
Unexpectedly high airway pressure needed to generate adequate tidal volume during IPPV.

Presentation
- High airway pressure, low tidal volume. Hypercarbia +/− hypoxia.
- Abnormal capnography.
- Circulatory collapse due either to hypoxia or to impaired venous return secondary to high intrathoracic pressures.

Immediate management
☑ 100% O_2.
☑ Consider context in which situation has arisen:
  - Has the patient's position changed?
  - Is there a pneumoperitoneum?
Is this anaphylaxis?
  - Any recent procedure (central venous line, regional block)?
  - Has difficulty been gradually worsening or is it of sudden onset?
☑ Examine chest for asymmetry.
☑ Auscultate lung fields for wheeze and/or decreased air entry.
☑ Exclude tension pneumothorax clinically.
☑ Switch to manual ventilation:
  - If ventilation is easy, look for a ventilator circuit problem.
  - If ventilation remains difficult, problem is in the anaesthetic circuit, catheter mount, filter, airway device, or patient.
  - Is the patient interfering with ventilator (coughing/breathing)?
  - Slow refilling of the reservoir bag, indicates impaired expiration (e.g. partial airway obstruction or bronchospasm).
☑ If circuit problem still suspected, change to manual ventilation with self-inflating bag connected directly to the airway device or new HME filter. Remember to maintain anaesthesia.
☑ Pass a suction catheter down the TT/SGA to confirm patency. Repeat laryngoscopy and pull TT back 2 cm under direct vision and try IPPV again. Replace TT if necessary.
- These points will isolate the cause to the patient, airway device, or circuitry.

Subsequent management
☑ Deepen anaesthesia/consider muscle relaxation if airway patency confirmed.
☑ Replace circuit if blocked or broken. Use self-inflating bag until new equipment available.
☑ If wheeze on auscultation, treat for bronchospasm (➲ p. 70).
☑ Exclude anaphylaxis (➲ p. 272) and discontinue potential drug precipitants.
☑ Bronchoscopy to exclude tracheobronchial obstruction (foreign body/ mucus or blood).

Investigations

CXR to exclude pneumothorax/incorrect TT position/pulmonary oedema/ARDS and pulmonary collapse. Treat as appropriate.

Risk factors

Pressure on diaphragm/chest wall—pneumoperitoneum, massive gastric distension, relaxant wearing off.

Exclusions/causes

- Incorrect fresh gas flow selection: on some anaesthetic machines there may be >1 FGF outlet.
- On some anaesthetic machines, incorrect switch placement between controlled and spontaneous ventilation modes.
- Incorrect ventilator settings (inappropriate alarm settings).
- Bronchoaspasm and anaphylaxis, haemo/pneumothorax, pulmonary oedema, fibrotic lung disease, ARDS.
- Airway secretions, blood, foreign body (including aspiration), laryngospasm with SGA.
- Equipment fault—kinked or occluded equipment (especially TT, or circuit). Bronchial intubation, cuff herniation, malpositioned SGA, blocked or incorrectly assembled breathing circuit.

Paediatric implications

- Laryngospasm and bronchospasm are far more common. Blockage of small tubes with secretions and bronchial intubation are also common.
- Oxygen reserves are less, so hypoxia develops rapidly.

Special considerations

- Early identification of the problem is aided by correctly set (and switched on) ventilator alarms.
- Total sudden obstruction is most likely to be blockage of circuit or airway (including displacement). May be anything from a small cap in filter to kinked tubing. By changing to a self-inflating bag directly attached to the TT, most of the circuit is bypassed. The TT/SGA can be removed and exchanged for a facemask.
- ⊕ See also 'Difficult mask ventilation', p. 80.

☹ Air/gas embolism

Definition

Presence of gas in the vascular system (arterial, venous, or both).

Presentation

- Sudden decreased or absent capnograph trace and decreased S_pO_2.
- Tachycardia, hypotension, loss of cardiac output, PEA cardiac arrest.

Immediate management

☑ 100% oxygen. Discontinue and do not restart nitrous oxide (expands embolus).
☑ Exclude PEA cardiac arrest and breathing circuit disconnection.
☑ If PEA arrest, exclude other causes (➲ see p. 11).
☑ Stop surgery, lower operation site below level of the heart, compress any bleeding points, and flood wound to prevent further air/gas entry.
☑ If arrest, left lateral head-down tilt.
☑ Attempt to increase venous pressure with fluids and vasopressors.
☑ CPAP and PEEP may help by raising venous pressure.
☑ Decompress pneumoperitoneum if present.
☑ Aspirate CVC, if present. Ideally tip of line should be in right atrium (i.e. within embolus). Do not delay resuscitation to site CVC, if not already present.

Subsequent management

☑ Inotropes may help to overcome increased pulmonary vascular resistance.
☑ Application of bone wax to exposed bone sinuses.
☑ Hyperbaric oxygen therapy (if practical) with paradoxical arterial emboli.

Investigations

Clinical diagnosis. Capnography, ABGs (hypoxaemia ± hypercapnia), CXR (pulmonary oedema), ECG (right heart strain and ischaemia).

Risk factors

- Surgical—wound above heart or surrounded by pressurized gas—neurosurgery, spinal surgery, shoulder surgery, neck surgery, vascular surgery, intramedullary nailing, major joint arthroplasty, laparoscopy, thoracoscopy, endoscopy.
- Anaesthetic—hypovolaemia, air within intravenous sets/pressurized infusions, central venous access, and removal of central venous catheters.
- Patient—patent foramen ovale (risk of paradoxical air embolus).

Exclusions
- Hypovolaemia, anaphylaxis, PEA cardiac arrest, breathing circuit disconnection, PE, pneumothorax.

Paediatric implications
Neonates—particular risk of paradoxical embolus via the foramen ovale. Although this closes functionally within 24 h of birth, it may not close anatomically until 3 months of age.

Special considerations
- Carbon dioxide is less dangerous than air due to rapid re-absorption.
- CPAP/PEEP increases intrathoracic pressure and CVP and may limit the size and progression of an embolus. However, the rise in right atrial pressure may cause a paradoxical embolus in a patient with a patent foramen ovale (present in 10–15% adults).
- Paradoxical embolus presents with CNS signs.
- No investigation is sensitive and specific. TOE is best. A combination of capnography, precordial Doppler, and clinical suspicion most practical.
- Other diagnostic signs include mill-wheel murmur and gas bubbles in retina.

Further reading
Muth, C.M., Shank, E.S. (2000). Primary care: gas embolism. *New England Journal of Medicine*, **342**, 476–82.

Airway

Jules Cranshaw and Tim Cook

☼ Unexpected difficult mask ventilation

Definition
Ineffective pulmonary gas exchange despite an optimal mask fit.

Facemask ventilation is difficult in ~1:20 cases and impossible in <1:1000. Most difficult mask ventilation is unanticipated. When anticipated, it actually occurs in ~1:5 cases.

Presentation
- No chest movement despite manual ventilation with a pressurized reservoir bag.
- Flat capnogram.
- Arterial oxygen desaturation.

Immediate management
- ☑ **Adequate oxygenation is the management goal**.
- ☑ Decide whether you can wake the patient. If rapid recovery of adequate spontaneous ventilation is likely, maintain CPAP with 100% oxygen at high flow and wake the patient. Ask an assistant to hold the oxygen 'flush' button.
- ☑ If rapid recovery of adequate spontaneous breathing is unlikely, deepen anaesthesia intravenously to exclude laryngospasm, straining, or breath-holding and stop coughing or spontaneous breathing against an obstructed airway. Preferably use propofol.
- ☑ If your anaesthetic plan was to administer a neuromuscular blocker, give it. Preferably, use rapid paralysis with suxamethonium (1.5 mg/kg) or rocuronium (1.2 mg/kg). **At every step, complete paralysis is more likely to help airway management than harm.**
- ☑ Aim for the best position for ventilation not laryngoscopy. In adults, start with the 'sniffing' ('flextension') position. Be prepared to try others. Flex the lower neck on the shoulders. Extend the head on the neck. Consider a 'head-elevated' position (ear level with manubrium) on pillow(s) or a 'ramped up' position if obese.
- ☑ Add chin lift or jaw thrust.
- ☑ Insert a correctly sized oral airway and consider a nasal airway but beware bleeding.
- ☑ Use 4- or 6-handed mask ventilation. Use your hands to obtain a seal and an assistant's to squeeze the bag. The tho-handed V-grip with the hands facing caudal is better than the C-grip with the hands facing each other. Use another assistant to apply two-handed jaw thrust. Slow, sustained pressure may be better than rapid, high pressure.
- ☑ Reduce or release cricoid force—be ready with suction.
- ☑ Insert an SGA; (remove cricoid force first) but do not use more than three attempts. If an attempt fails, consider different sizes, devices, and insertion methods. Use a different device at your last attempt.
- ☑ If SGA insertion improves oxygenation, pause and consider the options. If it is not safe to continue with an SGA, wake the patient or consider intubation via the SGA.

☑ If SGA insertion does not improve oxygenation, declare 'failed SGA insertion' and reattempt facemask ventilation with adjustments and adjuncts as just described. Prepare to intubate.

☑ If the final facemask attempt fails and a neuromuscular blocker has not yet been administered, rapidly fully paralyse with suxamethonium (1.5 mg/kg) or rocuronium (1.2 mg/kg). If a neuromuscular blocker has been given, ensure full paralysis.

☑ If still unable to oxygenate, declare 'failed mask ventilation' to the team and attempt tracheal intubation *with the optimal position for laryngoscopy and intubation.*

☑ If intubation fails, go to your plan for CICO (⊕ p. 88).

Subsequent management

☑ Make plans for managing the airway during emergence and extubation.

☑ Decompress the stomach if possible.

☑ Fully document any difficulties and strategies in notes. Set up an 'airway alert' for the future.

☑ Inform the patient verbally and in writing of difficulties. Advise them on future safe airway care. Notify databases and GP.

Risk factors

- Lack of preoxygenation. (Preoxygenation will not prevent DMV but will mitigate its impact.)
- Inexperience.
- Obesity, snoring, sleep apnoea, thick neck, beard, small jaw, absence of teeth, craniofacial abnormalities, neck radiotherapy, increasing age, male gender.
- Predictors: modified Mallampati classes 3 and 4, limited jaw protrusion.

Exclusions

If the reservoir bag fills, but the chest does not move on ventilation consider:

- suboptimal airway maintenance.
- blocked anaesthetic circuit, filter, catheter mount, mask, or airway device. Try a new self-inflating bag and a fresh mask. (⊕ See 'Equipment problems', p. 413.)
- inadequate anaesthetic depth. Partially preserved airway reflexes and 'straining' make ventilation difficult.
- laryngospasm (⊕ p. 104).
- unexpected upper airway pathology, e.g. tumour, cyst, abscess, foreign body (e.g. retained throat pack) (⊕ p. 219).
- unexpected lower airway pathology, e.g. tumour or extrinsic compression (⊕ p. 216).
- bronchospasm (⊕ p. 70).
- tension pneumothorax (uni-or bilateral) (⊕ p. 58).
- massive pleural effusion(s).
- unintentional hyperinflation by manual ventilation—let the patient expire fully.
- expiratory airway obstruction leading to gas trapping.

- gross aspiration (◑ p. 107).
- tracheoesophageal fistula.

If the reservoir bag does not fill, consider:
- have the gases been switched on?
- circuit, bag, or vaporizer leak.
- gas supply failure.

Paediatric considerations

- The same stepwise progression, techniques, and exclusions are appropriate.
- Try a shoulder roll if <2 years of age. Start with a neutral position initially if 2–8 y.
- Pass a gastric tube early. Gastric distention and its effects (vagal reflexes, difficult ventilation, and reflux) are more likely.
- Difficult intubation is less frequent in children. Intubation, after muscle relaxation, may be a more appropriate early strategy to improve the airway.
- If the S_pO_2 can be maintained >80% then reversal of neuromuscular blockade (if needed) and waking may be a safe option.
- If the S_pO_2 is <80% or there is bradycardia, paralyse and attempt intubation. If this fails, proceed to the paediatric CICO strategy (◑ p. 90).

Special considerations

- Adequate oxygenation is the goal but the adequate vs. harmful level and its duration is difficult to determine in any context. Pulse oximeters are not usually calibrated below 85% and tend to underestimate but oximetry may have a delay of more than 30 s. Isolated ECG changes with hypoxaemia under anaesthesia are not usually associated with acute adverse outcomes. However progressive bradycardia and cardiovascular failure associated with hypoxaemia should be interpreted as life-threatening.
- Successful insertion and function of an SGA will rescue >90% of cases. Choose and prepare your rescue SGA(s) before induction. Experience with the devices and their insertion methods matters. Second-generation devices generally have a better airway seal and may reduce the consequences of regurgitation and are therefore recommended.
- Get experienced help early but remember 'human factors' may be detrimental when many people arrive at an emergency.
- Cognitive aids may reduce the risk of human factors impeding treatment. The 'Vortex approach' emphasizes face mask ventilation, SGA insertion, and tracheal intubation but **not to fixate on any one** and to proceed to FONA when severe hypoxaemia occurs during airway management failure (for Vortex approach, ◑ see p. 89).
- Aim for stability. Try not to take great risks and actions which could make a stable situation much worse if there is only a small chance of success.
- There may have to be many hands working effectively and cooperatively near the patient: mask (2); jaw thrust (2); cricoid force (1) and bag (2).

- Difficult mask ventilation is associated with difficult intubation and probably with difficult SGA insertion. When mask ventilation fails, rescue by intubation is more likely to be difficult and fail too.
- Spontaneous breathing efforts against an obstructed airway may lead to post-obstructive pulmonary oedema during or after the event. This may accelerate or prolong hypoxaemia. (➲ See p. 68.)

Further reading

Adnet, F. (2000). Difficult facemask ventilation: an underestimated aspect of the problem of the difficult airway? *Anesthesiology*, **92**, 1217–18.

Chrimes, N. *The Vortex Approach*. Available at: http://vortexapproach.com

Frerk, C., Mitchell, V.S., McNarry, A.F., et al. (2015). Difficult Airway Society 2015 guidelines for management of unanticipated difficult intubation in adults. *British Journal of Anaesthesia*, **115**, 827–48.

Kheterpal, S., Healy, D., Aziz, M.F., et al. (2013). Incidence, predictors, and outcome of difficult mask ventilation combined with difficult laryngoscopy: a report from the multicentre perioperative outcomes group. *Anesthesiology*, **119**, 1360–9.

Langeron, O., Masso, E., Huraux, C., et al. (2000). Prediction of difficult facemask ventilation. *Anesthesiology*, **92**, 1229–36.

Nørskov, A., Rosenstock, C.V., Wetterslev, J., Astrup, G., Afshari, A., Lundstrøm, L.H. (2015). Diagnostic accuracy of anaesthesiologists' prediction of difficult airway management in daily clinical practice: a cohort study of 188064 patients registered in the Danish Anaesthesia Database. *Anaesthesia*, **70**, 272–81.

☼ Unanticipated difficult intubation

Definition

Unexpectedly difficult laryngoscopy or tracheal intubation during general anaesthesia.

Patients do not die from failure to intubate but failure to oxygenate. Strategies for managing unanticipated difficult intubation should be discussed at the team brief and the 'sign in' of the WHO Surgical Safety Checklist before anaesthetic induction.

Presentation

- Larynx not seen (but most failed intubations are not a Grade 4 laryngoscopic view—it is very rare).
- Only tip of epiglottis visible.
- Laryngeal view obstructed by airway pathology.
- Inability to insert a TT despite an adequate view.

Immediate management

See also Figure 4.1.

☑ Get experienced help urgently and the 'difficult airway trolley'.

☑ Ensure complete neuromuscular block.

☑ While oxygenation allows, optimize the laryngeal view by; lower neck flexion and upper neck extension; displacing the tongue laterally; adjusting or removing cricoid force; external laryngeal manipulation; backwards upwards rightwards pressure (BURP) on the thyroid cartilage.

☑ Maintain anaesthesia intravenously as required.

☑ If the epiglottis can be lifted with a grade 2b or 3a laryngeal view, aim a correctly bent TT introducer (or bougie) with a coudé-tip, between the epiglottis and posterior pharyngeal wall through the glottis, blindly if necessary. Beware airway trauma by passing an introducer too far and do not pass beyond 26 cm from the mouth in an adult. With the laryngoscope in place 'railroad' a small TT over the introducer. Rotate the TT tip over the larynx into the trachea. Remove the introducer. Confirm location with a normal capnogram and clinical examination during ventilation.

☑ If the epiglottis cannot be lifted or seen with grade 3b and 4 views, the 'blind' introducer technique is not recommended.

☑ If intubation fails because of a poor laryngeal view during direct laryngoscopy, a videolaryngoscope is recommended, the exact choice being determined by experience and training.

☑ Make no more than four attempts at laryngoscopy: fewer if you cannot improve the view. Reduce or release cricoid force. Try a small TT and bend the TT ± a stylet. The fourth attempt should be reserved for a more experienced operator.

☑ When desaturation occurs, mask ventilate with 100% oxygen. If unable, go to the difficult mask ventilation strategy (➲ p. 80).

☑ Each laryngoscopy risks airway trauma, CICO, recurrent desaturation, aspiration, cardiovascular instability, awareness, dental damage, difficult SGA insertion, and difficult extubation.

☑ If intubation is unlikely to succeed or maximum attempts are unsuccessful, declare 'failed intubation' to the team and proceed to Plan B (maintaining oxygenation via an SGA).

☑ Use a second-generation SGA with which you are experienced. Remove cricoid force during insertion. Have a maximum of three attempts, two with your first choice and the third with another type. Consider different sizes and insertion techniques.

☑ If oxygenation with the SGA is adequate, stop and think. Consider risks and benefits of options in context; waking the patient; intubation via the SGA using a flexible optical bronchoscope (FOB) ± Aintree intubating catheter; proceeding with the SGA; rarely— proceeding after tracheostomy or cricothyroidotomy.

☑ If you cannot adequately oxygenate declare 'failed SGA ventilation' to the team and proceed to Plan C (final attempt at facemask ventilation).

☑ Reconfirm complete neuromuscular block. Use all the positioning, techniques, adjuncts, and assistants from the difficult mask ventilation strategy in a final attempt to oxygenate.

☑ If you can oxygenate adequately then wake the patient unless this is not likely to be life-saving. This will require full reversal of neuromuscular block. Use sugammadex when appropriate. If you fail, declare 'cannot intubate cannot oxygenate'.

☑ Plan D is emergency FONA. Go to the CICO strategy. 'Scalpel' cricothyroidotomy is recommended (◑ p. 88).

Subsequent management

☑ Careful FOB inspection of the upper airway may be indicated.

☑ Plan for extubation. Airway trauma makes airway and lung contamination, laryngospasm, and obstruction more likely.

☑ Before extubation, make a plan for re-intubation. (◑ See 'Difficult extubation', p. 110.)

☑ Record a difficult intubation on/in notes; notify GP, databases, and patient (verbally and in writing) when fully recovered. Complete an 'airway alert'.

Investigations

• Capnography.
• Careful inspection of the airway after intubation.

Risk factors

• Inexperience.
• Previous difficult intubation.
• ITU, ED, obstetric units, and remote environments.
• Difficult mask ventilation.
• There are many predictors of difficult laryngoscopy but typically up to 90% of difficult intubations are not predicted.

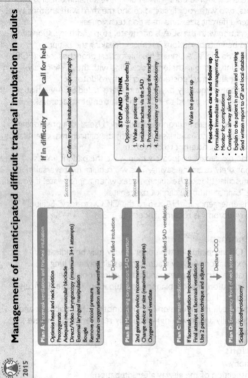

Figure 4.1 Management of unanticipated difficult tracheal intubation.

Reproduced from Difficult Airway Society 2015 guidelines for management of unanticipated difficult intubation in adults. C. Frerk, V. S. Mitchell, A. F. McNarry, C. Mendonca, R. Bhagrat, A. Patel, E. P. O'Sullivan, N. M. Woodall and I. Ahmad, Difficult Airway Society intubation guidelines working group. *British Journal of Anaesthesia*, 115 (6): 827–48 (2015)

The following text appears within the figure:

Management of unanticipated difficult tracheal intubation in adults

2015

Plan A: Facemask ventilation and tracheal intubation
- Optimise head and neck position
- Preoxygenate
- Adequate neuromuscular blockade
- Direct/Video Laryngoscopy (maximum 3+1 attempts)
- External laryngeal manipulation
- Bougie
- Remove cricoid pressure
- Maintain oxygenation and anaesthesia

If in difficulty → call for help

Succeed → Confirm tracheal intubation with capnography

→ Declare failed intubation

Plan B: Maintaining oxygenation: SAD insertion
- 2nd generation device recommended
- Change device or size (maximum 3 attempts)
- Oxygenate and ventilate

→ Declare failed SAD ventilation

STOP AND THINK
Options (consider risks and benefits):
1. Wake the patient up
2. Intubate trachea via the SAD
3. Proceed without intubating the trachea
4. Tracheostomy or cricothyroidotomy

Succeed → Wake the patient up

Plan C: Facemask ventilation
- If facemask ventilation impossible, paralyse
- Final attempt at facemask ventilation
- Use 2 person technique and adjuncts

→ Declare CICO

Plan D: Emergency front of neck access
- Scalpel cricothyroidotomy

Post-operative care and follow up
- Formulate immediate airway management plan
- Monitor for complications
- Complete airway alert form
- Explain to the patient in person and in writing
- Send written report to GP and local database

This flowchart forms part of the DAS Guidelines for unanticipated difficult intubation in adults 2015 and should be used in conjunction with the text.

- Individual predictors have low sensitivity and specificity. Multiple predictors may increase the odds of detecting difficulty.
- Predictors include modified Mallampati Class 3 or 4, thyromental distance <6.0 cm, mouth opening <2.5 cm, reduced upper cervical mobility, small jaw, large tongue, craniofacial abnormalities.
- Obesity modestly increases risk of difficulty but markedly increases speed of onset and severity of hypoxaemia.

Exclusions

- Inadequate anaesthesia and muscle relaxation.
- Poor patient positioning.
- Laryngoscope blade too short or long; difficult insertion causing unusual lie of the blade with poor view.
- Problems with TT shape or size (e.g. double lumen tubes).
- Laryngoscope light too dim or ambient light too bright.
- *Always exclude oesophageal intubation.*

Paediatric considerations

- The same stepwise progression, techniques, and exclusions are appropriate.

Special considerations

At the point of moving to Plan B, make an active decision if it is in the patient's best interests to wake or to continue with general anaesthesia and attempts to intubate. Consider:

- ease of oxygenation and ventilation via an SGA
- aspiration risk
- certainty of maintaining an adequate airway throughout surgery
- urgency of surgery
- the practicalities of waking the patient

Wake if oxygenation or ventilation is difficult, airway patency is precarious or there is a high aspiration risk, unless surgery is life-saving or waking is impossible.

Cognitive aids may lessen the risk of 'human factors' impeding best treatment. The Vortex approach emphasizes facemask ventilation, SGA insertion, and tracheal intubation but *not to fixate on any one technique* and to proceed to FONA before critical hypoxaemia occurs (→ p. 89).

Further reading

Chrimes, N. *The Vortex Approach*. Available at: http://vortexapproach.com
Cook, T.M., MacDougall-Davis, S.R. (2012). Complications and failure of airway management. *British Journal of Anaesthesia*, **109** Suppl 1, i68–i85.
Frerk, C., Mitchell, V.S., McNarry, A.F., et al. (2015). Difficult Airway Society 2015 guidelines for management of unanticipated difficult intubation in adults. *British Journal of Anaesthesia*, **115**, 827–48.
Nørskov, A.K., Rosenstock, C.V., Wetterslev, J., Astrup, G., Afshari, A., Lundstrøm, L.H. (2015). Diagnostic accuracy of anaesthesiologists' prediction of difficult airway management in daily clinical practice: a cohort study of 188 064 patients registered in the Danish Anaesthesia Database. *Anaesthesia*, **70**, 272–81.

☠️ Cannot intubate ... cannot oxygenate (CICO)

→ See also 'Cricothyroidotomy', p. 454.

Definition
The potentially lethal inability to oxygenate, despite optimum use of airway-opening manoeuvres, a facemask, and airway adjuncts, SGAs, and 100% oxygen at high positive pressure, combined with failed tracheal intubation.

Presentation
- Flat capnogram.
- No chest movement or breath sounds.
- Relentless desaturation.

Immediate management
☑ Call for help immediately but particularly for a specialist anaesthetist, intensivist, or surgeon with experience in cricothyroidotomy.
☑ Leave an SGA in place. It can be a route for exhalation and may improve identification of landmarks.
☑ Ensure complete neuromuscular block.
☑ Fully extend the head on the neck.
☑ Decide between two methods of cricothyroidotomy and ventilation according to available expertise:
   - 'Scalpel' cricothyroidotomy, inserting a narrow (4–6 mm ID) cuffed TT and conventional ventilation. This is the preferred approach.
   - Cannula cricothyroidotomy with a kink-resistant cannula <2 mm ID and jet (high pressure source) ventilation system using a 4 bar (400 kPa) oxygen source. **Beware complications (see next).** Experienced practitioners may convert a cannula to a TT using a Seldinger-based kit.
☑ If time allows, ultrasound may aid identification of the cricothyroid membrane.

Subsequent management
☑ Anaesthesia should be maintained intravenously.
NB: An emergency front of neck airway should not be undertaken lightly but it is wrong to wait until cardiac arrest. It may take minutes from decision to ventilation and delay is a feature of fatal cases. The 'Vortex approach' is a useful aide to prevent delay (see Figure 4.2).

'Scalpel' (previously 'surgical') cricothyroidotomy
☑ Beware endobronchial intubation when a TT is inserted through this unusually low level.
☑ Get a senior ENT surgeon urgently. Further airway surgery may be needed.

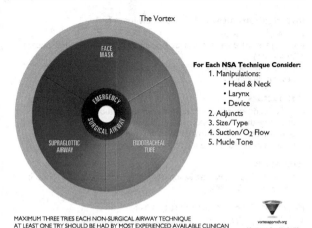

Figure 4.2 The Vortex Approach.
© Nicholas Chrimes 2016. Used with permission.

☑ Drain the stomach after a cuffed TT is secured. It may be distended, impair ventilation, and increase aspiration risk.

☑ Arrange critical care for complications (e.g. postobstructive pulmonary oedema, hypoxic encephalopathy, aspiration).

Cannula cricothyroidotomy with high pressure source ventilation ± conversion using a Seldinger technique

☑ Beware complications associated with cannulae and high airway pressure. A cannula provides no airway protection. If the upper airway is obstructed, restricted exhalation can cause sustained high intrathoracic pressure and cardiovascular compromise. Hypoventilation and hypercapnia also cause cardiovascular failure. High airway pressure and cannula displacement may cause tension pneumothoraces and subcutaneous emphysema. The latter can make examination and re-accessing the trachea difficult.

☑ With Seldinger technique-based kits, a cannula can be converted to a TT, typically 4–6 mm ID, which may be cuffed. A cuffed TT enables conventional ventilation. An uncuffed TT may make ventilation difficult if gas escapes via the upper airway. Occluding the SGA may help.

☑ A cannula is a short-term solution. At a suitable point a TT will have to be inserted.

Investigations after a TT has been inserted

- Arterial blood gases.
- CXR (exclude pneumothoraces, pneumomediastinum, endobronchial intubation).
- Careful endoscopic and radiographic examination for airway and oesophageal injury.

Risk factors

- Difficult and impossible mask ventilation and intubation occur more often together than alone.
- Both are associated with aspiration which may contribute to CICO.
- CICO may be consequence of traumatic intubation attempts.

Exclusions

- ➲ See 'Difficult mask ventilation' (➲ p. 80) and 'Unexpected difficult intubation', (➲ p. 84).

Paediatric considerations (ages 1–8)

- Call for experienced ENT assistance. If an experienced ENT surgeon is ready, rigid bronchoscopy and pressure-limited 'jet' ventilation or tracheostomy are preferable.
- If S_pO_2 <80% or there is bradycardia and no ENT surgeon is ready, ensure complete paralysis and perform a cannula cricothyroidotomy with a dedicated cannula of appropriate gauge and length. Perform a surgical cricothyroidotomy if cannula cricothyroidotomy fails.
- Use an adjustable pressure-limited 'jet' ventilator set initially at the lowest pressure. Increase pressure as needed to achieve adequate chest expansion. Allow complete expiration between breaths. An alternative is a 4 bar O_2 source with a flowmeter set in L/min to the child's age in years with a Y-connector to control ventilation. **Beware the consequences of upper airway obstruction (as just described). The flow rate may need to be reduced**.
- Decompress the stomach with a tube.

Special considerations

- In adults, perform a cricothyroidotomy not a tracheostomy whenever possible.
- Sometimes neck pathology (haematoma, infection, scarring) makes a lower approach safer.

Further reading

Cook, T.M., Nolan, J.P., Cranshaw, J., Magee, P. (2007). Needle cricothyroidotomy. *Anaesthesia*, **62**, 289–90.

Frerk, C., Mitchell, V.S., McNarry, A.F., et al. (2015). Difficult Airway Society 2015 guidelines for management of unanticipated difficult intubation in adults. *British Journal of Anaesthesia*, **115**, 827–48.

⚙ The partially obstructed airway presenting as an emergency

Definition

'Imminent' development of life-threatening airway obstruction in a patient presenting with a partially obstructed airway. This is particularly worrying when oxygenation or tracheal intubation will be difficult.

In extreme cases the only goal of airway management may be to immediately to 'rescue the airway' and prevent impending obstruction. Treatment of the obstructing lesion may occur at this time or as a seperate procedure.

Presentation

Acutely symptomatic tumour, trauma, inflammation, burn, foreign body, or surgical complication partially obstructing the airway. Presentation may be affected by the:

- Level—oral, supraglottic, laryngeal, mid-tracheal, and low tracheal. Several levels may be affected.
- Severity—increasing dyspnoea, positional or nocturnal dyspnoea, or dysphagia with anxiety, stridor, and acute dysphonia, expiratory noise (suggesting intrathoracic obstruction), accessory muscle use, hypoxaemia, and silent chest all suggest severe obstruction.

Immediate management

- ☑ Encourage the patient to adopt their best breathing position.
- ☑ Sustain adequate oxygenation with inspired oxygen. Humidified high flow nasal oxygen (HFNO) is frequently beneficial.
- ☑ Call for experienced, skilled anaesthetic and surgical help.
- ☑ Get any previous airway images and anaesthetic or surgical records describing strategies and difficulties.
- ☑ If indicated and time and severity allows, perform CT of the entire airway and nasendoscopy. (When oxygenation is impaired there is less time).
- ☑ Shrink a lesion if possible (corticosteroids, adrenaline, antibiotics, radiotherapy, chemotherapy, drainage of fluid by aspiration or blood by removing sutures or clips).
- ☑ Depending on the level of obstruction, involve ENT, maxillofacial, and thoracic surgeons in primary or back-up strategies to secure the airway.
- ☑ Rank strategies in order of risk to oxygenation.
- ☑ Favour strategies that will fail safely.
- ☑ Your three principal choices are: 'awake' or 'asleep'; spontaneous or controlled ventilation; oral/nasal tracheal intubation or FONA.
  - Get the difficult airway trolley. Include high flow oxygen delivery systems; CPAP; videolaryngoscopes, airway exchange catheters, transtracheal ventilation catheters with appropriate ventilation tools, rigid bronchoscopy. Heliox may improve gas flow but has an F_iO_2 of 0.21–0.3 unless supplemented.

Choices must reflect the:
- ability to preoxygenate successfully and prevent desaturation.
- dominance of difficult intubation or difficult ventilation.
- predicted ability to mask ventilate and likely efficacy of SGAs.
- degree of obstruction and mobility of lesion sitting and lying.
- risk of airway soiling (blood, pus, secretions, stomach contents).
- difficulty of FONA.
- ability to deliver general or local anaesthesia.

NB: Waking up does not always restore oxygenation; awake FOB intubation may fail or cause complications; surgery does not always provide a rapid route for oxygenation. Always decide clearly with your team how to proceed if 'Plan A' fails.

☑ **Develop an airway strategy. Weigh advantages and disadvantages of plans discussed below for different anatomical levels of obstruction. (Remember there may be more than one). For your patient, decide at least a Plan A and B.**

Obstruction above normal vocal cords where lesions impede intubation rather than gas flow

Awake FOB or videolaryngoscope-assisted intubation with local anaesthetic and supplemental oxygen

Strengths: you may see around obstructions; there may be team support if videomonitors are used; spontaneous ventilation and airway tone may be maintained.

Weaknesses: loss of view with secretions, blood, or pus; increased obstruction and dyspnoea during intubation; impairment of protective reflexes.

Relative contraindications: lesions likely to bleed on contact; a very narrow airway (the FOB may—rarely—cause complete obstruction—'cork in a bottle' effect).

Obstruction at or just below the vocal cords

Inhalational induction, laryngoscopy, and insertion of a small tracheal tube **(NB: 4.5 mm ID tubes typically have an OD >6 mm.)**

Strengths: adequate airway and upper oesophageal sphincter tone may remain. **Theoretically** obstruction leads to lightening of anaesthesia and thus airway improvement BUT there is little evidence that this is true.

Weaknesses: achieving adequate anaesthesia may take considerable time and increasing depth may worsen obstruction. Critical hypoxaemia may occur before any lightening and airway improvement. (You must have a 'Plan B'.)

Relative contraindications: severe obstruction especially when lying flat.

NB: TIVA with maintenance of spontaneous ventilation reduces airway stimulation and may have similar advantages to inhalational induction but is not as widely described and requires skill and experience.

Intravenous induction, paralysis, and insertion of a small tracheal tube, 'jet ventilation' catheter or rigid bronchoscope

Strengths: Induction, paralysis, and intubation is a familiar approach. An experienced and equipped team may establish temporary ventilation and oxygenation with specialist tools and treat a lesion immediately.

Weaknesses: Requires: up-to-date accurate knowledge of the dimensions of the restriction compared to the intended tube or catheter; adequate mask ventilation; laryngoscopy or rapid FOB-assisted intubation; experience and equipment for other approaches.

Relative contraindications: Severe obstruction. Predicted difficult mask ventilation, laryngoscopy, or intubation. Mobile masses that obstruct if 'blown' into the airway in inspiration or expiration.

Cricothyroidotomy (cannula, 'scalpel', or formal surgical)

Strengths: will bypass supralaryngeal and possibly laryngeal obstruction.

Weaknesses: insertion difficulty (misplacement, bleeding, blockage, uncertainty of location of cricothyroid membrane); cannula ventilation complications (subcutaneous emphysema, inadequate exhalation, barotrauma, device failure.)

Relative contraindications: overlying swelling, mass, thyroid, blood vessel, tracheal stent, major tracheal deviation. (Ultrasound may help.)

Awake tracheostomy

Identify patients for whom this is the lowest risk strategy BUT be aware it does not always succeed. You must have a 'Plan B'.

Obstruction at the tracheal level

Rigid bronchoscopy and 'jet ventilation'

Strengths: can act as a dedicated airway for assessment, oxygenation, ventilation, and surgery (resection, laser, or stent insertion).

Weaknesses: requires an experienced operator and team.

Relative contraindications: inadequate 'line-of-sight' for a rigid bronchoscope; severe trismus, cervical spine instability, or immobility.

Cardiopulmonary bypass

This is rarely an option in an emergency. It needs organization and time. Identify suitable cases and refer to a cardiothoracic unit early.

Subsequent management

☑ Use intravenous anaesthesia when delivery of volatile may be compromised.
☑ Use back-up strategies promptly. Prioritize oxygenation.
☑ Cricothyroidotomy is usually a temporary route. Make plans for a longer-term definitive airway as soon as feasible.
☑ Develop strategies for extubation. (➔ See 'Difficult extubation', p. 110.)

Investigations
- CXR, CT airway, nasendoscopy, airway ultrasound.

Risk factors
- Known airway pathology.
- Trauma and surgery to the neck and airway.
- Compressing neck masses (bleeding, oedema, postoperative swelling).
- Difficult intubation. This compounds difficulty with obstruction.
- Obesity. This hastens hypoxaemia.

Paediatric considerations
- Awake techniques are inappropriate for most children.
- Inhalational induction then insertion of a dedicated airway is an established strategy for FOB-guided intubation and treatment of obstruction.
- Children with airway difficulty desaturate fast and this demands experienced, skilled practitioners.
- Cricothyroidotomy is technically more challenging but the principles are as for adults (◑ p. 454).

Example strategies: Plan A is your first plan. Plan B is adopted if the decision is made to abandon Plan A

Options for oral and supraglottic lesions (e.g. trauma, burns, tumour, infection, surgical complications)
NB: There may be cases where insertion of an SGA may be safe, improve the supraglottic airway, facilitate FOB-guided intubation or surgical access, and enable ventilation—a 'dedicated' airway.
- Plan A: Awake FOB-guided intubation. Plan B: awake cricothyroidotomy or very rapid tracheostomy performed by an experienced surgeon who is scrubbed and prepared.
- Plan A: Awake cricothyroidotomy or tracheostomy. Even if not the chosen Plan A, a transtracheal ventilation catheter before another plan may provide some oxygenation and buy time. Plan B: Awake FOB-guided intubation.
- Plan A: Inhalational induction, laryngoscopy, and intubation. Plan B: Cricothyroidotomy or very rapid tracheostomy performed by an experienced surgeon who is scrubbed and prepared.

Laryngeal (e.g. stenoses, tumours, infection, burns, surgical complications)
- Plan A: Awake tracheostomy (below the first tracheal ring to avoid the lesion) particularly for severe airway distortion and fixed or friable lesions. Plan B: GA, rigid bronchoscopy and 'jet ventilation'.
- Plan A: Awake FOB-guided intubation with a small tracheal tube. Avoid if the lesion is friable or very narrow. The FOB will obstruct the airway as will surgical dilators. Plan B: GA and rigid bronchoscopy and 'jet ventilation'.
- Plan A: Inhalational induction, laryngoscopy (video preferred), and intubation. Plan B: GA, rigid bronchoscopy and 'jet ventilation'.

Mid-tracheal (e.g. bleeding into thyroid, trauma, surgical complication, tumour)
- Plan A: Intravenous induction, neuromuscular blockade, and early passage of a small tube, rigid bronchoscope or 'jet ventilation' catheter. FOB-guided inspection during insertion may be helpful. Plan B: Very rapid (low) tracheostomy performed by an experienced surgeon who is scrubbed and prepared but needs to be below obstructing lesion and bleeding or swelling may precipitate complete obstruction.
- Coughing can convert partial to complete obstruction. In the absence of anticipated upper airway problems, this may be a reason to avoid awake or inhalational techniques.

Low tracheal lesions (e.g. tumours, trauma, retrosternal goitre)
- Plan A: Intravenous induction, neuromuscular blockade, and early passage of a small tube, rigid bronchoscope or 'jet ventilation' catheter. FONA will not help. Transfer to a cardiothoracic centre may be the best option.

Mid- and low tracheal obstruction is a complex intrathoracic problem where Plan B may only be available in a cardiothoracic centre. Transfer must be balanced against the risks of transfer and organization time.

Further reading

Caplan, R.A., Benumof, J.L., Caplan, R.A., et al. (1993). Practice guidelines for management of the difficult airway. A report by the American Society of Anesthesiologists. Task force on Management of the Difficult Airway. *Anesthesiology*, **78**, 579–602.

Conacher, I. (2003). Anaesthesia and tracheobronchial stenting for central airway obstruction in adults. *British Journal of Anaesthesia*, **90**, 367–74.

Cook, T.M., Morgan, P.J., Hersch, P.E. (2011). Equal and opposite expert opinion. Airway obstruction of a retrosternal thyroid mass: management and prospective international expert opinion. *Anaesthesia*, **66**, 828–36.

Hung, O., Murphy, M. (2010). Context-sensitive airway management. *Anesthesia and Analgesia*, **110**, 982–83.

Mason, R.A., Fielder, C.P. (1999). The obstructed airway in head and neck surgery. *Anaesthesia*, **54**, 625–28.

Nouraei, S.A., Giussani, D.A., Howard, D.J., et al. (2008). Physiological comparison of spontaneous and positive-pressure ventilation in laryngotracheal stenosis. *British Journal of Anaesthesia*, **101**, 419–23.

Ovassapian, A., Yelich, S.J., Dykes, M.H.M., Brunner, E.E. (1983). Fibreoptic nasotracheal intubation—incidence and causes of failure. *Anesthesia and Analgesia*, **63**, 692–95.

Patel, A., Nouraei, S.A. (2015). Transnasal humidified rapid-insufflation ventilatory exchange (THRIVE): a physiological method of increasing apnoea time in patients with difficult airways. *Anaesthesia*, **70**, 323–29.

Patel, A., Pearce, A., Pracey, P. (2011). Head and neck pathology. In: Cook, T.M., Woodall, N., Frerk, C. (eds). *The 4th National Audit Project of the Royal College of Anaesthetists and the Difficult Airway Society: Major Complications of Airway Management in the UK*, pp. 143–54. London, UK: Royal College of Anaesthetists.

⑦ Rapid sequence induction

A 'classical' UK description

- Preoxygenation.
- Sequential rapid injection of an intravenous anaesthetic then suxamethonium chloride at a predetermined dose.
- 'Gentle' application of cricoid force while awake followed, after induction, by 'firm' pressure by a trained assistant.
- Intubation of the trachea with a cuffed TT at the earliest time likely to be successful, given the patient and properties and doses of the drugs injected.
- Avoidance of manual ventilation to reduce the risk of gastric inflation and regurgitation.

This classical description is often modified by the use of other muscle relaxants or co-administration of adjuncts.

An RSI is believed to reduce the likelihood of aspiration in patients at significant risk.

Immediate management

☑ A skilled assistant trained in applying cricoid force is needed.
☑ A tipping bed or trolley is mandatory.
☑ 20° head up tilt prolongs time to hypoxaemia.
☑ Check:
  - your team understands your plans for unexpected difficult intubation and ventilation.
  - suction, laryngoscopes (including videolaryngoscopes), TTs, cuffs, and rescue devices are working.
  - a large-bore IV cannula is connected to a running fluid infusion.
  - an active rigid sucker is at your right hand.
  - the patient's head and neck are optimally positioned for laryngoscopy.
  - the patient is fully preoxygenated: to an end tidal FiO2 of >0.9.
☑ Instruct the trained assistant to apply gentle cricoid force (10 N, 1 kg) as induction starts.
☑ Administer the predetermined dose of induction agent (preferably propofol) depending on the patient's body habitus and clinical condition.
☑ Immediately follow this with a predetermined dose of suxamethonium (1.5 mg/kg total body weight) or rocuronium (1.2 mg/kg lean body weight).
☑ Instruct the trained assistant to apply 3 kg of cricoid force (30 N) at loss of consciousness. This should have been practiced before the procedure.
☑ Avoid mask ventilation if unnecessary BUT gentle mask ventilation should be used when indicated (e.g. children, lung disease, obesity) to avoid, postpone, and reverse desaturation.

☑ Attempt laryngoscopy and intubation 45 s after administration of the neuromuscular blocker.

☑ Maintain cricoid force until the TT is inserted, cuff inflated, and its correct position confirmed by capnography and auscultation.

☑ If laryngoscopy is difficult, reduce and if necessary, remove cricoid force with suction immediately available. Reapply cricoid force if regurgitation occurs.

☑ If intubation is difficult, reduce and if necessary, remove cricoid force. Excessive force narrows the trachea and larynx.

☑ If intubation fails, reapply cricoid force. Follow (and clearly communicate) your predefined rescue plans.

☑ If your rescue plan is to insert an SGA, which should be ready, remove cricoid force to enable full insertion.

☑ NB: If intubation fails after suxamethonium administration, hypoxaemia is likely to occur before breathing returns. Assist ventilation.

Subsequent management

☑ Drain the stomach with a large-bore gastric tube.

☑ Following surgery, extubate awake and, classically in the lateral position, if aspiration risk remains (see DAS extubation guidelines, ➔ p. 110).

Indications

- RSI is indicated when there is increased risk of regurgitation at induction of anaesthesia (e.g. bowel obstruction, recent meal, symptomatic reflux, upper gastrointestinal haemorrhage,).

Exclusions

Avoid general anaesthesia (e.g. use regional techniques) or consider securing the airway before induction (awake intubation), particularly if the patient has features that suggest difficult laryngoscopy or intubation. Be aware topical anaesthesia can facilitate aspiration.

Paediatric considerations

- Young children are unlikely to cooperate with preoxygenation and cricoid force.
- Gently mask ventilate after induction to prevent hypoxaemia. This occurs more rapidly than in adults.
- Forces required for effective cricoid force in children are not established and the anatomy may be harder to define.
- Difficult laryngoscopy and tracheal intubation are less common in children.
- Use 2 mg/kg suxamethonium in infants; 1.5 mg/kg in older children.
- The risks associated with aspiration are still likely to be higher than those associated with performing an RSI.

Special considerations

Cricoid force

Training and practice are required: compressing a 50 ml syringe filled with air from 50 to 32 mls requires 3kg. One handed cricoid force is appropriate. One assistant cannot maintain constant force for more than 5 min. Poorly applied force may impair laryngoscopy and occlude the airway. The BURP manoeuvre (redirecting pressure on the thyroid cartilage Backwards, Upwards, and to the Right) may improve laryngoscopy but increases the risk of airway obstruction. In the rare event of vomiting (but not regurgitation), remove cricoid force to reduce the risk of oesophageal rupture.

Preoxygenation (denitrogenation) and per-oxygenation

This delays hypoxaemia. Normal breathing with an F_iO_2 of 1 for 3–5 min or until fractional end-tidal oxygen is >0.9 is ideal. Patients with lung disease require more time. A good facemask seal is essential to prevent oxygen dilution by entrained air. Four vital capacity breaths with the oxygen flush valve open can be used in an extreme emergency but has limitations.

Nasal oxygenation either at low flow (nasal cannulae) but preferably HFNO may reduce desaturation during prolonged intubation attempts but is less reliable in obesity.

Rocuronium

Rocuronium avoids some side effects of suxamethonium. Paralysis may last 50 min or more. Rapid reversal with sugammadex requires 16 mg/kg. However, reversal will not reverse mechanical obstruction nor restore spontaneous ventilation if suppressed by other agents. If reversal is one of your rescue plans, the right dose of sugammadex must be immediately available.

Use of opioids

An opioid may improve haemodynamic stability (e.g. for pre-eclampsia, IHD, raised ICP). The risks are hypopnoea and impaired preoxygenation (instruct the patient to breathe), prolonged apnoea despite reversal (antagonize with naloxone 400–800 µg IV) and nausea. The vomiting risk is small. A fast onset opioid such as alfentanil 10–30 µg/kg IV is suitable.

Nasogastric tube

An NG tube should be left in place and aspirated with gentle suction before induction and then left open to the atmosphere to normalize intragastric pressure.

Airway rescue

Inserting a rescue 'second-generation' SGA that provides good separation of the gastrointestinal and respiratory tracts is important. Early successful insertion is a priority. Experience with the chosen device therefore matters.

Evidence base and assumed safety of RSI

While there is little evidence that RSI improves safety, aspiration is the commonest cause of airway-related death in anaesthesia. It remains a clinical and medicolegal necessity in cases of high aspiration risk.

Further reading

Benumof, J.L., Dagg, R., Benumof, R. (1997). Critical hemoglobin desaturation will occur before return to an unparalyzed state following 1 mg/kg intravenous succinylcholine. *Anesthesiology*, **87**, 979–82.

Donati, F. (2003). The right dose of succinylcholine. *Anesthesiology*, **99**, 1037–8.

Frerk, C., Mitchell, V.S., McNarry, A.F., et al. (2015). Difficult Airway Society intubation guidelines working group. *British Journal of Anaesthesia*, **115**, 827–48.

Heier, T., Feiner, J.R., Lin, J., Brown, R., Caldwell, J.E. (2001). Hemoglobin desaturation after succinylcholine-induced apnea: a study of the recovery of spontaneous ventilation in healthy volunteers. *Anesthesiology*, **94**, 754–9.

Lin, C.W., Xue, F.S., Xu, Y.C., et al. (2007). Cricoid force impedes insertion of, and ventilation through, the ProSeal Laryngeal Mask Airway in anesthetized, paralyzed patients *Anesthesia and Analgesia*, **104**, 1195–8.

Morris, J., Cook, T.M. (2001). National survey of rapid sequence induction. *Anaesthesia*, **56**, 1090–7.

Vanner, R.G., Asai, T. (1999). Safe use of cricoid force. *Anaesthesia*, **54**, 1–3.

:☉: Oesophageal intubation

Definition
Unintended placement of a TT in the oesophagus.

Presentation
- An absent capnogram after attempted tracheal intubation and ventilation.
- An initially normal or low end-tidal CO_2 which rapidly diminishes with each breath.
- Progressive hypoxaemia after attempted tracheal intubation and ventilation. This can be considerably delayed by preoxygenation.
- Abnormal resistance or compliance with ventilation. Slow refilling of the reservoir bag due to absent expiration.
- Gurgling sounds in the epigastrium.
- A leak around the TT despite normal pressure and volume in the cuff.
- Regurgitation of gastric contents up the TT.

Immediate management
- ☑ Exclude cardiac arrest and severe bronchospasm (e.g. anaphylaxis) as a cause of abnormal capnogram.
- ☑ Check the breathing system quickly for ventilation failure.
- ☑ Stop ventilating when the diagnosis is suspected.
- ☑ Recheck the location of the TT by laryngoscopy.
- ☑ If in doubt, take it out and ventilate with oxygen by facemask or SGA to restore oxygenation.
- ☑ Reintubate the trachea and verify the TT position by direct observation of its passage through the vocal cords, capnography (the definitive test) and auscultation. Visualize the carina with a FOB if available.
- ☑ If intubation is difficult or fails, maintain oxygenation by ventilation with 100% oxygen and follow guidelines for unexpected difficult tracheal intubation (🔾 see p. 84).

Subsequent management
- ☑ Once the airway has been secured, decompress the stomach with a gastric tube.

Risk factors
- Difficulty in seeing the larynx at intubation.
- Difficulty in passing the TT into the trachea (blind use of a gum elastic bougie, adjuncts, or other blind tracheal intubation techniques).
- Intraoperative manipulation of the head or neck.
- Surgery or endoscopy involving a shared airway.
- Overconfidence and inexperience at intubation.
- Uncuffed TT.

Exclusions (all rarer than oesophageal intubation)

- Capnograph autocalibration, blocked or disconnected sampling line, or failure.
- Disconnection, obsrtruction or leak in the breathing system (⊃ p. 402).
- Ventilator failure (⊃ p. 405).
- Complete bronchospasm (including anaphylaxis) (⊃ pp. 70, 272).
- Tension pneumothorax—unilateral or bilateral (⊃ p. 66).
- Massive pulmonary embolus (⊃ p. 41).
- Kinked or obstructed TT.
- Failure to inflate or leaking TT cuff.
- Unintentional extubation.

Paediatric considerations

- Neonatal and infant TTs are prone to displacement. They are also more prone to softening, kinking, and obstruction.
- Gastric distension may make subsequent ventilation very difficult—consider early decompression.

Special considerations

- It is important to note that cardiac arrest is NOT a cause of a flat canogram. It produces an attenuated trace, which is improved by CPR. Auscultation of the chest and epigastrium may be unreliable and may lead to false reassurance.
- Late diagnosis of hypoxaemia is more likely in patients with pigmented skin.
- Difficult mask ventilation can push expired alveolar gas into the oesophagus and stomach. This may then lead to a brief period of CO_2 detection after oesophageal intubation.
- In experienced hands ultrasonography may be a modality to condirm correct tube position and exclude oesophageal intubation.

Further reading

Caplan, R.A., Posner, K., Ward, R.J., Cheney, F.W. (1990). Adverse respiratory events in anesthesia: a closed claims analysis. *Anesthesiology*, **72**, 828–33.

Clyburn, P., Rosen, M. (1994). Accidental oesophageal intubation. *British Journal of Anaesthesia*, **73**, 55–63.

Cook TM, Harrop Griffiths W. Capnography prevents avoidable deaths. No trace = Wrong place. *BMJ* 2019;364:l439 doi: 10.1136/bmj.l439

Cook, T.M., Woodall, N., Harper, J., Benger, J. (2011). Major complications of airway management in the UK: results of the 4th National Audit Project of the Royal College of Anaesthetists and the Difficult Airway Society. Part 2: intensive care and emergency department. *British Journal of Anaesthesia*, **106**, 632–42.

① Bronchial intubation

Definition
Unintentional passage of a TT beyond the carina.

Presentation
- Uneven chest expansion.
- Quieter breath sounds in the unintubated hemithorax.
- Unexpectedly high peak or plateau airway pressures or low tidal volumes in a pressure-limited ventilatory mode.
- Unexpectedly low or falling oxygen saturation but this may not be dramatic with a high F_iO_2.
- Variable effects on end-tidal CO_2 levels depending on the mode of ventilation (trace shape may be unchanged).

Immediate management
☑ Increase F_iO_2 to 100% if saturations are low or falling.
☑ Observe the chest and compare auscultation in both axillae.
☑ Check the length of the TT at the teeth is appropriate.
☑ Check there are no obstructions or kinks in the TT. Pass a suction catheter through the TT to verify patency.
☑ Observe the TT at the larynx with laryngoscopy, or the end of the TT with aN FOB. Reapply cricoid pressure, if appropriate. Deflate the cuff and withdraw the TT until breath sounds are heard bilaterally or the carina is identified through the FOB. Re-inflate the cuff.
☑ Auscultate the chest for the return of bilateral breath sounds during ventilation.
☑ Feel and measure the change in inspiratory pressure.
☑ Re-secure the tube. Note the length of the TT at the teeth.

Subsequent management
☑ Ensure adequate re-expansion of the non-ventilated lung. If bronchial intubation has been prolonged, this may require hand ventilation, CPAP, PEEP, recruitment manoeuvres, lateral positioning, or physiotherapy.
☑ Exclude ventilator-associated injury or barotrauma to the other lung.
☑ A chest X-ray may be sufficient to indicate re-inflation but in previously diseased lungs a CT may be needed.

Investigations
- FOB-guided visualization of carina.

Risk factors
- Inadequate check of TT depth after intubation.
- Length >21 cm at teeth in small females, >23 cm in larger patients.
- Emergency or difficult intubation.
- Intubation through an SGA.
- Inexperienced or non-anaesthetists.
- Paediatric patients in inexperienced hands.
- Uncut and preformed TTs (e.g. reinforced and RAE TTs).

- Manipulation of head or neck during patient positioning. Flexion advances a TT.
- Prone positioning.
- Surgery or endoscopy involving a shared airway (e.g. tonsillectomy).
- Pneumoperitoneum and head-down position. The carina moves cranially relative to the TT.
- Surgical manipulation of the trachea and bronchi.
- Aberrant tracheal or bronchial anatomy.
- Insertion of a TT through a tracheostomy or cricothyroidotomy.

Exclusions

- Breathing circuit obstruction (➲ p. 402). Switch to a new bag-valve-mask device.
- TT obstruction or kinking. Pass a catheter beyond the tip of the TT.
- Bronchospasm (➲ p. 70). This should be bilateral and associated with wheeze and sloping capnogram.
- Pneumothorax (➲ p. 66). Check bilateral expansion, percussion note, and position of trachea. Consider ultrasound.
- Large pleural effusion or haemothorax. Check percussion note. Strongly consider ultrasound.
- Complete or partial lung collapse. Consider if correct TT repositioning does not correct the problem. Consider inspection with FOB.
- Cuff herniation. Check cuff pressure. Pass a catheter beyond the tip of the TT. Considerinspection with FOB.
- Bronchial foreign body (➲ p. 216, including aspiration ➲ p. 107). TT repositioning does not correct this problem. Consider inspection with FOB.

Paediatric considerations

- Collapse and hypoxaemia occur more rapidly than in adults.
- There is an increased likelihood of bronchial intubation because:
  - the absolute length of the trachea is shorter.
  - uncuffed TTs may move more.
  - formulae for suggested TT insertion length are estimates only.
  - preformed tubes (e.g. RAE tubes) are often too long.

Further reading

Black, A.E., Mackersie, A.M. (1991). Accidental bronchial intubation with RAE tubes. *Anaesthesia*, **46**, 42–3.

Freeman, J.A., Fredricks, B.J., Best, C.J. (1995). Evaluation of a new method for determining tracheal tube length in children. *Anaesthesia*, **50**, 1050–2.

McCoy, E.P., Russell, W.J., Webb, R.K. (1997). Accidental bronchial intubation. An analysis of AIMS incident reports from 1988 to 1994 inclusive. *Anaesthesia*, **52**, 24–31.

☼ Laryngospasm

Definition

Abnormal narrowing or closure of the larynx by adductor muscles causing partial or complete airway obstruction usually in response to a noxious stimulus.

This section refers to laryngospasm during general anaesthesia. Laryngospasm can develop suddenly, silently, and without immediately obvious physical signs. Suspecting it in the context of common triggers and associations is important for early management before life-threatening rapidly progressive hypoxaemia develops. NB: Pulse oximetry lags behind real-time desaturation.

Presentation

- During spontaneous breathing:
  - stridor with partial laryngeal closure, silence with complete closure, respiratory distress, tracheal tug, suprasternal and intercostal recession, paradoxical movement of the chest and abdomen, unusually rapid hypoxaemia because of the cardiopulmonary effects of inspiratory efforts against high resistance.
  - Breath-holding. The diaphragm and abdominal muscles may contract tightly.
  - Difficult or impossible assisted ventilation via SGA or facemask.
  - Abnormal or flat capnogram.

Immediate management

- ☑ Stop or remove the stimulus causing laryngospasm.
- ☑ If possible, use measures to 'break it' before desaturation.
- ☑ Administer 100% oxygen at high flow.
- ☑ Apply continuous positive airway pressure via facemask or an SGA if correctly positioned and with a good airway seal.
- ☑ Apply considerable jaw thrust or anterior pressure on the postero-superior mandibular rami anterior to the mastoid processes (Larson's point) to 'break' laryngospasm by stimulation and airway clearance.
- ☑ Rapidly deepen anaesthesia with intravenous propofol. This may release laryngospasm and enable airway inspection.
- ☑ If desaturation begins, other measures have failed, you have doubts about the security of the airway or anxiety is high, administer a rapidly acting muscle relaxant.
- ☑ Make sure the airway is clear by laryngoscopy. Regurgitation may have triggered laryngospasm.
- ☑ If ventilation becomes easier, oxygenation improves, and the airway does not require protection, mask ventilation may be sufficient to maintain adequate oxygenation. If not, intubate.
- ☑ In the exceptional case of severe laryngospasm causing life-threatening hypoxaemia despite treatment, or where appropriate intubating drugs are unavailable, FONA may be life-saving (➲ p. 454).

Subsequent management

☑ Monitor for the development of post-obstructive pulmonary oedema. It may be fatal after the laryngospasm has resolved.

☑ Decompress the stomach.

☑ If intubation was required, plan for extubation in appropriate surroundings with monitoring, personnel, and equipment to manage recurrence. (➲ See 'Difficult extubation', p. 110.)

☑ Other drugs: doxapram (1–1.5 mg/kg IV), diazepam (1–2 mg IV in adults), lidocaine (0.5–1.5 mg/kg IV) and prophylactic magnesium sulphate (15 mg/kg over 20 min IVI) have been proposed to treat and prevent laryngospasm but may be suitable only in less severe cases.

Investigations

- Observe for late development of post-obstructive pulmonary oedema.
- CXR if concerned about possible aspiration or pulmonary oedema.

Risk factors

- Paediatric patients, especially younger children and infants.
- Light anaesthesia especially during induction and emergence.
- Soiling of the larynx with secretions/blood/gastric contents.
- Strong stimuli (e.g. anal stretch, cervical dilatation).
- Irritable airways (e.g. smokers, asthma, COPD, URTI).
- Tracheal extubation.
- Recurrent laryngeal nerve damage.
- Surgery to the larynx and upper airway.
- Barbiturate induction agents.
- Inhalational agents; desflurane > isoflurane > sevoflurane > halothane.
- Anaesthesia in very anxious patients.
- Insertion or removal of SGAs.
- Movement of the head and neck with SGAs *in situ*.

Exclusions

- Breathing circuit obstruction (➲ p. 413). Test with a new checked bag-valve-mask system.
- Supraglottic obstruction with the base of tongue, foreign body (e.g. surgical pack), clot, tumour, or oedema.
- Laryngeal obstruction; trauma (eg dislocated arytenoid cartilage), oedema, haematoma, tumour, or vocal cord paralysis (especially bilateral partial recurrent laryngeal nerve injury).
- Infraglottic airway obstruction; foreign body, gastric aspiration, clot, sputum, tumour, bronchospasm, tracheomalacia .
- Residual neuromuscular block.
- Breath-holding.
- Tension pneumothorax (➲ p. 66).
- Hyperventilation/anxiety.
- Hypocalcaemia and hypomagnesaemia (➲ p. 324, 328).

Paediatric considerations
- Laryngospasm is more common in children for many reasons.
- Hypoxaemia develops more quickly and management must be decisive and quick.
- Laryngospasm is a significant cause of paediatric anaesthesia-related bradycardia or cardiac arrest.
- Atropine is not a first line treatment for hypoxaemia-related bradycardia or cardiac arrest.

Special considerations
- Dose ranges of propofol and muscle relaxants vary, but in an airway crisis, give a dose that is going to be effective quickly.
- Suggested doses of propofol vary depending on the patient but 1 mg/kg is a guide.
- Suggested doses of suxamethonium vary from 0.1 to 2 mg/kg IV, depending on the age of the patient and the severity of hypoxaemia. If IV access is not immediately available, give 2–4 mg/kg suxamethonium IM/IO or into the tongue.
- Have atropine 10–20 μg/kg IV/IM/IO immediately available to prevent or treat any bradycardia caused by the stimulus that triggered laryngospasm (NOT hypoxaemia) particularly in children.
- Prolonged head-down position, prolonged prone position, massive fluid resuscitation, pre-eclampsia and anaphylactic reactions are all associated with laryngeal oedema that, on extubation, may resemble refractory laryngospasm.

Further reading
Larson, C.P. (1998). Laryngospasm—the best treatment. *Anesthesiology*, **89**, 1293–4.

ⓘ Aspiration during general anaesthesia or sedation

Definition

Entry of solid or liquid matter into the lower respiratory tract. The most common source is the upper gastrointestinal tract. Blood from the upper airway is another important cause.

Presentation

- It is important to distinguish regurgitation from aspiration. To confirm aspiration, matter should be seen entering the laryngeal inlet on laryngoscopy or found on suction (or rising up) a correctly located TT. This is unusual.
- Aspiration should be suspected during controlled ventilation if there is an unexpected rise in airway pressure, fall in chest compliance, or desaturation with crackles and wheeze on examination.
- During spontaneous ventilation, coughing, laryngospasm, dyspnoea, wheeze, and crackles may occur.
- Aspiration risk is highest during intubation and extubation.
- Immediately after a procedure, coughing, dyspnoea, wheeze, recession, crackles, hypoxaemia, and CXR changes consistent with aspiration pneumonitis suggest aspiration has occurred.
- Regurgitation may lead to aspiration so matter emerging from the mouth with an unprotected airway demands immediate action to prevent or reduce aspiration. Similarly, visible matter in the breathing tube of an SGA indicates aspiration has occurred or is likely. Matter visible in the drain tube of an SGA indicates regurgitation and actions should be taken to prevent, exclude, or reduce aspiration.

Immediate management

- ☑ Switch to 100% oxygen but avoid ventilating during airway clearance, within the limits of hypoxaemia.
- ☑ Clear the oropharynx with a rigid sucker to prevent further aspiration during subsequent airway manoeuvres.
- ☑ If an SGA is in use, distinguish between regurgitation and aspiration. Remove the SGA if you have evidence that it has failed to protect the larynx.
- ☑ Apply cricoid force if matter is presumed to be or is seen coming from the oesophagus.
- ☑ Tilt the patient >15° head down and extend the head on the neck. This aids drainage away from the larynx. The lateral position takes time, assistance, and makes airway manipulation more difficult.
- ☑ Rapidly paralyse (if not already paralysed) and as soon as possible, intubate.

☑ Use suction catheters to clear the trachea and bronchi. Consider FOB-guided suction.
☑ When the trachea and main bronchi are clear, re-establish an adequate lung volume and arterial saturation. Recruitment manoeuvres and PEEP may help. Use lung-protective ventilation. Bronchodilators may be indicated.
☑ Cancel elective surgery.
☑ Proceed with emergency surgery but complete as quickly as possible.
☑ NB: If vomiting, help the patient to turn on their side. Provide head-down tilt. Do not use cricoid force. It risks oesophageal rupture.

Subsequent management

☑ Do not confuse regurgitation with aspiration. Regurgitation precedes aspiration but the latter is not inevitable particularly if a TT or second-generation SGA is in use. When regurgitation occurs, it is important not to remove the TT or SGA before taking precautions to ensure this will not cause aspiration.
☑ Arrange critical care admission after massive aspiration, especially particulate. Blood clots can cause lethal airway obstruction and may require bronchoscopic (flexible or rigid) removal. Lethal complications may follow airway obstruction and pneumonitis.
☑ Some aspiration resolves rapidly, even during the procedure. Small amounts of blood rarely seem to cause problems. Extubation at the end may be safe. Observe continuously for at least 2 h in case symptoms and signs develop. Inform staff of your concerns and write in the notes.
☑ Prophylactic corticosteroids, antibiotics, or early bronchoalveolar lavage are not recommended.

Investigations

• CXR. Although often unremarkable in the first few hours, later films may show streaky and interstitial shadowing with regional or generalized hyperinflation. The right lower lobe is often affected after supine aspiration but any pattern may occur.

Risk factors

• Full stomach
• Inadequate starvation time
• Alcohol
• Abdominal pathology especially intestinal obstruction and upper GI bleeding
• Inadequate nasogastric drainage
• Significant trauma
• Opioid, anticholinergic, antidopaminergic agents and glucagon-like peptide analogues
• Latter half of pregnancy and up to 48 h post-partum
• Autonomic neuropathy (e.g. diabetes mellitus)
• Emergency procedures
• Blood or bleeding in the upper airway

- Raised intra-abdominal pressure (e.g. laparoscopic surgery)
- Ineffective cricoid force or poor application/premature release
- Difficult manual ventilation with inflation of the stomach
- Straining, coughing, or bucking on an SGA
- Hiccoughs
- Obesity
- Surgery in head-down or lithotomy position
- Extubation during light planes of anaesthesia
- Inadequate reversal of neuromuscular blockade
- Pharyngeal pouch or web
- Oesophageal pathology (stricture, tumour, achalasia, hiatus hernia, incompetent lower oesophageal sphincter)
- Impaired laryngeal reflexes
- Topical anaesthesia of larynx and trachea
- Neuromuscular disease affecting the larynx and/or the cough reflex
- Patients susceptible to residual anaesthesia or sedatives (e.g. frail elderly and young children)
- Not applying cricoid force when indicated
- Using an SGA in high-risk patients
- Deep sedation without airway protection

Exclusions

- Regurgitation without aspiration
- Misplacement, displacement, and cuff deflation of a TT or SGA
- Obstruction of breathing system or airway (➲ p. 413)
- Bronchospasm and anaphylaxis (➲ p. 70, 272)
- Foreign body aspiration (➲ p. 219)
- Acute pulmonary oedema (➲ p. 68)
- Pneumonia

Special considerations

- Ensure adequate starvation time. Use RSI when appropriate. Avoid GA in high-risk situations. Favour regional or local anaesthetic techniques without sedation.
- Buffering gastric acid preoperatively with sodium citrate, H_2 receptor antagonists, or proton pump inhibitors (given enough hours to take effect) does not reduce the risk of aspiration, but may reduce the severity of the consequences. This is not true for aspiration of particulate matter.

Further reading

Cook, T.M., Frerk, C. (2011). Aspiration of gastric contents and of blood. In: Cook, T.M., Woodall, N., Frerk, C. (eds). *The 4th National Audit Project of the Royal College of Anaesthetists and the Difficult Airway Society: Major Complications of Airway Management in the UK*, pp. 155–64. London, UK: Royal College of Anaesthetists.

Kluger, M.T., Visvanathan, T., Myburgh, J.A., Westhorpe, R.N. (2005). Crisis management during anaesthesia: regurgitation, vomiting and aspiration. *Quality and Safety in Health Care*, **14**, e4.

⚠ Difficult tracheal extubation

Definition

Extubation that risks acute airway, cardiorespiratory and other complications may be defined as difficult (➡ see 'Risk factors', p. 112).

Airway factors and comorbidities may indicate the patient's breathing and oxygenation will not be safe. Re-oxygenation, assisted ventilation, and airway management (including re-intubation) may also be difficult. Coughing and straining may cause problems raising venous, intracerebral, and intraocular pressure.

Presentation

• Difficult extubation should be anticipated.
• Beware acute airway trauma and chronic airway pathology, obesity, obstructive sleep apnoea, regurgitation, and cardiothoracic disease (extubation may cause bronchospasm, arrhythmia, myocardial ischaemia, and cardiac failure).
• Protracted prone or head-down positioning and fluid overload can cause airway oedema.
• Mandibular wires and 'halo' or internal cervical spine fixation may make re-intubation difficult.
• Hypothermia, acidosis, and coagulopathy may delay extubation.

Immediate management

☑ Plan extubation and related post-op care in 'at-risk' patients. The key decision is whether to extubate or postpone. Awake extubation should be the default where difficulty is anticipated but extubation is still planned. However, an 'advanced' technique may have advantages (➡ see '113 **Extubation techniques for 'at-risk' patients**);
  • 'deep' extubation
  • remifentanil-assisted extubation
  • changing the TT to an SGA
  • inserting an airway exchange catheter
☑ If extubation is not safe, wait until the risk is lower, or arrange a tracheostomy.
☑ Arrange an appropriate area with enough trained personnel, monitoring, and rescue equipment. Check your kit. Review and communicate your chosen plan and backups before extubation.
☑ If airway swelling or damage is a possibility consider direct inspection for oedema, haematoma, bleeding, blood clots, and laryngeal injury.
☑ Consider laryngeal nerve damage, if possible, and anticipate cord dysfunction after extubation.
☑ Clear the upper and lower airway with suction.
☑ Empty the stomach if indicated.
☑ Ensure full reversal of neuromuscular block. Sugammadex is more reliable after rocuronium than neostigmine.
☑ Assess recovery of TOF ratio using a quantitative monitor. Visual or tactile methods cannot reliably discriminate TOF ratios above 0.4.

☑ Re-establish and assess spontaneous ventilation.

☑ A cuff leak test may be performed. .Deflate the cuff. Consider postponing extubation if there is no leak around a TT during positive pressure inspiration. A large audible leak is reassuring but beware 'leak tests' are dependant on TT size and not specific nor sensitive for successful extubation.

☑ Review ease of ventilation, work of breathing, cardiovascular stability, and if indicated fluid balance, temperature, pH, and coagulation.

☑ Use a bite block to stop TT occlusion and related post-obstructive pulmonary oedema. If not already deflated, consider deflating the cuff if biting occurs.

☑ When there is high anxiety about upper airway obstruction after extubation, consider inserting a prophylactic subglottic cannula for oxygen delivery. Beware cannula misplacement, displacement, trauma, and barotrauma.

☑ Optimize patient position; decide between head up (e.g. obese) or left lateral head down (e.g. high risk of aspiration).

☑ Preoxygenate fully. Do not disconnect the circuit prior to extubation. Recruitment manoeuvres may improve oxygenation.

☑ Deflate the cuff and remove the TT with positive pressure to expel secretions.

☑ Monitor after extubation in an appropriate location until the risk of airway obstruction has passed.

Subsequent management

☑ Make efforts to continue oxygenation and support ventilation after extubation as required.

☑ Continue optimal positioning. Take care to avoid sedation with respiratory depression.

☑ Consider pre-existing, new indications and contraindications to CPAP, NIV, and HFNO.

☑ Nasopharyngeal airways may help obstructive sleep apnoea.

☑ Arrange physiotherapy if helpful. Good analgesia may be essential.

☑ Do not ignore increasing anxiety, agitation, and dyspnoea, even if there are no clinical signs.

☑ Re-intubate early with planning, equipment, and experienced staff. Avoid acting in extremis if at all possible.

☑ Document difficult extubation and strategies used (effective and ineffective).

☑ Complete alerts and communicate effectively, including in writing, with the patient and the GP.

☑ When indicated, advise of delayed effects of airway trauma (prolonged pain, hoarseness, dysphagia, and infection including neck and thorax).

Investigations

• FOB-guided inspection. Videolaryngoscopy. CXR will reveal soft-tissue injury and tube or AEC location. CT is more detailed.

Risk factors

Anaesthetic
- Failed anticipation, underestimation of difficulties, inadequate planning, over-confidence, inexperience.
- 'Light' anaesthesia and returning laryngeal reflexes.
- Laryngoscopy may have become more difficult as a result of surgery (e.g. surgical fixation of the cervical spine).
- Airway swelling (oedema, anaphylaxis, angioedema, prolonged prone position, airway and neck surgery, burns, haematoma).
- Previous difficult extubation (e.g. laryngospasm).
- Residual anaesthetics, opioids, neuromuscular blockade, and inadequate laryngeal reflexes.

Patient
- Obesity.
- Obstructive sleep apnoea (susceptibility to airway and respiratory compromise with opioids, sedatives, and anaesthetics).
- Chronic type 2 respiratory failure.
- Acute or chronic head and neck pathology.
- Previous surgery or radiotherapy for head or neck cancers.
- Raised ICP, IOP, severe cardiac or respiratory disease (including copious secretions).
- Fragile larynx (rheumatoid arthritis, tumour, radiotherapy changes).
- Fragile pharynx (pemphigus, pemphigoid, amyloid).
- Inadequate cough (chronic neuromuscular weakness, cerebrovascular event).
- Airway stenosis.
- Dysfunctional laryngeal reflexes.
- Cricoarytenoid joint dysfunction and vocal cord palsy.

Surgical
- Maxillofacial, major head and neck, and cervical spine surgery, especially with removal of normal venous or lymphatic drainage.
- Upper and lower airway surgery.
- Postoperative bleeding (ENT, airway, maxillofacial, thyroid, and carotid surgery).
- Prolonged head down or prone positioning.
- Recurrent laryngeal nerve injury (neck, thoracic).
- Lung atelectasis and collapse.
- Lung trauma, collapse, pneumothorax, large pleural effusion, haemothorax, thoracic surgery.

Exclusions
- Patients likely to require tracheostomy.

Paediatric considerations
- Techniques need to be chosen according to age and ability to cooperate.
- Complications of light anaesthesia and distress on emergence are more common.
- All but the smallest catheters obstruct a small child's airway and are unlikely to be tolerated.
- Upper respiratory tract infection is more common and associated with laryngospasm.

Extubation techniques for 'at-risk' patients

Awake extubation

- Awake extubation provides the safety of airway tone, reflexes, and respiratory drive. Consider for those at risk of aspiration, the obese, and some patients with a difficult airway. Explain the process preoperatively to prevent a perception of 'awareness'.

'Deep' extubation

- Consider only if airway management will be easy without significant aspiration risk. There is an increased risk of obstruction but reduced risk of coughing, bucking, straining, laryngospasm, and adverse cardiorespiratory stimulation.

Inserting an SGA under deep anaesthesia or neuromuscular blockade

- The 'Bailey manoeuvre' used a classic LMA inserted behind the TT before extubation. Effective insertion before TT removal reduces obstruction risk and provides some airway protection while avoiding the degree of stimulation of awake extubation. It is less appropriate if there is a regurgitation risk or potentially difficult re-intubation.

Remifentanil-assisted extubation

- A carefully titrated remifentanil infusion can suppress adverse stimulation during emergence. Safety relies on removal of other anaesthetics such that the patient is awake and cooperative while tolerating the TT. Delayed emergence, prolonged sedation, respiratory depression, airway obstruction, and aspiration with reduced airway reflexes are risks. It is less appropriate if there is a regurgitation risk or potentially difficult re-intubation. Topical or IV lidocaine may also reduce cough. Other cardiac suppressants (calcium channel blockers, magnesium, clonidine, dexmedetomidine, ketamine, and β-blockers) have their own advantages and disadvantages but less published relevant data.

Extubation over an AEC

- AECs should only be used with training and experience. Consider an AEC if re-intubation is both likely and going to be difficult. Local anaesthetic on the catheter and in the trachea enable it to be tolerated. Fix depth of insertion of the AEC meticulously. Oral insertion should never be >25 cm from the lips. Migration risks airway and oesophageal trauma. An AEC assists railroading TTs of ID >4 mm with a success rate of 90%. Oxygen administration through an AEC creaters a risk of barotrauma and death if it is placed or has migrated below the carina. If hypoxaemia is likely or developing, oxygen should preferably be administered by facemask, nasal cannulae, HFNO, or CPAP with airway-opening manoeuvres. In life-threatening circumstances, administer 1–2 L/min of oxygen via the AEC if the tip is known to be above the carina and there is a route for exhalation. Reliable re-intubation over the AEC is only possible after anaesthesia, muscle relaxation and with the assistance of direct or indirect laryngoscopy. Use of an AEC is less appropriate if there is a regurgitation risk. A staged extubation catheter includes a stiff wire to be left in the airway, with an AEC and then a TT to be railroaded over the wire if reintubation is needed. There is limited published experience with the staged extubation equipment.

Postponing extubation
- Risks may be so high that extubation should be postponed until they are reduced. These might be clinical (eg swelling that will resolve) or non-clinical (eg inadequate skilled help on site). If a patient is transferred to ICU there should be a written extubation plan and emergency re-intubation plan in the event of accidental extubation. Transfers must be carefully planned, staffed, and equipped. In ICU there should be appropriate monitoring, skilled staffing, and any necessary equipment immediately available for facilitating oxygenation, airway improvement (e.g. clip removers and wire cutters) and emergency re-intubation. All planned at-risk extubations should be supervised by an anaesthetist. Patients should remain starved.

Tracheostomy
- Tracheostomy should be considered if the airway is at risk for a considerable time due to comorbidities, surgery, or the extent of swelling or pathology.

Corticosteroids
- Corticosteroids (e.g. dexamethasone IV 0.15 mg/kg [max 4 mg] 6 hourly for 24 h) may reduce **inflammatory** oedema but will have no effect on a haematoma or oedema secondary to venous or lymphatic pressure. Topical or nebulized adrenaline works briefly. It is not recommended routinely.

Further reading

Axe, R., Middleditch, A., Kelly, F., Batchelor, T., Cook, T.M. (2015). Macroscopic lung barotrauma during oxygenation and ventilation via an airway exchange catheter. *Anesthesia and Analgesia*, **120**, 355–61.

Cavallone, L., Vannucci, A. (2013). Extubation of the difficult airway and extubation failure. *Anesthesia and Analgesia*, **116(2)**, 368–83.

Duggan, L.V., Law, J.A., Murphy, M.F. (2011). Brief review: supplementing oxygen through an airway exchange catheter: efficacy, complications, and recommendations. *Canadian Journal of Anaesthesia*, **58(6)**, 560–8.

Popat, M., Mitchell, V., Dravid, R., Patel, A., Swampillai, C., Higgs, A. (2012). Difficult Airway Society Guidelines for the management of tracheal extubation. *Anaesthesia*, **67**, 318–40.

☢ Airway fire

Definition

Ignition of an airway device (e.g. TT, jet ventilation catheter), swab or tissue by a laser or diathermy.

The preoperative briefing must include communication of any increased fire risk, its reduction by specific anaesthetic and surgical techniques, and how to manage a fire. Syringes containing 50 mL 0.9% sodium chloride should always be immediately available during airway surgery where fire is a risk.

Presentation

- Visible burning in or smoke from the surgical field.
- Usually recognized by the surgeon first.

Immediate management

- ☑ Stop the laser or diathermy.
- ☑ Turn off anaesthetic gas flow or supplementary oxygen. Stop ventilation.
- ☑ Disconnect any airway device from the breathing system.
- ☑ Clamp the end of the device to reduce airflow to the burning area.
- ☑ Remove any burning or damaged airway device and retain for subsequent examination of completeness.
- ☑ Flood any burning area remaining in the airway with 0.9% sodium chloride solution.
- ☑ Extinguish the fire completely.
- ☑ Maintain anaesthesia intravenously throughout.
- ☑ Do **NOT** ventilate immediately. Delaying ventilation will reduce oxygen flow to any hot area or debris and avoid blowing debris distally.
- ☑ Remove any swabs or packs from the airway.
- ☑ Remove debris from the accessible airway with rigid suckers and forceps under direct vision or videolaryngoscopy.
- ☑ Remove debris from the infraglottic airway with large-bore suction catheters, forceps, and a fibreoptic bronchoscope with a large working channel. Rigid bronchoscopy may be better.
- ☑ Restart anaesthetic gases and ventilate when the airway is clear, first with air and later with just enough oxygen to maintain adequate saturation. (Consider the possibility of remaining hot debris distally.)
- ☑ Intubate early to prevent oedema jeopardizing the airway.
- ☑ Use temporary transtracheal jet ventilation if intubation is impossible.
- ☑ Arrange urgent FOB evaluation of the trachea. This may guide cricothyroidotomy or tracheostomy.

Subsequent management

☑ Consider deferring extubation. Laryngospasm, progressive airway oedema, and complete airway obstruction are possible complications. Further bronchoscopic evaluation may be advisable. ARDS may develop slowly. Critical care admission should be considered in all cases to maintain the airway and support gas exchange.

☑ When extubation is planned, ensure this occurs in an appropriate high-care area with suitable monitoring, personnel, and equipment to enable rapid re-intubation if required.

☑ Consider high-dose intravenous corticosteroids (e.g. dexamethasone 0.5 mg IV (maximum 8 mg) 6 hourly for six doses) to reduce oedema.

☑ Arrange early referral to a specialist centre for management of scarring and stenosis.

Investigations

• Flexible and rigid bronchoscopy.

Risk factors

• Fire requires fuel, a gas that supports combustion and ignition. The fuel is any material that burns, the supporting gas may be oxygen or nitrous oxide, and ignition may be provided by a laser or diathermy (particularly unipolar). Argon plasma may be safer.

• During laser use the risk is increased by:
  • use of inappropriate equipment (e.g. normal TT, tracheostomy tube or jet catheter).
  • misuse of appropriate equipment (e.g. use of air rather than 0.9% sodium chloride in the TT cuff).
  • high inspired oxygen or nitrous oxide concentrations.
  • an inadequate cuff seal.
  • flammable material in the airway (e.g. swabs that have been allowed to dry).

Exclusions

• The normal smoke 'plume' released during laser activity—but remember the 'plume' and burned tissue may still ignite in oxygen.

Paediatric considerations

• Relatively little airway oedema can result in a significant reduction in gas flow.

Special considerations

• If HFNO is used during airway surgery, including during apnoea, diathermy and laser should not be used because of the risk of fire.

• Stopping airflow often stops or reduces burning. During laser use, avoid nitrous oxide and use the lowest F_iO_2 possible to achieve adequate oxygen saturation. Use a carrier gas that does not support combustion, such as nitrogen or helium if possible.

• On ignition, airway devices channel smoke, hot gas, and debris distally. Anticipate a significant lower airway burn.

- Filling the TT cuff with 0.9% sodium chloride and placing flame-retardant wet packs around uncuffed TTs before supraglottic surgery may reduce the risk of an airway fire. Protocols must be in place.
- Methylene blue added to the 0.9% sodium chloride in the TT cuff may make a cuff breach obvious just before any oxygen-rich carrier gas reaches the upper airway.
- Practising airway fire drills may increase the speed of decision-making in a crisis, but efficient communication between the surgeon and the anaesthetist is essential. Most oxygen-enriched fires occur so fast that even the quickest response from the operating team cannot prevent patient burns.

Further reading

FDA. *Alerts and Notices*. Available at: https://www.fda.gov/radiation-emitting-products/radiation-safety/alerts-and-notices

Kitching, A.J., Edge, C.J. (2003). Lasers and surgery. *British Journal of Anaesthesia. CEPD Reviews*, **8**, 143–6.

Patel, A. (2002). Anaesthesia for endoscopic surgery. *Anaesthesia and Intensive Care Medicine*, 201–5.

Paediatrics

Daniel Lutman

☠ **Neonatal resuscitation and transition support of babies at birth**

Definition
Resuscitation of the newborn infant at delivery.

Presentation
- Floppy, blue, or pale newborn, apnoeic or gasping respiration, bradycardia.

Immediate management
(See Figure 5.1, newborn life support algorithm, ➜ p.121.)
☑ Dry and wrap baby. Maintain temperature (36.5–37.5°C).
☑ Assess colour, tone, breathing, heart rate.
☑ Open airway (neck in neutral position).
☑ Give five inflation breaths (2–3 s, 30 cmH₂O).
☑ Reassess heart rate, confirm chest movement.
☑ If ventilation inadequate:
  - reposition airway.
  - repeat inflation breaths.
  - reassess heart rate.
☑ If still no response:
  - inspect oropharynx and suction if necessary.
  - consider intubation (see Table 5.1 for endotracheal sizing).
  - repeat inflation breaths.
☑ After 30 s of effective ventilation if the heart rate <60 bpm and not increasing:
  - start chest compressions at a rate of 120/min.
  - Three chest compressions to one breath (synchronized).
☑ Reassess heart rate every 30 s.
☑ If heart rate increasing, stop chest compressions. Continue ventilation if not breathing.
☑ If heart rate still <60 bpm, continue ventilation and chest compressions.
☑ If no response, consider giving drugs (see Table 5.2):
  - insert umbilical venous catheter, intraosseous, or other venous access.
  - give adrenaline IV or IO (0.1–0.3 mL/kg 1:10 000).
  - give sodium bicarbonate intravenously (2–4 mL/kg 4.2%).
  - if still no response, give glucose IV (2.5 mL/kg 10%).
  - if baby is pale or white, give a rapid infusion of 10–20 mL/kg 0.9% saline or O-neg (CMV-negative) blood as volume expansion.

Subsequent management
☑ If the response to resuscitation is prompt and the baby is pink, vigorous, and crying, hand to parents.

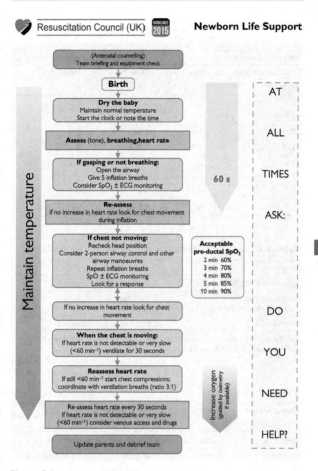

Figure 5.1 Newborn life support.
Reproduced with the kind permission of the Resuscitation Council (UK).

☑ If there are NO signs of life after 10 min of continuous adequate resuscitation with ventilation, cardiac compressions, drugs, and volume expansion, discontinuation of resuscitation should be discussed with a senior paediatrician.
☑ Record Apgar scores (see Table 5.3).

Table 5.1 Endotracheal tube diameters and lengths according to gestation and weight

50th centile weight by gestation		Tube diameter and length at the lip	
Gestation (weeks)	Body weight (kg)	Diameter (mm)	Length (cm)
23/24	0.5	2.5	6
26	0.75	2.5	6.5
27	1.0	2.5	7
30	1.5	2.5	7.5
33	2.0	2.5–3.0	8
35	2.5	3.0	8.5
37	3.0	3.0–3.5	9
40	3.5	3.5	9.5
	4.0	3.5–4.0	10

Table 5.2 Doses and routes for resuscitation drugs in the newborn

Drug	Dose	Route
Adrenaline 1:10 000	0.1–0.3 mL/kg	Intravenous/IO
Sodium bicarbonate 4.2% (0.5 mmol/mL)	2–4 mL/kg (1–2 mmol/kg)	
Glucose 10%	2.5 mL/kg	Intravenous/IO
Volume expander (Group O-neg., CMV-neg. blood or 0.9% saline)	10–20 mL/kg	Intravenous/IO

Table 5.3 Apgar scores

Clinical feature	Score		
	0	1	2
Colour	Pale/blue	Body pink, extremities blue	Pink
Heart rate	Absent	<100 bpm	>100 bpm
Response to stimulation	Nil	Some movement	Cry
Muscle tone	Limp	Some flexion of extremities	Well flexed
Respiratory effort	Absent	Poor respiratory effort or weak cry	Good

Reproduced with permission from Apgar, V. (1953). A proposal for a new method of evaluation of the newborn infant. *Curr. Res. Anesth. Analg.* 32 (4): 260–7. Copyright © 1953 International Anesthesia Research Society. doi:10.1213/00000539-195301000-00041.

Subsequent management

☑ If the response to resuscitation is prompt and the baby is pink, vigorous, and crying, hand to parents.
☑ If there are NO signs of life after 10 min of continuous adequate resuscitation with ventilation, cardiac compressions, drugs, and volume expansion, discontinuation of resuscitation should be discussed with a senior paediatrician.
☑ Record Apgar scores (see Table 5.3).

Risk factors

- Fetal distress, instrumental delivery, meconium-stained liquor.
- Maternal opioid administration, general anaesthetic.
- Multiple births, preterm delivery, shoulder dystocia.

Exclusions

- Hypovolaemia—baby remains very pale despite good ventilation and reasonable heart rate. Give 20 mL/kg O-negative blood via the umbilical vein (0.9% saline if blood not available). May need to be repeated.
- Diaphragmatic hernia—difficult to establish lung inflation, displaced apex, scaphoid abdomen. Pass wide-bore nasogastric tube and empty the stomach. Intubate to avoid further mask ventilation.
- Pneumothorax—tension pneumothoraces can develop during resuscitation. Poor air entry on one or both sides. Heart sounds quiet. If condition too critical to await X-ray, needle anterior chest wall, second intercostal space, mid-clavicular line, aspirating air using 20 mL syringe and three-way tap.
- Hydrops fetalis—many causes of this condition. Infants are born with severe generalized oedema and may have ascites, pleural, or pericardial effusions. Poor response to resuscitation may be improved by draining effusions and ascites with a needle or cannula.
- Congenital complete heart block. Baby has good colour, tone, and respiration but heart rate remains around 60 bpm. Good pulses. No further resuscitation is needed. Transfer to neonatal unit for further investigation.
- Macerated stillbirth. No heart beat detectable at any stage after birth. Skin sloughage, abdominal discoloration. Baby has been dead *in utero* for some time. Further resuscitation attempts are futile.

Special considerations

Meconium aspiration

- Most infants with meconium-stained liquor are in good condition. If baby is vigorous, no further airway management is required.
- If baby is floppy, with absent or poor respiratory effort, ventilation should be initiated within the first minute as just described.
- Tracheal intubation should be performed to assist ventilation rather than to suction the airway.
- Routine intubation and suction has not been shown to improve outcome and is now recommended only if obstruction is suspected.

Prematurity
- Wrapping a preterm infant in food-grade plastic wrapping immediately after birth greatly reduces the risk of hypothermia.
- Maintaining temperature 36.5 to 37.5°C is important.
- For most preterm infants, inflation pressures of 20–25 cmH$_2$O are adequate.
- Consider CPAP to support respiration.
- Most infants of 28 weeks' gestation or fewer require treatment with surfactant. Early administration is more effective than later treatment.

Maternal opioids
- Naloxone is not a drug of resuscitation.
- Establish effective ventilation first.
- Consider naloxone if infant remains depressed.
- 200 µg (60 µg/kg) dose intramuscularly for term infants.

Oxygen therapy
Ventilation may be initiated with air, if the clinician is concerned regarding the effects of hyperoxia in the preterm infant. Unless the infant responds immediately to air, additional oxygen should be given.
Pulse oximetry should be used to guide therapy and avoid hyperoxaemia.

Reasons to transfer to SCBU
- Ongoing requirement for respiratory support.
- Major congenital abnormality.
- Prematurity.

Further reading
Resuscitation Council (UK) (2015). *Resuscitation and Support of Transition of Babies at Birth*. London, UK: Resuscitation Council. Available at: https://www.resus.org.uk/resuscitation-guidelines/resuscitation-and-support-of-transition-of-babies-at-birth/

☠ Paediatric basic life support

Definition
- Maintenance of the airway and support of respiration and circulation without the use of equipment:
  - infant—under 1 y.
  - child—1 y to puberty.

Presentation
- Unresponsive child, signs of breathing and circulation absent.
- Primary cardiac arrest uncommon.
- Ventricular fibrillation less than 10% of cases.

Immediate management
(➲ See Figure 5.2, 'PBLS algorithm', p. 126.)
  Check child's responsiveness:
☑ gently stimulate, 'Are you alright?' (children with suspected spine injuries should not be shaken).
If responding:
☑ leave in position, check condition, reassess regularly.
If not responding:
☑ open airway by tilting the child's head and lifting the chin, do not push on soft tissues under the chin as this may block the airway, avoid head tilt if spinal injury suspected—use jaw thrust.

Airway
☑ Keep airway open. Look, listen, and feel for breathing by putting your face to the child's face and looking along the chest.

Breathing (<10 s for assessment)
☑ If the child is breathing normally, turn on side, watch for continued breathing.
☑ If not breathing or irregular breathing pattern, remove any obvious airway obstruction, do not perform a blind finger sweep, give five rescue breaths (of 1 sec duration).

Circulation pulse (<10 s for assessment)
☑ Look for signs of life and check pulses:
  - child—carotid
  - infant—brachial
☑ If pulse >60 bpm, continue rescue breathing until the child starts to breathe.
☑ If pulse <60 bpm or absent (or uncertain), start chest compressions and continue rescue breaths.

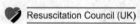

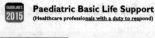

Resuscitation Council (UK) · GUIDELINES 2015 · **Paediatric Basic Life Support**
(Healthcare professionals with a duty to respond)

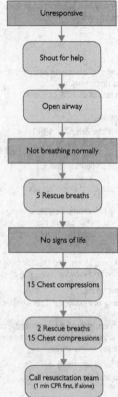

Figure 5.2 Paediatric basic life support (PBLS) algorithm (Healthcare professionals with a duty to respond).

Reproduced with the kind permission of the Resuscitation Council (UK).

Subsequent management

☑ Calling for help is vital, but if only one rescuer is present undertake resuscitation for 1 min before going for assistance.
☑ If resuscitation is successful, transfer to hospital/ICU. There may be a continuing risk of further cardiorespiratory arrest *en route*.
☑ Obtain IV/IO access as soon as is practical.

Risk factors

Primary respiratory and cardiovascular disease, metabolic disease, immersion in water, choking, trauma, haemorrhage, electrocution, sepsis.

Exclusions

Hypoxia—respiratory obstruction, drowning, poisoning, toxic gases, electric shock.

Special considerations

- Immersion in cold water:
  - BLS should be continued until the core temperature is above 32°C.
  - VF may be persistent at lower body temperatures.

Rescue breaths

Child

☑ Head tilt and chin lift.
☑ Pinch nose closed, open mouth, and maintain chin lift.
☑ Blow steadily into mouth while watching the chest rise.
☑ Take your mouth away and observe the chest fall—maintain the head tilt and jaw lift.
☑ Repeat 5 times.

Infant

☑ Head tilt and chin lift.
☑ Cover the nose and mouth with your mouth. This may be difficult in a larger infant and mouth to nose with the mouth held closed may be more effective.
☑ Blow steadily into mouth and nose over 1 s, watching the chest rise.
☑ Take your mouth away and observe the chest fall—maintain head tilt and jaw lift.
☑ Repeat 5 times.

Chest compressions

Child

☑ Place the heel of one hand over the lower half of the sternum.
☑ Lift your fingers to avoid pressing on the child's ribs.
☑ Keep your arm straight, press vertically down on the sternum.
☑ Depress the chest by one-third of its depth.

☑ Release and repeat at a rate of 100–120 compressions per min.
☑ After 15 compressions, tilt the head, lift the chin, and give two effective breaths.
☑ Continue compressions and breaths in a ratio of 15:2.
☑ Children over the age of 8 may need the adult two-handed compression technique.

Infant
☑ Place the tips of two fingers one finger breadth below a line between the nipples.
☑ Press down on the sternum and depress the chest by about 4 cm.
☑ Release and repeat at a rate of 100–120 compressions per min.
☑ Continue compressions and breaths at a 15:2 ratio.
☑ If there is more than one rescuer, then an alternative technique in an infant is:
  • encircle the chest with both hands, placing both thumbs over the lower half of the sternum, one finger's breadth below a line between the nipples.
  • press down on the sternum with both thumbs to about 4 cm.
  • the second rescuer delivers rescue breaths.

Foreign body obstruction
  (See Figure 5.3, 'FBAO algorithm'.)
☑ Encourage coughing because this is the most effective way of relieving obstruction caused by FBs in the airway.
☑ Active interventions to dislodge an FB are indicated when coughing attempts become ineffective or breathing is inadequate.
☒ Blind finger sweeps in the mouth are contraindicated as the FB may be impacted/pushed further into the airway.

Conscious with an ineffective cough
☑ Position the child prone with his head lower than his chest and his airway open.
☑ Deliver up to five sharp blows to the middle of the back between the shoulder blades.
☑ If the FB is not dislodged, then proceed to perform five anterior thrusts (chest for infants, abdominal for child >1 y).
☑ Chest thrust—place the infant supine with the head lower than the chest and the airway open.
☑ Deliver up to five sharp chest thrusts to the sternum, using the same technique as for chest compressions.
☑ Abdo thrust—stand or kneel behind child, encircle the torso with your arms, clench your fist and place it between umbilicus and xiphisternum. Grasp your fist and pull inwards and upwards.
☑ The aim is to relieve obstruction with each blow/thrust rather than to deliver all five blows/thrusts.
☑ After chest or abdominal thrusts, check the mouth for evidence of dislodged FB. Remove any debris carefully.

Unconscious with ineffective cough
☑ Open the mouth: attempt removal of an obvious foreign body with single finger sweep.
☑ Reassess airway and breathing.
☑ If still obstructed, continue with BLS by opening airway, giving five rescue breaths, and commencing CPR (➜ see 'Paediatric BLS', p. 125).

Reassess airway and breathing:
☑ continue with BLS.

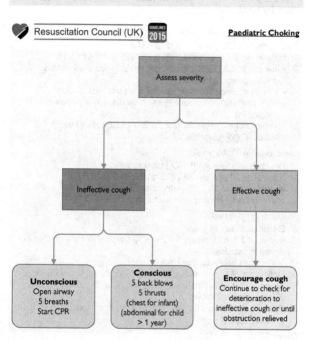

Figure 5.3 Paediatric FBAO treatment.
Reproduced with the kind permission of the Resuscitation Council (UK).

Further reading
UK Resuscitation Council Guidelines. Available at: https://www.resus.org.uk

☠ Paediatric advanced life support

Definition
Application of advanced skills to support vital organ function.

Presentation
- Asystolic arrest, rarely VF/VT, in response to hypoxia, trauma, sepsis, cardiac disease, metabolic derangement or vagal stimulation.
- Cardiac arrest in children is usually secondary to hypoxia—not an acute primary event.

Immediate management
(See Figure 5.4, PALS algorithm, ➲ p. 131.)
☑ Initial management is as BLS (➲ see p. 125 and Figure 5.2).
☑ After establishing CPR and calling for help, assess rhythm using cardiac monitor/defibrillator:
  - infants may need pads or paddles front and back of chest.
  - child pads should be placed just below the right clavicle and in left axillary line.
☑ Rhythm is often 'non-shockable' (PEA/asystole) but may be 'shockable' (VF/pulseless VT).

Non-shockable (PEA/asystole)
☑ Drugs should be given IV/IO (not tracheal).
☑ Adrenaline 10 μg/kg IV/IO (0.1 mL/kg of 1 in 10 000).
☑ Repeat cycles of 10 μg/kg adrenaline/3–5 min CPR.
☑ Briefly reassess rhythm after each cycle of 2 min CPR.

Shockable (VF/pulseless VT)
☑ Defibrillate once (4 J/kg).
☑ Resume CPR immediately for 2 min without reassessing rhythm or feeling for a pulse.
☑ Then pause briefly to check the monitor.
☑ Defibrillate (4 J/kg) if still in VF/VT and resume CPR immediately.
☑ Repeat cycles of defibrillation, CPR, and 10 μg/kg adrenaline every 3–5 min (about 2 cycles).
☑ A standard AED may be used for children either attenuated (<8 y) or in adult mode (>8 y).

During CPR
☑ Consider reversible causes (4Hs & 4Ts):
  - Hypoxia
  - Hypovolaemia
  - Hypo/hyperkalaemia
  - Hypothermia
  - Tension pneumothorax
  - Tamponade
  - Toxic/drug ingestion
  - Thromboemboli

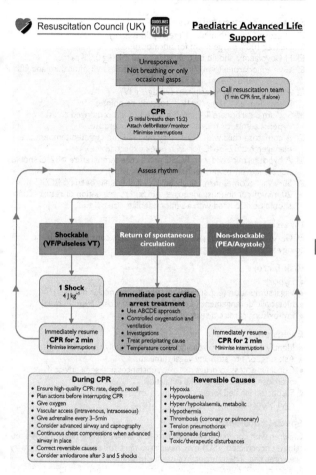

Figure 5.4 Paediatric advanced life support (PALS).
Reproduced with the kind permission of the Resuscitation Council (UK).

Subsequent management

- ☑ Effective CPR with minimal interruptions is key.
- ☑ Deliver 100% oxygen, aim for normocapnia.
- ☑ Hypovolaemia should be treated with 20 mL/kg 0.9% saline.
- ☑ Give amiodarone (5 mg/kg IV) for VF/pulseless VT after third and fifth shocks (dilute in 4 mL/kg 5% glucose).
- ☑ Atropine if a vagal precipitant (20 µg/kg IV)
- ☑ Magnesium 25–50 mg/kg IV if 'torsade de pointes'.
- ☑ Sodium bicarbonate 1–2 mL/kg 8.4% IV for a prolonged arrest, hyperkalaemia, or tricyclic antidepressant overdose.
- ☑ A comatose child with ROSC may benefit from targeted temperature management 32–36°C for 24 h (seek expert advice).
- ☑ A hypothermic child with ROSC and a core temperature >32°C should not be actively rewarmed (seek expert advice).
- ☑ Survival becomes increasingly unlikely if there has been no ROSC after 20 min of continuous, adequate, APLS; discontinuation of resuscitation should be discussed with a senior paediatrician.

Investigations

ECG, ABGs, FBC, U&Es, glucose, clotting screen, consider COHb and toxicology screen (depending on history).

Risk factors

- Hypoxia
- Vagal stimulation (e.g. surgical traction on the ocular muscles)
- Metabolic derangement (e.g. diabetic ketoacidosis, hypothermia)
- Pre-existing cardiac disease

Exclusions

- Identify causes of hypoxia and treat immediately.
- Ask surgeons to stop any vagal stimulation.
- Consider access to drugs or toxic substances and seek advice if overdose suspected. Smoke inhalation.
- Suspected inhaled foreign body in an arrested child may need urgent rigid bronchoscopy.

Special considerations

Children with congenital heart defects (e.g. univentricular heart, Fallot's tetralogy, uncorrected VSD) may have large right-to-left shunts as pulmonary pressures rise. Try to maintain systemic pressure.

Extracorporeal membrane oxygenation may be of benefit either in refractory arrest or after ROSC in a setting where it is immediately available.

Intraosseous access

(See also intraosseous access, ➔ p. 492.)

All recommended resuscitation drugs can be given by this route. Recommended sites for insertion:
- Anterior surface of the tibia, 2–3 cm below the tibial tuberosity (avoiding the epiphyseal plate).
- Anterolateral surface of the femur, 3 cm above the lateral condyle.

Further reading

UK Resuscitation Council Guidelines. Available at: https://www.resus.org.uk

☠ Drowning

Definition

- **Drowning**—a process resulting in primary respiratory impairment from submersion/immersion in a liquid medium (ILCOR definition).

Presentation

History of immersion in a fluid with respiratory or cardiorespiratory arrest. May be profoundly hypothermic. There may be associated trauma—involve the paediatric trauma team.

Immediate management

Basic life support

☑ Consider cervical spine injury. The neck should be immobilized by in-line stabilization.
☑ If resuscitation equipment is available, give oxygen via bag/valve/mask.
☑ There is a risk of aspiration of gastric contents, early intubation is desirable.
☑ Consider a rapid sequence induction.
☑ Pass a gastric tube to decompress the stomach and also allow gastric lavage.

Advanced life support

☑ If core temperature is <30°C, withhold adrenaline and other resuscitation drugs.
☑ Core temperature 30–35°C, double the drug dose interval.
☑ If VF is present, three shocks with CPR should be given, but further defibrillation attempts should be withheld until core temperature reaches 30°C.

Active re-warming

Resuscitation is unlikely to be successful unless the core temperature can be increased >32°C. Institute rectal or (preferably) oesophageal temperature monitoring.

☑ Remove all wet clothing and dry the patient.
☑ Use forced warm-air blanket and warm all IV fluids.
☑ If possible, warm the ventilator breathing circuit or use a circle system with soda-lime and low fresh gas flow to warm inspired gas (NB: reduced CO_2 production in hypothermia).
☑ Gastric or bladder lavage with 0.9% saline at 40–42°C.
☑ Peritoneal lavage with potassium-free dialysate at 40–42°C 20 mL/kg/15 min cycle.
☑ Extracorporeal circuit with blood re-warming.

Secondary survey

☑ Complete a secondary survey for other injuries

Subsequent management

☑ Aim to optimize recovery from the hypoxic CNS injury.
☑ Manage associated trauma.
☑ Supportive therapy in an intensive care unit.
☑ Regular tracheal toilet and culture of aspirate.
☑ Consider antibiotic therapy.
☑ Physiotherapy and follow-up chest X-ray.

Investigations

ABGs, blood glucose, electrolytes, core temperature with **low-reading thermometer** (e.g. thermistor probe), CXR, blood cultures, CT C-spine.

Risk factors

- Children playing near water. Accidental injury resulting in immersion, exposure to poisons (e.g. pesticides or toxic gases) near waterways or farmyard slurry.
- History of non-accidental injury.

Exclusions

- Diving accidents with head injury
- Exposure to toxic waste and chemicals in water
- Poisoning
- Deliberate harm (non-accidental injury)

Special considerations

- Three-quarters of drowning victims survive intact if they receive immediate BLS when removed from the water.
- Longer exposures reduce the chance of survival; a submersion of less than 10 min has a higher chance of a good outcome.
- Return of spontaneous ventilatory effort soon (a few minutes) after commencing resuscitation is a good prognostic sign.
- Adult data suggests 0.5% patients will have a cervical spine injury.
- Profound hypothermia (after cold water immersion) may preserve vital organ function but predisposes to ventricular fibrillation, which may be refractory to treatment until re-warming has occurred to above 32°C.
- The myocardium is unresponsive to drugs at temperatures <30°C, so if core temperature is <30°C withhold adrenaline and other resuscitation drugs. Accumulation of drugs occurs peripherally with standard ALS dose intervals, so >30°C use lowest recommended doses and double the dose interval.
- Submersion causes initial apnoea and bradycardia due to vagal stimulation (diving reflex). Continuing apnoea leads to hypoxia and reflex tachycardia. Further hypoxia produces severe acidosis. Eventually breathing resumes (the 'break-point') and fluid is inhaled, causing immediate laryngeal spasm. Eventually this spasm subsides with profound hypoxia; water and debris are inhaled. Subsequent hypoxia and acidosis lead to bradycardia and arrhythmia, culminating in cardiac arrest.

Further reading

Mackway Jones, K., Molyneux, E., Phillips, B., Wieteska, S. (eds) (2001). *Advanced Paediatric Life Support: The Practical Approach*, 3rd edition. London, UK: BMJ Books.
UK Resuscitation Council Guidelines. Available at: https://www.resus.org.uk

☠ Acute severe asthma

(See also bronchospasm, ➔ p. 70.)

Definition
Severe bronchospasm caused by reversible narrowing of hyper-reactive inflamed airways.

Presentation
- **Acute severe**—any one of:
  - PEFR 33–50% best or predicted, S_pO_2 <92%, pulse >125 bpm (>5 y) or >140 bpm (2–5 y), respiration >30 breaths/min (>5 y) or >40 breaths/min (2–5 y).
- **Life-threatening**—any of the following in a patient with acute severe asthma:
  - PEFR <33% best or predicted, S_pO_2 <92% or P_aO_2 <8 kPa (60 mmHg), normal P_aCO_2 (4.6–6 kPa [35–45 mmHg]), hypotension, exhaustion, confusion, or coma, silent chest, cyanosis, poor respiratory effort.
- **Near-fatal**—raised P_aCO_2 and/or requiring mechanical ventilation
  - confused or drowsy, maximal use of accessory muscles, exhausted, S_pO_2 <92% in air, heart rate >140 bpm and unable to talk, bradycardia is preterminal sign.

Immediate management
☑ 100% O_2.

Acute severe
☑ Salbutamol 10 puffs via inhaler and spacer ± facemask or nebulized salbutamol (2.5–5 mg).
☑ Prednisolone PO 20 mg (2–5 y), 30–40 mg (>5 y) or IV hydrocortisone (<1 y 25 mg, 1–5 y 50 mg,; 6–12 y 100 mg four times daily).
☑ Repeat salbutamol every 20–30 min, add ipratropium bromide 250 µg nebulized every 20–30 min.

Life-threatening
☑ Salbutamol nebulized 2.5–5 mg.
☑ Ipratropium bromide nebulized 500 µg (2–12 y 250 µg).
☑ IV hydrocortisone (<1 y 25 mg, 1–5 y 50 mg, 6–12 y 100 mg four times daily).
☑ Repeat bronchodilators every 20–30 min.
☑ Consider IV bronchodilators; salbutamol, aminophylline, and magnesium sulphate.

Subsequent management
☑ If improving—monitor S_pO_2, nebulizers 3–4 hourly, oral prednisolone for 3 days, transfer to respiratory ward once stable.

☑ If deteriorating despite medical therapy:
- salbutamol as a single dose IV (1 month–2 y 5 µg/kg; 2–18 y 15 µg/kg, maximum 250 µg),
- then by infusion of 1–2 µg/kg/min, dose adjusted according to response and heart rate—monitor for lactic acidosis.
- aminophylline 5 mg/kg loading dose (not if already on theophylline) then 1 mg/kg/h (<9 y), 800 µg/kg/h (9–16 y) IV infusion.
- continue nebulizers every 20 min.
- IV magnesium sulphate 50 mg/kg over 30 min (max. 2 g).

☑ If impending respiratory failure: intubate, ventilate, and transfer to PICU once stable (caution: see special considerations).

Investigations
- S_pO_2, peak expiratory flow (PEFR) or FEV_1 (>5 y)
- If critical: ABGs, CXR, lactate, serum theophylline level

Risk factors
- History of asthma with previous acute admissions
- Respiratory tract infection
- Trigger exposure (e.g. stress, cold, exercise, smoke, allergen)
- Prematurity and low birth-weight infants

Exclusions
- Consider other causes of wheeze:
  - bronchiolitis or croup
  - aspiration of foreign body—asymmetry on auscultation
  - epiglottitis—rare since introduction of HIB vaccine
  - pneumonia—primary cause of wheeze or trigger of asthma attack
  - tracheomalacia
  - anaphylaxis

Special considerations
- IPPV may be difficult in severe asthma with very high airway pressures (30–40 cmH_2O), sloping expiratory capnograph trace, and small tidal volumes. Hand ventilation may be necessary. Consider permissive hypercapnia if single system disorder (aim for arterial pH of 7.25).
- Try PEEP 5–7 cmH_2O and slow respiratory rates/long expiratory times to avoid dynamic hyperinflation.
- Volatile anaesthetic agents all cause bronchodilatation and may be useful *in extremis*. Attention should be given to scavenging of waste gas.
- These children are usually dehydrated, so induction of anaesthesia for intubation should be preceded with a fluid load of 20 mL/kg of crystalloid. Slow administration of drugs is preferable, but rapid sequence induction may be required in non-fasted patients.
- Consider ketamine 1–2 mg/kg.
- Avoid histamine releasing drugs like morphine or atracurium.
- If an inotrope is required, consider adrenaline by infusion.
- If sedation is adequate postintubation intensive physiotherapy can be very beneficial.

Table 5.4 PEFR by height

Height (cm)	PEFR (L/min)
120	215
130	260
140	300
150	350
160	400
170	450
180	500

- **Peak expiratory flow rate in children**—this is a simple method of measuring airway obstruction and will detect moderate or severe disease. It is measured using a standard Wright peak flow meter (see Table 5.4):

  Expected PEFR (L/min) = [height (cm) − 80] ×5

Further reading
British Thoracic Society/Scottish Intercollegiate Guidelines Network. *Asthma.* Available at: https://www.brit-thoracic.org.uk/quality-improvement/clinical-resources/asthma/

:⚙: Stridor

Definition
- Harsh respiratory noise produced by airway obstruction.
- Inspiratory stridor implies laryngeal/nasal/pharyngeal pathology.
- Expiratory stridor implies tracheal/bronchial (intrathoracic).
- Biphasic stridor implies subglottic or glottic pathology.

Presentation
- Stridor, increased work of breathing suprasternal, intercostal, or subcostal recession and increased use of accessory muscles.
- Signs of deterioration and need for urgent intervention—hypoxia, fatigue, or decreasing conscious level, increased work of breathing.
- Impending respiratory failure may also be heralded by a reduction in work of breathing (exhaustion) and less stridor (more complete obstruction).
- Beware the disinterested child.

Immediate management
- ☑ Allow the child to sit quietly on the parent's lap in a comfortable position.
- ☑ Observe closely without interference.
- ☑ Assess severity of respiratory distress and plan for most likely underlying cause.
- ☑ Supplemental oxygen can result in falsely reassuring S_pO_2 readings in severe obstruction.
- ☑ Consider EMLA® or tetracaine gel 4% (Ametop®) for intravenous access.
- ☑ Consider nebulizing 0.5 mL/kg 1 in 1000 adrenaline (up to 5 mL).
- ☑ If condition deteriorating, prepare for intubation.

Anaesthesia for the child with the obstructed airway
- ☑ Call for senior anaesthetist and senior ENT help.
- ☑ Inhalational induction in theatre in a quiet environment.
- ☑ Consider antisialagogue (atropine 20 µg/kg IV—min 100 µg, max 600 µg).
- ☑ 100% O_2 and sevoflurane
- ☑ May induce on parent's lap or sitting if airway best maintained in that position.
- ☑ Apply CPAP via facemask once tolerated.
- ☑ Adequate depth of anaesthesia will take a long time to achieve!
- ☑ Maintain spontaneous breathing but check if you can ventilate with the bag. If yes, **gently** assist inspiration if necessary, but avoid gastric distension.
- ☑ Once patient is sufficiently anaesthetized—direct laryngoscopy without muscle relaxant.
- ☑ Intubate if possible—may need much smaller tube than anticipated in croup (do not pre-cut the ETT).

☑ Intubation may be difficult in epiglottitis—look for air bubbles from glottic opening. Use a bougie and railroad tube over it.
☑ If emergency IV access required remember intraosseous route can be quickly established.
☑ If obstruction persists following successful intubation: try advancing the tube (mediastinal mass/foreign body), consider a blocked tube (tracheitis), try prone ventilation (mediastinal mass).
☑ The vast majority of children with stridor can be intubated by an experienced anaesthetist; occasionally rigid bronchoscopy in the hands of an experienced ENT surgeon may be life-saving.

Subsequent management
☑ Once intubated, maintain anaesthesia (IV morphine and midazolam infusion or inhalational agent while in theatre).
☑ Consider dexamethasone 0.6 mg/kg IV if not already given.
☑ Transfer to PICU.
☑ Cefotaxime 50 mg/kg IV 6-hourly or ceftriaxone 50 mg/kg IV daily (epiglottitis).
☑ Extubation: dexamethasone often given (0.25 mg/kg IV 6-hourly 2 or 3 doses) at least 6 h prior to extubation. A small leak around the ET tube at a pressure of 20 cmH$_2$O should be observed before attempting extubation.
☑ Soft-tissue X-rays usually add no useful information. Even with a leak, oedema may require re-intubation in some cases.

Investigations
Check S$_p$O$_2$ on air and 100% oxygen.

Risk factors
• Croup most likely acute cause in United Kingdom.
• High degree of overlap in clinical presentation.
• Supplementary oxygen may be falsely reassuring as a child in severe respiratory distress may be pink in oxygen until preterminal.

Exclusions
• Croup—harsh barking cough, febrile, miserable but well.
• Epiglottitis—toxic, no cough, low-pitched inspiratory and expiratory stridor, and drooling.
• Foreign body—sudden onset, previously well, coughing, choking, aphonia, and drooling. Rarely visible on X-ray.
• Anaphylaxis—swelling of face and tongue, wheeze, urticarial rash.
• Retropharyngeal abscess—high fever, hyperextension of neck, dysphagia, pooling of secretions.
• Bacterial tracheitis—toxic, tender trachea (vigilance is required if intubated—mucopurulent membrane can block ET).
• Pre-existing stridor—congenital abnormality, laryngomalacia, or subglottic stenosis.

:☠: Anaphylaxis

(See also 'Adult anaphylaxis', p. 272.)

Definition

- A severe, life-threatening, generalized, or systemic hypersensitivity reaction.
- This definition includes IgE- and non-IgE-mediated reactions.

Presentation

- Commonly—stridor, wheeze, cough, desaturation, respiratory distress, ECG changes, cardiovascular collapse, and clinical signs of shock.
- Less commonly—oedema, rash, and urticaria.
- Consider when compatible history of severe allergic-type reaction with respiratory difficulty and/or hypotension, especially if skin changes are present.

Immediate management

- ☑ Call for help.
- ☑ 100% O_2.
- ☑ Adrenaline 1 µg/kg slow IV given incrementally with ECG monitoring until hypotension resolves (1:10 000 solution).
- ☑ OR IM adrenaline (1:1000 solution) is less arrhythmogenic:
  - 12+ y: 500 µg (0.5 mL).
  - 6–12 y: 250 µg (0.25 mL).
  - >6 months–6 y: 120 µg (0.12 mL).
  - <6 months: 50 µg (0.05 mL).
- ☑ Antihistamine: chlorphenamine:
  - 12+ y: 10 mg IM or slow IV.
  - 6–12 y: 5 mg IM or slow IV.
  - 6 months–6 y: 2.5 mg IM or slow IV.
  - <6 months: 250 µg/kg IM or slow IV.
- ☑ Hydrocortisone:
  - 12+ y: 200 mg IM or slow IV.
  - 6–12 y: 100 mg IM or slow IV.
  - 6 months–6 y: 50 mg IM or slow IV.
  - <6 months: 25 mg IM or slow IV.
- ☑ Repeat doses of adrenaline may be given at 5 min intervals as necessary, further fluid boluses may be needed.
- ☑ Consider adrenaline IV infusion (0.05–0.5 µg/kg/min).

Subsequent management

- ☑ Remove precipitant if practicable.
- ☑ Volume expansion with sodium chloride 0.9% 20 mL/kg.
- ☑ Bronchodilators, e.g. salbutamol inhalers/nebulizers, as per protocol for acute severe asthma (p. 136) if bronchospasm severe and unresponsive to adrenaline.

☑ Catecholamine infusion as CVS instability may last several hours—adrenaline or noradrenaline 0.05–0.5 µg/kg/min.

☑ Check ABGs, consider bicarbonate—up to 1 mmol/kg 8.4% sodium bicarbonate (1 mmol = 1 mL) if pH less than 7.1.

Investigations
Take clotted blood samples for mast cell tryptase (early, 1–2 h, and 24 h samples).

Risk factors
- Previous allergic reaction; particularly history of increasingly severe reactions.
- History of asthma or atopy.
- Penicillin, radiographic contrast media, some foods (especially nuts). Cross-sensitivity means that previous exposure is not always necessary (e.g. latex and bananas).
- Intravenous administration of antigen increases risk.

Exclusions
- Primary cardiovascular disease (e.g. congenital heart disease in the newborn)
- Sepsis (with rash)
- Latex allergy
- Tension pneumothorax
- Acute severe asthma (history of asthma, previous admissions)
- Airway obstruction (e.g. foreign body aspiration)

Special considerations
- Never give undiluted adrenaline 1:1000 IV. IM adrenaline carries less risk of provoking potentially life-threatening arrhythmias, but may be poorly absorbed if perfusion is compromised, such that the dose may be ineffective. IV adrenaline may cause arrhythmia, but given slowly with full ECG monitoring, may be more effective in profound anaphylactic shock.
- Chlorphenamine and steroids take hours to achieve any benefit—omission in immediate management is acceptable.
- Chlorphenamine is not suitable for neonates.
- Absence of a circuit/airway filter increases the risk of exposure to aerosolized latex particles.
- Report adverse drug reactions to MHRA (℡ http://www.mhra.gov.uk).
- All patients with anaphylaxis should be referred to an allergy clinic (℡ https://www.bsaci.org).

Further reading
Harper, N.J., Dixon, T., Dugué, P., et al.: Association of Anaesthetists of Great Britain and Ireland (2009). Suspected anaphylactic reactions associated with anaesthesia. *Anaesthesia*, **64**, 199–211.
UK Resuscitation Council Guidelines. Available at: https://www.resus.org.uk

:✪: Major trauma

Definition

Serious injury to head/chest/abdomen/pelvis/spine.

Presentation

- A history is the key to understanding the severity and pattern of injuries.
- There is considerable time pressure initially. A protocolized multidisciplinary approach, which prioritizes the treatment of immediately life-threatening injuries, has improved outcomes.
- After this initial 'Primary survey' a detailed 'Secondary survey' aims to completely identify all the injuries.
- Children and infants often have a greater compensatory reserve than adults, resulting in a tendency to underestimate the severity of injuries.
- Treatment priorities are a clear airway, adequate ventilation, avoidance of hypoxia, and hypotension.

Immediate management

☑ ABC—100% O_2.

☑ Place two large-bore cannulae or obtain intraosseous access. Do not waste time if peripheral veins are not available.

☑ Intubation after rapid sequence induction may be required to protect the airway (GCS <8 or trend in the GCS motor component), and avoid hypoxia (respiratory failure developing). Protect the cervical spine—assume spinal damage and use in-line stabilization or a hard collar.

☑ Unconscious patients must be ventilated, preferably using muscle relaxants. Aim for normocapnia.

☑ Hypovolaemia as evidenced by tachycardia and poor capillary refill should be treated with fluid boluses of 20 mL/kg crystalloid (Hartmann's solution or 0.9% saline). Use colloid if the initial response to crystalloid is poor. Blood should be given as the third fluid bolus if there is no improvement.

☑ Avoid fluid overload in head-injured patients, but ensure perfusion with an adequate mean arterial pressure. There may be large blood loss from scalp wounds or into the subdural space in patients with head injuries, particularly infants.

☑ Thoracentesis or pericardiocentesis may be required urgently.

☑ An orogastric tube and urinary catheter should be placed routinely.

Subsequent management

☑ Secondary survey looking at all systems for signs of injury. Vital signs and neurological status (disability) should be reassessed continually.

☑ All patients need ventilation, oxygenation, and cardiac output problems addressed before transfer to CT or PICU. The clinician undertaking a transfer must have a clear understanding of the risk of the journey and the benefit of the transfer in order to make the correct stabilization decisions.

☑ Seizures in the context of traumatic brain injury: consider phenytoin infusion.

☑ If non-accidental injury is suspected, contact Child Protection Service (usually via a consultant paediatrician).

Investigations

• FBC, U&Es, glucose, crossmatch ABGs, clotting
• X-ray—C-spine, CXR, pelvis, thoracic/lumbar spine
• Ultrasound—checking for abdominal free fluid
• CT scan
• Peripheral X-rays

Risk factors

• Pedestrians most at risk, then cyclists and vehicle passengers.
• Head injury accounts for 40% of trauma deaths in children.

Exclusions

• Non-accidental injury in cases of apparent accidental trauma, particularly head injury. 'Shaken baby' syndrome.
• Poisoning, deliberate or accidental in cases of coma or fitting.

A = Airway
B = Breathing
C = Circulation
D = Disability (neurological assessment)
E = Exposure (remove clothes to assess—BUT keep warm)

Disability is assessed initially using **AVPU**:

A = Alert
V = responds to **V**oice
P = responds to **P**ain
U = Unresponsive

The GCS can be used in children over 4 y of age (see Glasgow coma scale, ➲ p. 194).

Further reading

Mackway Jones, K., Molyneux, E., Phillips, B., Wieteska, S. (eds) (2001). *Advanced Paediatric Life Support: The Practical Approach*, 3rd edition. London, UK: BMJ Books.

:Ö: Burns

➲ SEE ALSO burns in adults, p. 426

Definition

Dry burn or scalding injury ± smoke inhalation.

Presentation

- Obvious thermal injury—remove all clothing where possible.
- Smoke deposits, carbonaceous sputum, airway obstruction, or bronchospasm suggest airway/lung damage, and early intubation should be considered before oedema makes this very challenging.
- Hypovolaemia soon after burn injury is probably due to other causes, such as bleeding (e.g. from falls, injuries sustained while escaping the fire or blast).
- A multidisciplinary paediatric trauma team should manage all but the most straightforward cases.

Immediate management

☑ ABC—100% O_2.
☑ Airway assessment. If in doubt, intubate. Use uncut tied ET tube to allow for facial oedema.
☑ Analgesia essential—IV morphine 100 µg/kg titrated and repeated as required. Consider ketamine 0.5–1 mg/kg.
☑ Two large-bore IV cannulae or IO access. Consider femoral central line (avoids risk of pneumothorax). Initially Hartmann's or 0.9% saline 20 mL/kg for hypovolaemia—repeat as required if signs of hypovolaemia (capillary refill >2 s; low blood pressure). Urine output should be >1–2 mL/kg/h. NB: Burn fluid formulae are not used at this stage.
☑ Consider inhalational induction with sevoflurane if airway involvement could make the airway or intubation difficult.

Subsequent management

☑ Measure COHb. Use 100% oxygen until COHb <10%. The risk/benefit of hyperbaric oxygen is not clear.
☑ Cyanide antidote may be required (sodium nitrite 3% solution 4–10 mg/kg, plus sodium thiosulphate 50% solution 400 mg/kg [max 12.5 g]). Monitor methaemoglobin level (should remain <10%).
☑ Urinary catheter to guide fluid balance (urine output >2 mL/kg/h).
☑ Wound care—infection is a significant cause of mortality. Keep the burn wound covered with 'clingfilm', sterile towels, or dressings.
☑ Antibiotic prophylaxis according to local protocol.

Fluid therapy

- Burn depth and area are assessed during the secondary survey. This assessment can be used to guide fluid therapy during subsequent management. NB: Formulae for fluid therapy are only a guide, and

frequent reassessment of circulatory status and urine output are required.
- Special charts that take into account changes in relative surface area with age (e.g. Lund and Browder, Figure 5.5) can be used to assess the burn area. The 'rule of nines' (see p. 428) cannot be applied to children below 14 years of age. For extensive burns, count unburnt area using the patient's palmar surface area (including fingers) = 0.8% BSA.
- Dry, waxy/leathery, insensitive burns that DO NOT BLEED on pinprick are full thickness. Full-thickness burns can easily be confused with normal skin.
- Patients with partial-thickness burns greater than 10% BSA or 5% full thickness require IV fluid in addition to basal fluid requirement. This additional fluid can be calculated using different formulae (seek expert advice), e.g. Parkland—4 mL × Weight kg × % Burn SA (mL).
- 50% of this volume is given in the first 8 h following the burn injury. Controversy exists as to the relative benefit of crystalloid or colloid, but crystalloid is now more commonly used. Subsequent fluid therapy is guided by urine output.

Investigations

S_pO_2, ABGs, Hb, COHb, cyanide level (>100 ppm may be fatal), U&Es, glucose, G&S, myoglobin (particularly in electrical burns), chest radiograph if inhalation.

Risk factors

- 70% are preschool children, greatest risk 1–2 years of age.
- Most fatal burns in house fires are due to smoke inhalation. Other injuries are often sustained while attempting to escape the fire.
- Cyanide poisoning in house fires due to burning plastics and wool.
- Common causes of burns in children include hot drinks, hot baths (infants), cooking oil.
- Electrical burns.

Exclusions

Non-accidental injury (NAI)—burns may have a 'glove or stocking' appearance due to limb, or whole-body, immersion in a hot bath. 'Cold burns' (contact with deep frozen objects), delay in seeking help, vague history, and the combination of healing and fresh injuries should also lead to suspicion of NAI. If NAI is suspected, contact the Child Protection Service (usually via a consultant paediatrician).

Criteria for transfer to a burns unit

- More than 10% partial or any full-thickness burns.
- Burns to special areas, e.g. face, hands, and perineum.
- Lack of facilities to manage burn wounds of <10% BSA.
- Lack of expertise at the receiving hospital (e.g. paediatric team).

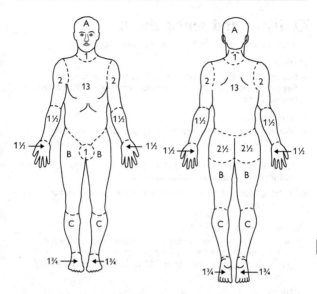

Relative percentage of area affected by growth (age in years)

	0	1	5	10	15	Adult
A: half of head	9½	8½	6½	5½	4½	3½
B: half of thigh	2¾	3¼	4	4½	4½	4¾
C: half of leg	2½	2½	2¾	3	3¼	3½

Figure 5.5 Assessing extent of burns—Lund and Browder charts.

Reproduced from Lund, C. C., Browder, N. C. (1944). The estimation of areas of burns. *Surgery Gynecology & Obstetrics* (now *Journal of the American College of Surgeons*), 79:352–58. © 2019 by the American College of Surgeons. Published by Elsevier Inc. All rights reserved.

Special considerations

- Small area electrical burn—may be internal organ damage and myoglobinuria.
- Psychological damage.
- Careful and complete documentation in NAI cases.

Further reading

Peltier, P.J., Purdue, G., Shepherd, J. (2001). *Burn Injuries in Child Abuse*. Rockville, MD: US Department of Justice, National Criminal Justice Reference Service.
University of Washington (2011). *Pediatric Burn Injuries*. Available at: https://www.depts.washington.edu/pccm/3-pediatric%20burns%2011.pps

☼ Sepsis and septic shock

(See also description of adult treatment of sepsis, ➲ p. 373.)

Definition
- **Sepsis**—acute organ dysfunction secondary to infection.
- **Septic shock**—sepsis plus vasopressor requirement in the absence of hypovolaemia.

Presentation
- **'Warm' shock**—low blood pressure, especially low diastolic, tachycardia, vasodilated with short capillary refill time, often high cardiac output.
- **'Cold' shock**—normal or low blood pressure, tachycardia, prolonged capillary refill, often low cardiac output state.

Early recognition and fluid administration is the key intervention that improves outcome.

Immediate management

☑ If the child is febrile and unwell, but conscious with an adequate circulation, give oxygen; obtain vascular access, baseline investigations, give maintenance fluid, and observe for signs of impending septic shock.

Septic shock
☑ Recognize impaired mental status and perfusion.
☑ Deliver oxygen and assess airway (BLS).
☑ 20 mL/kg crystalloid (not containing glucose) boluses titrated to improvement in haemodynamics.
☑ Measure lactate level.
☑ Correct hypoglycaemia/hypocalcaemia, give antibiotics.
☑ Contact a PICU for advice as soon as severe sepsis is identified.
☑ If the shock persists and hepatomegaly or chest crackles develop start peripheral or IO dopamine (5–15 µg/kg/min), intubate (ketamine/suxamethonium/fentanyl), establish central and arterial access and give more fluid or blood to target Hb 100 g/L.
☑ Fluid-refractory, dopamine-resistant shock:
  - warm shock—noradrenaline (0.1–1.0 µg/kg/min).
  - cold shock—adrenaline (0.1–1.0 µg/kg/min).
  - titrate the inotropes to clinical endpoints and $S_{cv}O_2$ saturations >70%.
  - Consider dobutamine (5–15 µg/kg/min) or milrinone (0.25 to 0.75 µg/kg/min) for refractory cold shock.
  - management should be guided by advice from the local PICU.

Consider
☑ Hydrocortisone 1 mg/kg 6-hourly if there is adrenal insufficiency.
☑ 4.5% human albumin may be used after initial boluses of crystalloid.
☑ Support coagulation with plasma therapies and platelets.

☑ Profound acidosis should be corrected with 8.4% sodium bicarbonate (4.2% in neonates). Give half the correction based on base deficit (if pH <7.1) and repeat ABGs:

Full correction (mL) = weight × 0.3 × base deficit.

☑ Avoid hypoglycaemia.
☑ Antibiotics:
- neonates—ampicillin 30 mg/kg 6-hourly (8-hourly if aged <7 days), plus gentamicin 2.5 mg/kg 8-hourly (12-hourly if aged <7 days); monitor blood levels.
- older children—cefotaxime 50 mg/kg 6-hourly IV, or ceftriaxone 50 mg/kg daily.
- Consider clindamycin for toxic shock syndromes.
- ECMO for refractory shock.

Subsequent management
☑ Do not perform lumbar puncture if risk of raised ICP.
☑ If raised ICP is suspected, mannitol (0.5–1.0 g/kg) or furosemide (1 mg/kg) to 'buy time'. The patient should be catheterized.

Investigations
Hb, U&Es, glucose, clotting, ABGs, calcium, magnesium, phosphate, blood cultures

Risk factors
- Exposure to Gram-positive or -negative bacteria, *Listeria spp.*, *Rickettsia spp.*, fungi, and viruses, particularly herpes.
- Immune system deficiency, surgery, and chronic illness.

Exclusions
- Hypovolaemia from any cause.
- Primary cardiac disease (e.g. cardiomyopathy); congenital cardiac defects (e.g. undiagnosed ventricular septal defect with heart failure).
- Anaphylaxis.
- Poisoning.

Special considerations
- The shocked child with no obvious haemorrhage should be treated as sepsis until another cause is found.
- Rash in meningococcal disease does not always develop immediately. A careful survey for purpuric spots is mandatory. A small number of cases have no rash.
- Bleeding into mucosal surfaces may indicate DIC.
- Fever may not be present in babies. A temperature >38°C is significant.
- Deteriorating level of consciousness, irritability, hypertonia/hypotonia warrant immediate investigation.

Meningitis
- A petechial or purpuric rash may occur not only with meningococcal meningitis but also with *Haemophilus* spp. and pneumococcus (*Streptococcus pneumoniae*).
- Meningitis may be bacterial or viral. Bacterial meningitis is more common in neonates and infants. Viral meningitis is usually less severe, with fever, headache, and neck stiffness, but may mimic bacterial meningitis:
  - newborns—Group B β-haemolytic streptococcus, Gram-negative bacteria (*Escherichia coli; Pseudomonas* spp.), *Listeria* spp.
- Infants >3 months and children—*Haemophilus influenzae, Streptococcus pneumoniae, Neisseria meningitidis*, TB, fungi, viruses (usually enteroviruses), coxsackie-, and echoviruses.
- Consider meningitis in any infant or child with an altered level of consciousness or coma, particularly with fever and a high white cell count.
- Common signs—fever, lethargy, irritability, decreased appetite, vomiting, headache, photophobia, altered consciousness, convulsions, neck stiffness. Signs of raised ICP—bulging fontanelle, papilloedema, altered pupils. Focal signs (e.g. hemiparesis) suggest tumour or ischaemia.
- Steroids are indicated in *H. influenzae* and *S. pneumoniae* meningitis to reduce hearing loss due to eighth nerve damage. There is no indication for routine steroid use in viral meningitis or encephalitis.

Encephalitis
- Rarer than meningitis. Most common presentation is altered level of consciousness/coma, headache, nausea, and vomiting. Herpesvirus infection may present with convulsions, often focal. Fitting may be difficult to control. Varicella infection characteristically involves the cerebellum (ataxia).
- Common pathogens—herpes simplex and zoster, Epstein–Barr virus, cytomegalovirus, measles, mumps, varicella, enteroviruses, adenoviruses.
- Consider cephalosporin, a macrolide and acyclovir + CT scan if the patient is sick and aetiology uncertain.

Further reading

Dellinger, R.P., Levy, M.M., Rhodes, A., et al. (2012). Surviving Sepsis Campaign: international guidelines for management of severe sepsis and septic shock. *Critical Care Medicine*, 41(2), 580–637.

Levin, D.L., Morris, F.C. (eds) (1997). *Essentials of Paediatric Intensive Care*, 2nd edition. Edinburgh, UK: Churchill Livingstone.

Macnab, A.J., Macrae, D.J., Henning, R. (eds) (2001). *Care of the Critically ill Child*. Edinburgh, UK: Churchill Livingstone.

Useful data

Paediatric ET tube sizes and length

For emergency intubations consider using a cuffed tube one size smaller than calculated in Table 5.5. Be aware that below a size 4 this may compromise the ID available for gas exchange and secretion removal.

Normal values

For a list of normal values for paediatric anaesthesia see Table 5.6.

Table 5.5 Paediatric ET tube sizes and length

Age	Weight (kg)	ID (mm)	ED (mm)	At lip (cm)	At nose (cm)
Newborn	<0.7	2.0	2.9	5.0	6
Newborn	<1.0	2.5	3.6	5.5	7
Newborn	1.0	3.0	4.3	6	7.5
Newborn	2.0	3.0	4.3	7	9
Newborn	3.0	3.0+	4.3	8.5	10.5
Newborn	3.5	3.5+	4.9	9	11
3 months	6.0	3.5	4.9	10	12
1 year	10	4.0	5.6	11	14
2 years	12	4.5	6.2	12	15
3 years	14	4.5	6.2	13	16
4 years	16	5.0	6.9	14	17
6 years	20	5.5	7.5	15	19
8 years	24	6.0	8.2	16	20
10 years	30	6.5	8.9	17	21
14 years	50	7.5	10.2	19	23

ET tube size: (age/4) + 4; ET tube length (oral): (age/2) + 12; ID, internal diameter; ED, external diameter.

Drug formulary

See Table 5.7 for useful drug doses and Table 5.8 for infusions for paediatric anaesthesia.

Table 5.6 Normal values

Age	Weight (kg)	Pulse (bpm)	Mean BP (mmHg)
Term	3.5	95–145	40–60
3 months	6.0	110–175	45–75
6 months	7.5	110–175	50–90
1 year	10	105–170	50–100
3 years	14	80–140	50–100
7 years	22	70–120	60–90
10 years	30	60–110	60–90
12 years	38	60–100	65–95
14 years	50	60–100	65–95

Age <9 years: weight (kg) = (age + 4) ×2; Age >9 years: weight (kg) = approximately 3× age.

Table 5.7 Useful drug doses

Adrenaline	IV: 1 µg/kg (0.01 mL/kg of 1:10 000) increments
	IM: 10 µg/kg (0.1 mL/kg of 1:10 000 or 0.01 mL/kg of 1:1000)
	ETT: 100 µg/kg (0.1 mL/kg of 1:1000)
	Infusion: 0.05–1 µg/kg/min
Aminophylline (not if on oral theophylline)	Load 5 mg/kg IV over 1 h
Amiodarone	5 mg/kg IV centrally (or peripherally in emergency)
Atracurium	0.5 mg/kg IV then 0.1 mg/kg as required
Atropine	10–20 µg/kg IV (min. 100 µg, max. 600 µg)
Bicarbonate (sodium)	1 mmol/kg IV
Chlorphenamine	1 month–1 y — 250 µg/kg (avoid in neonates) IM/Slow IV
	1–5 y — 2.5–5 mg IM/Slow IV
	6–12 y — 5–10 mg IM/Slow IV
Calcium chloride 10%	0.1–0.2 mL/kg slow IV
Calcium gluconate 10%	0.3–0.5 mL/kg slow IV
Dantrolene	1 mg/kg repeated until improvement (max. 10 mg/kg/24 h)

Table 5.7 (Contd.)

Dexamethasone	0.15 mg/kg/dose (max 10 mg) 6-hourly PO/IV
Diazepam	0.3 mg/kg IV/IO; 0.5 mg/kg PR
Fentanyl	1–2 µg/kg
Furosemide	0.5–1 mg/kg
Glucose	Hypoglycaemia: 2.5 to 5 mL/kg 10% glucose
	Hyperkalaemia: 10% glucose 5 mL/kg/h and insulin 0.05 to 0.1 units/kg/h
Glycopyrronium	5–15 µg/kg IV
Ketamine	Anaesthesia: 1–2 mg/kg IV, 5–10 mg/kg IM
	Sedation/analgesia: 0.5 mg/kg then 4 µg/kg/min IV infusion
Lidocaine	Nerve block: max. 3 mg/kg
Lorazepam	Status epilepticus: 0.1 mg/kg IV
Magnesium	25–50 mg/kg IV slowly
Mannitol	0.25–0.5 g/kg IV
Midazolam	Sedation: 0.1–0.2 mg/kg IV, up to 0.3 mg/kg nasal, 0.5 mg/kg PO (use IV solution in juice or buccal suspension)
Mivacurium	0.1–0.2 mg/kg IV
Morphine	0.1–0.2 mg/kg IV
Naloxone	Opioid overdose: 100 µg/kg IV/IM/SC—then 10 µg/kg/h
	Reversal in anaesthesia: 0.5–1 µg/kg IV increments repeated as necessary
Neostigmine	Reversal of neuromuscular blockade: 50–100 µg/kg IV
Nitric oxide	1–20 ppm (0.1 L/min of 1000 ppm added to 10 L/min gas = 10 ppm)
Noradrenaline	0.05–0.5 µg/kg/min IV infusion; via a central line. Can be given peripherally only for very short periods due to profound vasoconstriction.
Phenytoin	20 mg/kg IV (not greater than 1 mg/kg/min) (therapeutic range = 10–20 mg/L)
Propofol	2–5 mg/kg IV
Remifentanil	Up to 1 µg/kg IV, then 0.05–0.25 µg/kg/min IV infusion
Rocuronium	0.6–1.2 mg/kg IV, then 0.1–0.2 mg/kg IV as required
Salbutamol	2.5 mg nebule 2–6 hourly, 15 µg/kg over 10 min IV then 1–5 µg/kg/min
Suxamethonium	2 mg/kg IV (child), 3 mg/kg (neonate)
Thiopental	2–5 mg/kg IV slowly (up to 7 mg/kg in status epilepticus)
Tramadol	1–2 mg/kg IV
Vecuronium	0.1 mg/kg IV then 20–50 µg/kg IV as required

Table 5.8 Infusions

Adrenaline, Noradrenaline	300 µg/kg in 50 mL of 5% glucose
	1 mL/h = 0.1 µg/kg/min
	Dose range: 0.05–1 µg/kg/min (0.5–10 mL/h)
	Peripherally in emergency, change to central venous line when available
Dobutamine, Dopamine	3 mg/kg in 50 mL of 5% glucose
	1 mL/h = 1 µg/kg/min
	Dose range: 3–20 µg/kg/min (3–20 mL/h)
	Peripherally in emergency, change to central venous line when available
Atracurium	Dose range: 0.5 mg/kg then 300–600 µg/kg/h

Obstetrics

Mark Scrutton and Michael Kinsella

☠ Maternal collapse

Definition
Acute maternal cardiovascular collapse/respiratory failure after 20 weeks in pregnancy.

Presentation
- Collapse in late pregnancy—usually during labour, postpartum, or intraoperatively.
- Shock, respiratory distress, impaired consciousness, convulsions.

Immediate management
☑ ABC—100% O_2.
☑ Position—minimize compression of the inferior vena cava by the uterus. If external cardiac massage (ECM) required, displace uterus to the left by manually retracting uterus laterally; otherwise turn full left lateral unless obstetric management precludes this.
☑ Intubate as soon as possible to prevent aspiration and ensure effective alveolar ventilation in presence of diaphragmatic splinting. If there is a delay in intubation, consider cricoid pressure.
☑ Persisting gas exchange impairment in the presence of adequate alveolar ventilation and circulation may indicate pulmonary oedema, pulmonary or amniotic fluid embolus, or pulmonary aspiration.
☑ Initial rapid intravenous fluid infusion if the diagnosis is unclear. If bleeding is present, do not delay giving blood (O-negative if patient-specific blood not immediately available).
☑ Vasopressor—consider ephedrine for α- and β-effects, phenylephrine or metaraminol for α-effect—the choice may depend on maternal heart rate. If these do not produce a response use adrenaline 100 µg IV and then escalating doses. Adrenaline causes placental vasoconstriction but should not be avoided on this account.
☑ Cardiac arrest—perform perimortem Caesarean section (CS) within 5 min of arrest unless there is return of adequate circulation; prepare for this immediately.

Subsequent management
☑ The condition of the fetus, if undelivered, must be assessed as soon as possible. Delivery of a compromised baby must be coordinated with stabilization of the mother.
☑ Further investigation and treatment, and transfer to operating theatre or ITU, will depend on the cause.

Investigations
ECG, ABGs, U&Es, coagulation tests. If indicated investigate for pulmonary embolus (PE) following local protocol. Echocardiogram.

Risk factors

- Venous return and cardiac output are impaired by haemorrhage, IVC compression, and high regional anaesthesia. These causes augment each other.
- Vasovagal bradycardia and asystole may occur.

Exclusions/Causes

- Aortocaval compression—rapid improvement in lateral position.
- Hypovolaemia—obstetric examination to check for internal bleeding (intrauterine or extrauterine); will respond to adequate volume replacement—CVP guidance may help. Consider echo if readily available.
- High regional block—check sensory level, arm motor power, and breathing; hypotension should respond to vasopressors given early and in liberal doses; intubation and ventilation may be necessary.
- Eclampsia—cardiovascular system returns to normal or hypertension after convulsion; possible respiratory impairment if pulmonary aspiration has occurred.
- Local anaesthetic toxicity—prodromal symptoms, convulsions; bupivacaine may produce torsade de pointes VT, prolonged cardiac depression. Treat with Intralipid® (❸ see p. 248).
- Pulmonary embolism—may have history suggestive of DVT or other risk factors; ECG changes (S_I Q_{III} T_{III}, sinus tachycardia, and/or new RBBB). Radiological investigations as per local protocol (e.g. V/Q or CT pulmonary angiogram—CTPA).
- Cardiac disease—variable presentation, echocardiogram as soon as possible to identify myocardial dysfunction, valve lesions, establish cardiogenic or non-cardiogenic cause for pulmonary oedema.
- Anaphylaxis—temporal relationship to drug administration; bronchospasm may be prominent; final diagnosis by serum tryptase assay.
- Amniotic fluid embolus; variable presentation but most commonly includes respiratory failure; also cardiovascular collapse, coagulopathy, and convulsions. Diagnosis is by exclusion and lack of response to treatment.
- Drug error (e.g. thiopentone or a muscle relaxant).

Special considerations

- Cardiac arrest in pregnant women is rare. The team leader must be aware of the importance of early perimortem CS.
- A significant degree of body/pelvic lateral tilt is required to relieve compression of the IVC in situations of cardiovascular collapse—much greater than the 15° required during routine CS. Lateral tilt during CPR is therefore not practical—for example the maximum amount of thoracic tilt consistent with effective ECM is 27°. Current advice is to use manual uterine displacement to the left.
- Cricoid pressure and early intubation are necessary because of increased risk of aspiration. Normal P_aCO_2 in term pregnancy is 4.0 kPa. Variable-performance oxygen masks achieve lower F_iO_2 in pregnant than non-pregnant women.

- Blood volume is increased by 20% in term pregnancy, therefore blood loss is initially better tolerated than in non-pregnant subjects.
- The use of alpha-adrenergic agonists during resuscitation unresponsive to adrenaline is currently under debate. In the event of cardiovascular collapse after extensive regional anaesthesia, standard resuscitation doses of vasopressors may not be effective.
- CPR provides little blood flow to the fetus, and delivery of the fetus by CS within 5 min is recommended to enhance maternal resuscitation by relieving IVC compression. The larger the pregnant uterus, the greater the degree of IVC compression. Perimortem CS is recommended at >20 weeks' gestation.
- The postpartum application of abdominal aortic compression should be considered, diverting flow to the brain and heart. It may also help to control uterine haemorrhage.

Treatment of severe local anaesthetic toxicity

⮑ See also p. 248.
☑ Call for help.
☑ ABC—100% oxygen: early oxygenation essential.
☑ Control seizures with benzodiazepine, thiopental, or propofol.

If cardiovascular collapse:
☑ CPR.
☑ Give bolus Intralipid® 20% 1.5 mL/kg over 1 min.

(105 mL for 70 kg patient)
☑ Start IV infusion of Intralipid® 20% at 15 mL/kg/h.

(1050 mL/h for 70 kg patient)
☑ If circulation is not restored repeat bolus twice at 5 min intervals then increase infusion rate to 30 mL/kg/h.

(2100 mL/h for 70 kg patient)
☑ Continue infusion until circulation restored and stable.

Further reading

AAGBI safety guideline. *Management of Severe Local Anaesthetic Toxicity*. Available at: https://www.aagbi.org/sites/default/files/la_toxicity_2010.pdf

☼ Intrauterine fetal resuscitation

Definition

- Measures to maximize fetal oxygenation in response to acute fetal compromise, usually during labour. The aim is to restore uteroplacental oxygen delivery and fetoplacental (umbilical) blood flow.

Presentation—indications/urgency

- Severity of acute fetal compromise should be communicated to the anaesthetist by the obstetrician.
- Severe compromise needing immediate delivery is often indicated by sustained fetal bradycardia.
- Less severe compromise is associated with:
  - late or complicated variable decelerations.
  - sinusoidal heart rate pattern.
  - tachycardia with absent variability.
  - pH <7.2.

Immediate management

- ☑ Syntocinon—switch off.
- ☑ Position—full left lateral; continue for transfer. If fetal heart rate remains severely abnormal try right lateral or knee–elbow position for possible cord compression.
- ☑ Tocolysis—terbutaline 0.25 mg subcutaneous.
- ☑ Oxygen—15 L/min via tight-fitting Hudson mask with reservoir bag.
- ☑ Fluid—1 L Hartmann's solution rapid infusion (unless contraindicated, e.g. pre-eclampsia etc).
- ☑ Consider IV ephedrine (6 mg) if low blood pressure/after labour, regional analgesia.
- ☑ NB: electronic fetal monitoring should be re-started in theatre and maintained as long as possible.

Subsequent management

- ☑ Delivery of the fetus may be necessary if resuscitation is ineffective. The obstetrician will determine whether this is possible vaginally or by CS. Urgency of CS is categorized as either:
  1. immediate threat to life of woman or fetus.
  2. maternal or fetal compromise which is not immediately life-threatening.
     - Decision-making on the mode of anaesthesia for category 1 CS will vary case by case and unit by unit (% see also 'Category 1 Caesarean section', p. 175).

Investigations

- Obstetric examination to assess cervical dilation, cord prolapse.
- Fetal scalp blood sampling if fetal heart rate pattern is improving.

Risk factors

- Factors associated with irreversible disruption of fetal oxygenation making urgent fetal delivery more likely include:
  - suspected placental abruption/separation
  - umbilical cord prolapse with abnormal fetal heart rate
  - uterine scar dehiscence
  - fetal haemorrhage (e.g. from vasa praevia)

Exclusions

- Fetal bradycardia may be an early warning of significant maternal hypotension related to regional analgesia and other rare causes of maternal collapse.

Special considerations

- Care with IV fluid in women with pre-eclampsia.
- Terbutaline may be contraindicated in some women with cardiac disease.
- Maternal cardiovascular compromise that reduces uteroplacental oxygen delivery will affect the fetus. The management is the same as intrauterine fetal resuscitation, except for tocolysis.

Umbilical cord prolapse

- ☑ Maintain manual upward displacement of presenting part.
- ☑ Reposition into left semi-prone position or knee–elbow (former better for transport and regional anaesthesia induction).
- ☑ Gently replace cord into the vagina.
- ☑ Give oxygen by mask at maximum flow rate.
- ☑ Give terbutaline 0.25 mg subcutaneously (0.5 mL).
- ☑ If delivery not immediately possible: insert size 14 Foley catheter into the bladder and blow up the balloon; instil 500 mL warmed sterile solution through the catheter and then clamp it (manual displacement may now be discontinued).
- ☑ Check fetal heart rate. Prepare for:
  - **abnormal**—Category 1 CS—general anaesthesia is likely to be required.
  - **normal**—Category 2 CS—spinal or epidural top-up may be considered.

Further reading

Thurlow, J., Kinsella, S.M. (2002). Intra-uterine resuscitation: active management of fetal distress. *International Journal of Obstetric Anaesthesia*, **11**, 105–16.

☼ Severe haemorrhage

Definition
- **Primary**—acute peripartum blood loss from uterus or genital tract of over 1000 mL.
- **Secondary**—blood loss from uterus or genital tract of over 1000 mL occurring between 24 h and 12 weeks postpartum.

Presentation
- Hypovolaemic shock—systolic BP <90 mmHg, pulse rate >120 bpm, decreased level of consciousness, decreased peripheral perfusion.
- Blood loss frequently underestimated.
- Total blood volume increases by 20% in pregnancy, so symptoms and signs are often masked, but decompensation may be rapid.

Investigations
- FBC, clotting screen (including fibrinogen), cross-match.
- Consider thromboelastography (TEG/ROTEM)—but note that parturients have different 'normal' values.

Risk factors
- Antepartum haemorrhage (abruption/placenta praevia)
- Prolonged labour
- Multiparity
- Previous CS, uterine surgery, uterine anomaly (e.g. fibroids)
- Multiple pregnancy, large baby, polyhydramnios
- Previous postpartum haemorrhage
- Coagulation disorder

Exclusions
- Hypotension associated with vagal stimulation, e.g. uterine inversion or products of conception sitting in the cervical os.

Immediate management
- ☑ Call for help.
- ☑ ABC—100% O_2.
- ☑ Establish two 14 G IV cannulae.
- ☑ 2000 mL IV crystalloid/colloid.
- ☑ Activate major haemorrhage protocol.
- ☑ Group-specific red cells (consider O-negative).
- ☑ Tranexamic acid: 1 g IV stat followed by 1 g IV if bleeding ongoing after 30 minutes or recurs within 24h.
- ☑ Give coagulation factors—earlyIn severe haemorrhage or disseminated intravascular coagulation (DIC), cryoprecipitate or fibrinogen concentrate are preferred to fresh frozen plasma (FFP) as FFP can dilute fibrinogen levels which are raised in pregnancy. .
- ☑ If likely cause is uterine atony or retained products, consider oxytocin 5–10 IU **slow** IV (NB: causes vasodilatation that may exacerbate

hypovolaemia), ergometrine 500 µg IM, misoprostol 400–1000 µg
PR/SL, carboprost 250 µg IM (may provoke bronchospasm). See
oxytocic drugs, Table 6.1.
☑ Bimanual compression.
☑ Transfer to theatre for EUA while resuscitation is in progress—do
not delay.
☑ Use vasopressors as required (ephedrine 6 mg, phenylephrine 25–50
µg, or adrenaline 5–10 µg).
☑ General anaesthesia may be indicated in haemorrhage—RSI is
mandatory. Regional anaesthesia is relatively contraindicated, but
occasionally considered in some situations, e.g. epidural *in situ* in a
stable patient.

Subsequent management
☑ Arterial line, central line, and urinary catheter after definitive treatment
started.
☑ Continue to monitor FBC and clotting.
☑ Warm fluid (rapid infusion system).
☑ Warm patient.
☑ During laparotomy, consider aortic compression if haemorrhage is
excessive.
☑ Target Hb may be >70 g/L in this group due to the fact that re-
bleeding within the first 24 h postpartum is not uncommon.
☑ Aim for fibrinogen >2 g/L.
☑ Once stabilized the patient should be transferred to an obstetric HDU
or ITU for further monitoring.

Special considerations
• Haemorrhage may be concealed or difficult to quantify in obstetrics and
is commonly underestimated.
• Following severe abruption or amniotic fluid embolus, fulminant DIC
may occur. This will require large quantities of clotting factors.
• Maintaining fibrinogen levels with cryoprecipitate or purified fibrinogen
particularly important.
• Recombinant activated factor VII has been used with success in several
cases of massive obstetric haemorrhage. Make every effort to correct
other abnormalities first (FFP/cryo/platelets/red cells).

Autotransfusion (cell salvage)
• Cell salvage techniques are used increasingly in obstetrics.
• Contamination with amniotic fluid does not appear to contraindicate cell
salvage techniques.
• Likely to become a 'standard of care'.

Interventional radiology
☑ In situations where significant haemorrhage predicted (e.g. placenta
accreta) consider prophylactic intra-arterial access that allows occlusion
of the uterine arteries if required.

Table 6.1 Oxytocic drugs

	Dose	Side effects
Oxytocin Carbetocin	5 IU slow IV injection 10 IU/h IV infusion 100 IU slow IV injection	Vasodilatation → hypotension. Tachycardia. Possibly increased pulmonary vascular resistance
Ergometrine	500 μg IM injection	Vasoconstriction → hypertension. Bradycardia. Nausea and vomiting. Contraindicated in pre-eclampsia
Misoprostol	400–1000 μg PR/SL	Flushing, hyperthermia, diarrhoea
Carboprost	250 μg IM/intrauterine (one dose every 15 min, max. 8 doses)	Hypertension. Bronchospasm (severe if accidental IV injection)

Syntometrine® contains 5 IU oxytocin and 500 μg ergometrine in 1 mL solution. All oxytocic drugs are potentially dangerous in maternal cardiac disease and should only be used with caution.

☑ Although unlikely to be helpful in acute massive haemorrhage, emergency interventional radiology may help in situations of persistent moderate haemorrhage.

Further reading

Collins, P.W., Bell, S.F., deLloyd, L, Collis, R.E. (2019). Management of postpartum haemorrhage: from research into practice, a narrative review of the literature and the Cardiff experience. *International Journal of Obstetric Anesthesia*, 37, 106–117.

Esler, M.D., Douglas, M.J. (2003). Planning for hemorrhage. Steps an anesthesiologist can take to limit and treat hemorrhage in the obstetric patient. *Anesthesiology Clinics of North America*, **21**, 127–44.

Mousa, H.A., Alfirevic, Z. (2003). Treatment for primary postpartum haemorrhage. *Cochrane Database of Systematic Reviews*, **1**, CD003249.

Su, L.L., Chong, Y.S., Samuel, M. (2007). Oxytocin agonists for preventing postpartum haemorrhage. *Cochrane Database of Systematic Reviews*, **3**, CD005457.

☣ **Amniotic fluid embolus**

Definition
- Severe reaction to entry of amniotic fluid into maternal circulation.

Presentation
- Diagnosis is by exclusion. Presents as respiratory failure with dyspnoea, hypoxaemia, hypotension, and circulatory collapse.
- Early phase of transient pulmonary hypertension and right heart failure is followed by left ventricular dysfunction.
- DIC is likely. Convulsions secondary to cerebral hypoxia.

Immediate management
- Mortality is high and prolonged CPR may be needed.
- Both increased pulmonary vascular resistance and left ventricular failure can occur.
- Coagulopathy may be prominent; order cryoprecipitate (fibrinogen), FFP and platelets along with blood.
- Treatment is supportive.
- Consider urgent delivery of the baby by CS.

Oxygenation
- ☑ Call for help. ABC assessment.
- ☑ 100% Oxygen. Intubate and ventilate if necessary.
- ☑ Consider PEEP/CPAP.

Haemodynamic support
- ☑ See 'Maternal collapse' (⊕ p. 156).
- ☑ IV fluids and vasopressors to support blood pressure.
- ☑ Left uterine displacement.
- ☑ Surgical delivery of fetus and control of bleeding.

(Post-delivery) uterine tone and bleeding reduction
- ☑ See 'Severe haemorrhage' (⊕ p. 161).
- ☑ Bimanual uterine massage/compression.
- ☑ Oxytocin, carbetocin, ergometrine, carboprost, misoprostol (see oxytocic drugs, Table 6.1).
- ☑ Expect coagulopathy—ensure blood products are available.
- ☑ Consider cell salvage and use a fluid warmer.
- ☑ Consider Rusch balloon/B-Lynch suture.
- ☑ Consider radiological embolization/hysterectomy.

Subsequent management
- ☑ A haematologist should be involved at an early stage.
- ☑ Appropriate radiological investigation (e.g. V/Q or CTPA) to exclude PE.
- ☑ Echocardiogram to exclude specific cardiac lesions and quantify left and right ventricular impairment, and pulmonary hypertension.

- AFE has a 50% mortality, only 15% overall will survive without neurological impairment.

Investigations
- FBC, U&Es, coagulation, echocardiogram.

Risk factors
- Induction of labour.
- Multiple pregnancy.
- Caesarean section.
- Older ethnic minority women.

Exclusions
- Hypovolaemia—obstetric examination to check for internal bleeding (intrauterine or extrauterine), will respond to adequate volume replacement, whereas with AFE there will be continuing circulatory depression after normal circulating volume is restored.
- Pulmonary embolus—history of risk factors; no coagulopathy.
- Eclampsia—recovery once convulsion is finished, possibly followed by hypertension. No pulmonary gas exchange problem in the absence of pulmonary aspiration.
- Local anaesthetic toxicity—temporal relationship to LA administration, prodromal symptoms, convulsions, prolonged cardiac depression, but no gas exchange impairment.
- Cardiac disease—variable presentation, echocardiogram ASAP.
- Anaphylaxis—temporal relationship to drug administration; bronchospasm, gas exchange impairment not marked; final diagnosis by serum tryptase assay.
- Drug error (e.g. thiopentone or a muscle relaxant).

Further reading
Knight, M., Tuffnell, D., Brocklehurst, P., Spark, P., Kurinczuk, J.J.; UK Obstetric Surveillance System (2010). Incidence and risk factors for amniotic-fluid embolism. *Obstetrics and Gynecology*, **115**, 910–17.

☼ Severe pre-eclampsia

Definition
- Hypertension ≥160/110 mmHg and proteinuria +++ (≥300 mg/24 h).
- May also include:
  - Headache, visual disturbance, epigastric pain
  - Hyper-reflexia
  - Platelet count <100 × 10^9/L
  - Abnormal LFTs

Presentation
- Increased blood pressure after 24 weeks' gestation and/or proteinuria, oedema, headache, visual disturbances, and epigastric pain.

Investigations
- FBC, coagulation, U&Es, LFTs, urate.
- Urine protein:creatinine ratio (PCR).
- Repeat 6-hourly.

Risk factors
- Nulliparity.
- New partner.
- Afro-Caribbean race.
- Underlying maternal condition (e.g. hypertension, renal disease, diabetes, obesity, antiphospholipid syndrome, cardiac disease).

Exclusions
- Pre-existing hypertension.
- Renal or hepatic disease.
- Acute fatty liver of pregnancy.

Immediate management: hypertension

First-line agent: labetalol
☑ Ensure no contraindications: exclude asthma.

Oral therapy
☑ Oral therapy 200 mg stat dose.
☑ Repeat oral 200 mg dose if not controlled at 30 min.
☑ If BP not controlled 30 min after second dose or oral therapy is not tolerated, commence intravenous therapy.

Intravenous therapy
☑ Bolus of 50 mg.
☑ BP should be controlled within 5 min.
☑ Repeat at 5 min intervals to a maximum dose of 200 mg or until BP controlled.
☑ Commence labetalol infusion at 20 mg/h.
☑ Double infusion rate every 30 min to maximum 160 mg/h.

Second-line agent: nifedipine
☑ Indicated if labetalol fails or is contraindicated.
☑ 10 mg oral (not sublingual).
☑ Repeat after 30 min if BP not controlled.

Third-line agent: hydralazine
☑ 5 mg IV bolus.
☑ Repeat at 15 min.
☑ Infusion 5–15 mg/h.

Immediate management: prevention of eclampsia
Magnesium
☑ Loading dose 4 g IV over 5–15 min.
☑ Infusion 1 g/h IV for 24 h minimum.
☑ Further 2 g IV bolus if eclamptic seizure occurs.
☑ NB: In the event of magnesium overdose causing cardiorespiratory compromise, give 1 g calcium gluconate IV (10 mL of 10% solution). (➲ See also p. 326.)

Subsequent management
☑ Team approach involving senior obstetrician, obstetric anaesthetist, and midwife.

Aims of treatment
☑ Stabilize **before** delivery—may take several hours.
☑ Control hypertension.
☑ Prevent eclampsia.
☑ Timely delivery of baby.

Fluid balance
☑ Fluid restrict—1 mL/kg/h background. Replace losses.
☑ Hourly fluid balance measurement. Tolerate oliguria.
☑ 'Fluid challenges' of more than 250 mL should only be given with care—consider CVP guidance.

Anaesthetic management
Analgesia in labour
• Epidural analgesia indicated to prevent surges in blood pressure associated with pain of contractions.
• Epidural analgesia should not be used to treat hypertension.
• Uncorrected platelet count <50 × 10^9/L is a relative contraindication to regional anaesthesia; between 50 and 100 × 10^9/L, consult local protocol/consultant advice.
• Platelet function as well as platelet count may be reduced in pre-eclampsia.

Regional anaesthesia for CS
• Preferred to general anaesthesia.
• No clear advantage between single-shot spinal, combined spinal–epidural, or epidural—choice should be made according to clinical situation.

General anaesthesia
- Call for senior help early.
- Patient is frequently not fasted.
- Anaesthetic drugs may potentiate the effects of antihypertensive agents and interact with magnesium.
- Airway oedema may complicate intubation.
- Obtund pressor response to intubation and extubation (see Table 6.2).
- HDU monitoring postoperatively—airway oedema may worsen following extubation.

Special considerations
- Indications for ITU: respiratory, renal, liver failure.

Table 6.2 Methods of obtunding pressor response to intubation and/or extubation

Alfentanil	7.5–10 µg/kg
Magnesium sulphate	30 mg/kg
Esmolol	0.5 mg/kg
Labetalol	0.5 mg/kg
Lidocaine	1 mg/kg

Further reading

Ramanathan, J., Bennett, K. (2003). Pre-eclampsia: fluids, drugs, and anesthetic management. *Anesthesiology Clinics of North America*, **21**, 145–63.

Santos, A.C., Birnbach, D.J. (2003). Spinal anesthesia in the parturient with severe pre-eclampsia: time for reconsideration. *Anesthesia and Analgesia*, **97**, 621–22.

The Magpie Trial Collaboration Group (2002). Do women with pre-eclampsia, and their babies, benefit from magnesium sulphate? The Magpie Trial: a randomised placebo-controlled trial. *Lancet*, **359**, 1877–90.

:☠: Eclampsia

Definition
Tonic–clonic seizure associated with pre-eclampsia (● see p. 166).

Presentation
- Approximately 33% of seizures occur before labour, 33% during labour, and 33% in the puerperium.
- Seizures may occur over a week after delivery.

Investigations
- FBC, coagulation, U&Es, LFTs, urate.
- Urine protein:creatinine ratio (PCR).

Risk factors
- Pre-eclampsia
- Nulliparity
- New partner
- Afro-Caribbean race
- Underlying maternal condition (e.g. hypertension, renal disease, diabetes, obesity, antiphospholipid syndrome, cardiac disease)

Exclusions
Epilepsy or other intracerebral events not associated with pre-eclampsia.

Immediate management
- ☑ Call for help.
- ☑ ABC—100% O_2.
- ☑ Left lateral recovery position.
- ☑ Do not attempt to insert airway or hand ventilate.
- ☑ If undelivered, assess fetal condition once emergency situation over.
- ☑ Magnesium sulphate 4 g IV over 5–15 min followed by 1 g/h infusion.
- ☑ For recurrent seizures give further IV bolus of 2 g magnesium—consider measuring plasma levels.
- ☑ **Do not give diazepam for the first fit**.

NB: Average length of first fit in eclampsia is 90 s. If seizure persists, consider diazepam, thiopental, or propofol once anaesthetist present. Consider other causes of fits, including intracranial haemorrhage.

Subsequent management
- ☑ Delivery should be undertaken when the mother's condition has stabilized.
- ☑ Control severe hypertension (>160/110 mmHg) with intravenous labetalol or hydralazine according to local protocol (● see p. 166).
- ☑ Consideration should be given to the possibility that the fit was precipitated by an intracranial bleed—full neurological examination mandatory. Consider CT/MRI imaging.

☑ Mode of delivery is contentious. Consultant obstetrician and anaesthetist should be informed in all cases.
☑ If fetal distress severe and failing to respond to intrauterine resuscitation (⮕ see p. 159), urgent delivery may be considered but may compromise maternal safety.

Further reading

Eclampsia Trial Collaborative Group (1995). Which anticonvulsant for women with eclampsia? Evidence from the Collaborative Eclampsia Trial. *Lancet*, **345**, 1455–63.

☢: Total spinal

● See also 'Total spinal', p. 258

Definition

Cardiorespiratory collapse caused by direct action of local anaesthetic on high cervical nerve roots and/or brainstem.

Presentation

- May vary from rapid maternal loss of consciousness and collapse to gradual rise of block, causing difficulty in breathing and/or respiratory failure before loss of consciousness.
- Tingling of hands and difficulty speaking are important warning signs of an ascending block (● see p. 258).
- Bradycardia and hypotension.
- Fetal bradycardia.

Investigations

- Examine to exclude other causes of collapse. Assess fetus if undelivered.

Risk factors

- Accidental dural puncture (recognized and unrecognized).
- Accidental subdural placement of epidural catheter.
- Large or rapid epidural top-ups (e.g. for category 1 CS).
- Spinal injection with epidural *in situ*.
- Epidural top-up after recent spinal injection.

Exclusions

- Other causes of maternal collapse (e.g. PE, amniotic fluid embolus, cardiological, neurological, anaphylaxis, drug error).

Immediate management

☑ Call for help.
☑ Reassure patient and partner.
☑ ABC—100% O_2. Intubation will be required. If conscious, the patient will need a general anaesthetic (reduce doses).
☑ Support blood pressure and circulation with incremental IV doses of ephedrine 6 mg, phenylephrine 25–50 μg, or adrenaline 5–10 μg. Vasopressor infusions may be required.
☑ Deliver baby if appropriate (difficulty stabilizing mother or non-recovering fetal compromise).
☑ If ALS unsuccessful, baby should be delivered by 5 min.
☑ Once resuscitated, anaesthetic agents will be required to keep mother asleep while block resolves.

Subsequent management

- Block will often recede in under 1 h, but may persist for several hours.
- Persisting high block—transfer to ITU until extubated.

Further reading

Yentis, S.M., Dob D.P. (2001). High regional block—the failed intubation of the new millennium? *International Journal of Obstetric Anaesthesia*, **10**, 159–61.

⨀ Accidental dural puncture

Definition
Accidental passage of an epidural needle through dura mater and arachnoid mater into the CSF.

Presentation
- Immediate—CSF through Tuohy needle or epidural catheter.
- Early—high block or total spinal (➲ see p. 171).
- Late—post-dural puncture headache.
- Rarely—epileptiform fit, subdural haematoma.
- Incidence 0.5–4%.

Investigations
- Assess temperature and glucose content of fluid leaking through Tuohy needle or catheter. If warm and containing glucose, it is likely to be CSF.

Risk factors
- Moving target
- Increased BMI
- Inexperienced operator
- Rotating the Tuohy needle once in the epidural space
- Previous spinal surgery
- Previous dural puncture
- ? Loss of resistance to air
- ? Sitting position

Exclusions
- Other causes of headache—simple, meningitis, hypertension, subarachnoid haemorrhage.

Immediate management
- ☑ Consider threading the epidural catheter into the CSF or re-site epidural a space above.
- ☑ Regardless of eventual positioning of epidural catheter, all further top-ups or infusions must be given by the anaesthetist.
- ☑ Accidental dural puncture no longer mandates instrumental delivery—second stage should be managed normally.
- ☑ Patient should be followed up after delivery.
- ☑ If CS becomes necessary, top-ups down the epidural catheter (regardless of eventual position) or *de novo* single-shot spinal both carry increased risk of high block or total spinal.

Postdural puncture headache (PDPH)
Features
- Incidence— >80% (16 G Tuohy needle), 1% (25 G pencil-point spinal needle).

- Tends to occur within 72 h of dural tap.
- Rarely occurs before 12 h.
- Postural—relieved by lying down.
- Worse with mobilization.
- Fronto-occipital headache.
- May be incapacitating.
- Transiently relieved by abdominal compression (diagnostic test).
- Neck stiffness common.
- Photophobia.
- Occasional cranial nerve involvement: tinnitus, diplopia.

Treatment

Early

☑ Bolus (20 mL) or infusion (1000 mL/8 h) of 0.9% saline down epidural catheter has been reported as being effective in some cases.

☑ 'Prophylactic' blood patch injected down epidural catheter before the headache occurs has been reported as effective, but headache more likely to re-occur when compared to 'delayed' blood patch. (NB: Do not do this if catheter has been placed into CSF.)

Intermediate

☑ Keep patient well hydrated.

☑ Regular simple analgesics—paracetamol, NSAIDs, and oral morphine if severe.

☑ Caffeine may provide temporary relief. 50 mg tablets orally up to 1-hourly prn (max. 300 mg in 24 h).

☑ Several other therapeutic agents, including ACTH and sumatriptan, have been tried, but results have been disappointing.

Epidural blood patch

- Considered the definitive treatment.
- Initially reported as over 90% effective, results now suggest that long-term success rate may be as low as 30%.
- Success improved by delaying until at least 24 h post-dural tap, siting the patch at the same level as the tap or one level below, and injecting greater than 15 mL of autologous blood.

Further reading

Reynolds, F. (1993). Dural puncture and headache. *British Medical Journal*, **306**, 874–6.

Sprigge, J.S., Harper, S.J. (2008). Accidental dural puncture and post dural puncture headache in obstetric anaesthesia: presentation and management: a 23-year survey in a district general hospital. *Anaesthesia*, **63**, 36–43.

Obstetric Anaesthetists Association. OAA Guidelines for Treatment of Obstetric Post-Dural Puncture Headache. (2019) Available at: https://www.oaaanaes.ac.uk/assets/_managed/cms/files/Guidelines/New%20PDPH%20Guidelines.pdf

Sudlow, C., Warlow, C. (2003). Epidural blood patching for preventing and treating post-dural puncture headache (Cochrane Review). *The Cochrane Library*, **2**, CD001791.

Turnbull, D.K., Shepherd, D.B. (2003). Post-dural puncture headache: pathogenesis, prevention and treatment. *British Journal of Anaesthesia*, **91**, 718–29.

:⚙: Category 1 Caesarean section

Caesarean urgency scale

1. Immediate threat to life of woman or fetus.
2. Maternal or fetal compromise, no immediate threat to life.
3. No maternal or fetal compromise, requires early delivery.
4. At a time to suit the woman and maternity services.

Presentation

- Usually for acute fetal compromise (➲ see also 'Intrauterine fetal resuscitation', p. 179).
- Commonest maternal indication is antepartum haemorrhage.

Preoperative preparation

- Rapid preoperative assessment—allergies, medication, past anaesthetics, general health, recent food or drink, airway assessment.
- Intravenous access if not already established. Start fast crystalloid infusion prehydration, or colloid/blood for hypovolaemia.
- Premedication—sodium citrate 0.3 M 30 mL PO. Intravenous ranitidine 50 mg and metoclopramide 10 mg may be given if there is time.
- Supine with left uterine displacement using a wedge or lateral table tilt. If there is no delay in starting anaesthesia and surgery, this position may be used on arrival in the operating theatre. However, full left lateral position is associated with least aortocaval compression and should be used if there will be a delay.
- Preoxygenation should be started immediately on positioning on the operating table. Use high oxygen flow and tight mask fit.

Choice of anaesthesia

- General anaesthesia is the quickest to establish but is associated with more life-threatening maternal complications and early neonatal depression. The factors that must be identified rapidly to inform the choice of anaesthetic are: the urgency (communicate with surgeon), maternal preference (communicate with mother), and specific contraindications or difficulties (brief history as mentioned plus preoperative examination of airway, body mass index, spine, and coagulation status). If regional anaesthetic is attempted, a time limit must be imposed and conversion to GA performed once this is exceeded.
- Management of the woman with an epidural *in situ* varies. Epidural anaesthesia is less reliable than spinal. A selective approach is outlined in Figure 6.1. Spinal doses may have to be adjusted in the presence of an epidural (➲ see 'Spinal after epidural', p. 176).
- The rate of GA conversion of regional anaesthesia in category 1 CS is significantly higher than in less urgent cases—be prepared!

General anaesthesia

($\ominus$ See also 'Rapid sequence induction', p. 96; $\ominus$ 'Failed intubation—obstetrics', p. 180.)

- Formal preoxygenation before GA involves breathing 100% oxygen from a well-fitting anaesthetic mask for 3 min. Computer modelling suggests 2 min is adequate for pregnant women.
- Maintain 100% inspired oxygen until delivery if there is fetal compromise, increase inspired inhalation agent concentration to compensate for lack of N_2O.

Spinal

- In urgent cases, a 'rapid sequence spinal' may be appropriate. After spinal insertion, the patient should be placed immediately supine with left lateral displacement.
- The addition of lipophilic opioid (25 µg fentanyl or 0.3 mg diamorphine) reduces discomfort or pain for a given level of sensory block, but the spinal should not be delayed if the drug cannot be rapidly obtained.

Rapid sequence spinal

☑ Deploy other staff for intravenous cannulation and monitoring—don't inject spinal until cannula secured.
☑ Preoxygenate during attempt.
☑ 'No touch' technique—gloves only. Apply antiseptic skin preparation solution immediately, wipe off any liquid if not dry when equipment ready.
☑ Local infiltration not mandatory.
☑ Add fentanyl 25 µg if there is time; if not consider increased dose of bupivacaine.
☑ Only one attempt at spinal unless obvious correction allows a second.
☑ If necessary, start surgery when block ≥ T10 and ascending—be prepared to convert to GA. Keep mother informed.

Spinal after epidural

- Sensory block level is higher for a particular spinal dose if administered after an epidural. This effect is greater with recent (<30 min) large-volume top-ups (volume effect) using concentrated local anaesthetic (addition-of-block effect). Dangerously high spinal blocks requiring respiratory support are more common after epidural (1:50) versus spinal alone (<1:4000) ($\ominus$ see 'Total spinal', p. 171). It is thought that this risk is greater if the epidural has been topped up recently. Many anaesthetists reduce the spinal dose by 20–40% if administering after a recent epidural 'Caesarean section' top-up.

Epidural top-up

- There is no conclusive data on the best solution(s) to use. Meta-analysis suggests quickest onset local anaesthetic is lidocaine + adrenaline 1 in 200 000, improved by adding fentanyl 100 µg. Sodium bicarbonate 8.4% (2 mL per 20 mL of lidocaine, 0.2 mL per 20 mL of bupivacaine) is often added as well.

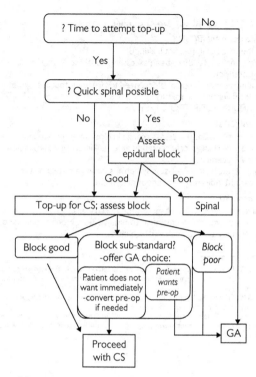

Figure 6.1 Category 1 Caesarean section.

- Mixtures will take longer to prepare than simple solutions, and the preparation time must be considered in this situation where seconds count.
- The safest practice is to give a slow fractionated top-up in the operating theatre with full monitoring. This may be too slow for category 1 CS. Consider starting the epidural top-up in the labour room and give the full top-up under close observation (Box 6.1). If dural puncture has occurred or was suspected, do not top-up in the labour room.
- Have available:
  - free-running drip
  - vasopressors
  - oxygen supply and method to ventilate lungs
- Standard total volume for top-up is 20 mL. Consider reduction to 15 mL if the block is high or dense or the woman is of short stature.
- Top-up in left lateral position (right lateral if fetal heart rate problems on left).

Box 6.1 **Epidural top-up checklist**

Safety assessment (30 s)
☑ Is the epidural in (i.e. not leaking)?
☑ Is it spinal?—Has there been excessive motor block, recurrent hypotension?
☑ Is it intravenous?—poor block, need for frequent top-ups, symptoms of local anaesthetic toxicity.
☑ PERFORM ASPIRATION TEST.

Test dose (60 s)
☑ Give 3 mL; wait 30 s; assess change in block (e.g. any 'global' subjective change, cold sensation at S1, ankle dorsiflexion) indicating spinal placement.
☑ Give 3 mL; wait 30 s, assess symptoms (strange taste, tinnitus, sedation) indicating intravenous placement.

Main dose (90 s)
☑ Give remainder while observing for any changes.
☑ Stay with woman and maintain communication. Monitor pulse and BP. Be prepared to deal with high block.

Further reading

Hillyard, S.G., Bate, T.E., Corcoran, T.B., Paech, M.J., O'Sullivan, G. (2011). Extending epidural analgesia for emergency Caesarean section: a meta-analysis. *British Journal of Anaesthesia,* **107,** 668–78.

Kinsella, S.M., Girgirah, K., Scrutton, M.J.L. (2010). Rapid sequence spinal for category 1 urgency Caesarean section: a case series. *Anaesthesia,* **65,** 664–9.

Royal College of Obstetricians & Gynaecologists (2010). *Classification of Urgency of Caesarean Section.* Available at: https://www.rcog.org.uk/en/guidelines-research-services/guidelines/good-practice-11/

① Problems during Caesarean section

Severe hypotension
⊃ See also p. 29.
- Regional anaesthesia:
  - An interaction between mid-thoracic block, IVC compression ± hypovolaemia may reduce venous return, cardiac output, and systemic blood pressure.
  - Classically this induced a vasovagal reaction with bradycardia. However, bradycardia now more commonly occurs with normal or high blood pressure during α-adrenergic agonist vasopressor treatment (phenylephrine or metaraminol).
  - Once a severe reaction is established, it may not resolve until delivery of the baby. This situation may require large doses of vasopressors including an agent to increase heart rate (β-agonist, ephedrine, or adrenaline; anticholinergic, glycopyrronium). If there is likely to be a delay in delivery, use the full lateral position.
- Other causes include anaphylaxis to antibiotic (⊃ see p. 272), reaction to oxytocin or general anaesthetic drugs, undiagnosed cardiac disease, amniotic fluid embolus (⊃ see p. 164), and others.

Acute uterine relaxation (tocolysis)
- This may rarely be requested by the obstetrician where delivery is difficult.
- GTN IV is the drug of choice (50 μg boluses—double the dose if effect is poor). Dilute 1 mg/mL solution 1 in 20 = 50 μg/mL. Other tocolytic agents either have too slow an onset or too protracted a duration. The use of general anaesthesia with inhalational agents to produce tocolysis is obsolete, although this effect may be utilized if GA is being used for other indications.

Haemorrhage
⊃ See p. 161.
Inhalational agents interfere with uterine contraction. If haemorrhage occurs during CS under general anaesthetic, consider switching to intravenous anaesthesia with propofol.

Nausea and vomiting
During CS with regional anaesthesia this may be related to a decrease in cardiac output and hypotension. Before delivery this usually responds to a vasopressor and optimizing position, whereas after delivery blood loss must be excluded.

Failed intubation
⊃ See p. 84; p. 180.

Endobronchial intubation
⊃ See p. 102.

Pre-eclampsia
⊃ See p. 166.

:O: Failed intubation—obstetrics

(➔ See also 'Unanticipated difficult intubation', p. 84.)

Definition
Failure to intubate trachea during rapid sequence induction.

Presentation and incidence
- Rapid sequence induction of general anaesthesia for CS.
- Incidence 1:400.
- The problems of failed intubation during other obstetric surgery are much reduced compared to CS, and are not discussed specifically.

Immediate management
See Figure 6.2.
- ☑ Not more than two attempts at intubation unless special circumstances.
- ☑ Call for help.
- ☑ Maintain oxygenation—ventilate with mask + oropharyngeal airway OR LMA[a] as appropriate. Reduce/remove cricoid pressure if necessary.
- ☑ Oxygenation possible—decide whether to wake/continue.[b]
- ☑ Oxygenation not possible—'Can't intubate, can't oxygenate' situation[c]—perform front-of-neck procedure using needle or surgical cricothyroidotomy.

Notes:
[a] Second-generation supraglottic airway device (LMA ProSeal, LMA Supreme, i-gel) is preferred to first generation. Suction the oesophageal port or pass gastric tube after placement.
[b] Before induction plan whether to wake/continue in the event of failed intubation—multifactorial decision depends on patient, fetus, anaesthetist, and clinical circumstances; only continue if essential OR safe to do so.
[c] CICO—consider reversible factors—excessive cricoid pressure, laryngeal spasm. Consider risk/benefit of a second dose of suxamethonium or non-depolarizing neuromuscular blocker in the specific circumstance. Don't give if going to wake up; administration advised before front-of-neck procedure.

Subsequent management
If continuing anaesthesia:
- ☑ Maintain cricoid pressure if possible
- ☑ Decide on spontaneous/positive pressure breathing
- ☑ Decide on paralysed/unparalysed
- ☑ Decide on inhalational or intravenous anaesthesia.
  - Get a second pair of hands/senior anaesthetist for any advanced airway techniques to intubate/second anaesthetic.
  - Blind intubation through an LMA should be avoided.

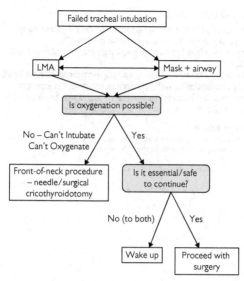

Figure 6.2 Failed intubation algorithm.

If waking:

☑ Maintain cricoid pressure if possible
☑ Decide whether to turn left lateral/continue supine.
☑ Options for surgery are regional technique or an awake intubation using fiberscope/videolaryngoscope/LMA.

Risk factors

- Psychological:
  - urgency
  - highly stressful situation and environment
- Anaesthetic technique:
  - cricoid pressure/rapid sequence induction
- Anatomical:
  - tissue oedema (particularly in pre-eclampsia)
  - increased BMI
  - large breasts
- Physiological:
  - reduced functional residual capacity and increased oxygen consumption results in rapid desaturation despite preoxygenation
  - increased intra-abdominal/intragastric pressure and reduced lower oesophageal sphincter tone result in reduced 'barrier pressure' increasing likelihood of aspiration

Special considerations
- Rapid sequence induction: pay attention to detail—particularly preoxygenation, positioning, and cricoid pressure.
- Likelihood of a failed intubation requiring a front-of-neck procedure is 1:50.
- Likelihood of a failed intubation resulting in maternal death is 1:100.
- Training and familiarity with appropriate equipment is essential.
- Regular failed intubation drills are essential; this may use low- or high-fidelity simulation.

Further reading
Obstetric Anaesthetists' Association/Difficult Airway Society (2015). *Obstetric Failed Tracheal Intubation Guideline 2015*. Available at: https://www.oaa-anaes.ac.uk

☼ Placenta praevia & low lying placenta

(➲ See also 'Severe haemorrhage in obstetrics', p. 161.)

Definition (current)

Placenta praevia: the placenta lies over the internal os.
Low lying placenta: the placental edge is within 20mm of the internal os after 16 weeks.

Presentation

- Elective or emergency lower segment CS (LSCS).
- Diagnosis may already have been made antenatally.
- Painless revealed antepartum haemorrhage.

Causes of haemorrhage

- Premature antenatal partial separation of the placenta.
- Increased blood supply to lower segment at site of uterine incision.
- Placental site is supplied by underdeveloped spiral arteries in thin walled lower segment that is unable to contract effectively.
- Placenta accreta spectrum (5% if no previous LSCS, 25% if placental site overlies incision from one previous LSCS, 50% if placental site overlies incision from two or more previous LSCS).

Investigations

- FBC, clotting, group & save or cross-match.

Risk factors

- Previous CS.

Immediate management

- ☑ Two anaesthetists, 14 G IV access with rapid infusion equipment, 4 units blood cross-matched and in theatre.
- ☑ If significant antepartum haemorrhage, resuscitation, and LSCS occur simultaneously—use O-negative or group-specific blood as appropriate. Activate the Major Haemorrhage Protocol.
- ☑ Use call salvage.
- ☑ Administer blood and blood products early.
- ☑ Senior obstetrician must be present.
- ☑ Consider regional anaesthesia if cardiovascularly stable. Combined spinal–epidural preferable as operation may be prolonged.
- ☑ Consider intra-arterial, central venous, and cardiac output monitoring, particularly if actively haemorrhaging or if increased risk of placenta accreta (e.g. anterior placenta praevia with previous LSCS scar).
- ☑ If GA required, use rapid sequence induction. Consider TIVA/TCI, as avoiding volatile anaesthetics may help uterine contraction.
- ☑ Oxytocin 5 IU slow IV for delivery of placenta followed by infusion of 30–40 IU over 4 h.
- ☑ Early recourse to ergometrine 500 µg IM, misoprostol 400–1000 µg PR/SL, or carboprost 250 µg IM or intramyometrial.

Subsequent management

☑ If intraoperative haemorrhage persists, surgeon should consider B-Lynch suture. Hysterectomy may be required.

☑ HDU monitoring following LSCS—increased chance of postpartum haemorrhage.

Special considerations

• USS, CT, and MRI have all been used to try to identify presence and severity of placenta accreta or percreta. None of them has proved highly predictive of intraoperative haemorrhage or outcome.

• Preoperative radiological placement of intrailiac balloon catheters has been reported as effective in several cases. However, this requires specialist skills and equipment in semi-elective/elective situations, and may provoke fetal distress.

• Successful postoperative radiological embolization has been reported. Again, specialist skills and equipment are required.

Further reading

Parekh, N., Husaini, S.W., Russell, I.F. (2000). Caesarean section for placenta praevia: a retrospective study of anaesthetic management. *British Journal of Anaesthesia*, **84**, 725–30.

Placenta Praevia and Placenta Accreta: Diagnosis and Management (Green-top Guideline No. 27a) (2018) https://www.rcog.org.uk/en/guidelines-research-services/guidelines/gtg27a/ (accessed 9:12:19)

☼: Retained placenta

(➔ See also 'Severe haemorrhage in obstetrics', p. 161.)

Definition

Retention of some or all of placenta and/or membranes following vaginal delivery requiring examination and removal under anaesthetic.

Presentation

- Occurs in 0.5–1% of all deliveries.
- May be associated with minimal blood loss or with major ongoing haemorrhage depending on the degree of separation and the amount of uterine tone.
- The placenta should always be inspected after delivery to ensure that large fragments are not missing. In any significant postpartum haemorrhage with uterine atony, EUA to exclude retained placenta must be considered.
- Retention of some placental tissue is relatively common. This usually presents as minor persistent vaginal bleeding over days/weeks after delivery requiring ERPC (evacuation of retained products of conception) as an elective/urgent procedure. However, it may present as significant primary (up to 24 h) or secondary (24 h–6 weeks) postpartum haemorrhage.

Investigations

- FBC, clotting, group & save.

Exclusions

- Uterine atony without retained products of conception.
- Genital tract trauma.

Immediate management

- ☑ Intravenous access with 14 G cannula.
- ☑ Fluid resuscitation if appropriate.
- ☑ G&S—cross-match if blood loss >500 mL and continuing.
- ☑ Consider oxytocin (5 IU slow IV), ergometrine (500 μg IM), carbetocin (100 μg IV) to help deliver placenta.
- ☑ Catheterize and empty bladder.
- ☑ Transfer to theatre for EUA if placenta remains undelivered or if haemorrhage significant. Do not delay EUA to resuscitate patient. NB: Even if haemorrhage minimal, do not delay transfer to theatre as sudden severe haemorrhage may occur at any time.
- ☑ Regional anaesthesia preferred—top-up epidural if *in situ* or establish spinal anaesthesia. Block to T6 required.
- ☑ If regional technique contraindicated or cardiovascularly unstable, give GA with rapid sequence induction.

Subsequent management

- ☑ Give postoperative Syntocinon infusion for 4 h minimum.
- ☑ Consider further dose of ergometrine 500 µg IM, misoprostol 400–1000 µg PR/SL, or carboprost 250 µg IM or intramyometrial, if uterine atony persists despite evacuation of uterus.
- ☑ Consider invasive monitoring ± fluid responsiveness monitoring if haemorrhage greater than 1000 mL.
- ☑ Consider HDU/ITU monitoring post-op.

Further reading

Broadbent, C.R., Russell, R. (1999). What height of block is needed for manual removal of placenta? *International Journal of Obstetric Anaesthesia*, **8**, 161–4.

Tandberg, A., Albrechtsen, S., Iversen, O.E. (1999). Manual removal of the placenta. Incidence and clinical significance. *Acta Obstetricia et Gynecologica Scandinavica*, **78**, 33–6.

☼ Ruptured ectopic pregnancy

Definition
Abnormal placentation of fetus in uterine cornu or fallopian tube causing pain and subsequent rupture of cornu or tube.

Presentation
- Usually from 6 to 12 weeks of pregnancy.
- Sudden onset of left or right iliac fossa pain associated with a positive pregnancy test.
- May be associated with severe cardiovascular compromise or collapse.
- May be diagnosed by pelvic USS.

Investigations
- FBC, clotting, group & save.

Risk factors
- Previous ectopic pregnancy.
- Previous tubal surgery.
- Previous pelvic infection.

Exclusions
- Other pelvic/lower abdominal surgical causes (e.g. appendicitis, tubo-ovarian abscess).

Immediate management
- ☑ 14 G IV access. (NB: Even apparently 'stable' ectopics may suddenly decompensate.)
- ☑ FBC, G&S—cross-match 4 units if cardiovascularly compromised.
- ☑ Resuscitate and operate simultaneously.
- ☑ GA with rapid sequence induction once abdomen has been surgically prepared—GA may precipitate sudden cardiovascular collapse.
- ☑ GA may require modification if cardiovascularly compromised—consider ketamine.
- ☑ If cardiovascularly unstable, laparoscopy usually inappropriate.
- ☑ Consider cell salvage. (Cell salvage has been used successfully in laparoscopic cases.)
- ☑ Consider intra-arterial and central venous monitoring ± fluid responsiveness monitoring.
- ☑ Consider HDU/ITU post-op. (NB: Most patients with ruptured ectopics are young and fit and will recover rapidly so long as surgery is not delayed.)

Subsequent management
- ☑ Correct anaemia and coagulopathy.
- ☑ PCA and local anaesthetic blocks if open surgery.
- ☑ HDU/ITU until stable.

Neurology/neurosurgery

Katharine Hunt and Manni Waraich

☼ **Raised intracranial pressure**

Definition

Intracranial pressure (ICP) >25 mmHg.

Presentation

- Clinical signs of acute rises in ICP include deteriorating conscious level, sluggish or unequal pupil responses progressing to non-reactivity, hypertension and bradycardia, loss of consciousness, and death. Chronic rises in ICP cause pressure headache, vomiting, and papilloedema.
- ICP >25 mmHg measured by intraparenchymal microtransducer or external ventricular drain—the latter measures CSF pressure in lateral ventricles and this is the 'gold standard' for ICP measurement.
- Identification of abnormal ICP waveforms—these are often triggered by phasic cerebral vasodilatation in response to a fall in CPP, and terminated by rises in blood pressure:
  - plateau ('A') waves are paroxysmal rises to 50–100 mmHg (usually on a high baseline pressure) and last for several minutes (up to 20 min).
  - 'B' waves are shorter lived fluctuations lasting about a minute and peaking at 30–35 mmHg.
  - abnormal ICP waveforms reflect reduced intracranial compliance.

Investigations

- ICP monitoring, invasive cardiovascular monitoring, regular ABGs, core temperature.
- Consider CT scan if acute rise in ICP or altered clinical state.
- Sodium levels and osmolality.

Risk factors

- Head injury (⊃ p. 192), Intracranial haematoma (⊃ p. 196, 199)
- Anoxic brain injury
- Intracranial infections, tumour

Immediate management

- ☑ Sedation and analgesia to control cerebral metabolic rate and minimize blood pressure surges.
- ☑ Mechanical ventilation to maintain P_aO_2 >13.3 kPa (100 mmHg) and P_aCO_2 4.0–4.5 kPa (30–34 mmHg).
- ☑ Nurse in 20–30° head-up position with neck in neutral position and unobstructed neck veins (avoid ETT ties).
- ☑ Maintain adequate CPP (>60 mmHg)
- ☑ Mannitol 20% (0.5 g/kg) or other osmotic agent such as hypertonic saline (1.8 % or 3%). Hypertonic saline should be administered via a central line at a dose of 3 ml/kg. Serum Na+ levels should be checked regularly.

Subsequent management

☑ Maintain CPP >60 mmHg to ensure adequate cerebral perfusion (➲ see 'Management of head injury', p. 193 by volume resuscitation and inotropes/vasopressors.

☑ Treat blood pressure if above the upper limit of autoregulation (mean BP >130 mmHg) to minimize vasogenic brain swelling, using short-acting drugs such as labetalol or esmolol.

☑ Moderate hyperventilation to P_aCO_2 4.0–4.5 kPa (30–34 mmHg)should be avoided since overzealous hyperventilation may worsen cerebral ischaemia by further reduction of critically low cerebral blood flow.

☑ Treat pyrexia. Aim for normothermia with target temperature management systems.

☑ Although moderate hypothermia (target temperature 34- 35C)has not been shown to improve outcome in recent prospective randomized trials, modest reductions in temperature can be effective in reducing ICP resistant to maximal medical management

☑ Mannitol (0.5 g/kg), usually as a 20% solution or hypertonic saline (1.8% or 3%).

☑ CSF drainage via a ventricular catheter is an efficient method of reducing ICP but is an invasive procedure and not without risk.

☑ Barbiturate infusion may be effective in intracranial hypertension refractory to other therapies.

Decompressive craniectomy (removal of bone flap) with enlargement of the dura (duraplasty) is a therapeutic option for intracranial hypertension refractory to conventional therapy.

Special considerations

• There is no merit in persisting with therapies such as mannitol if they have no, or only a short-lasting, effect.

Further reading

Forsyth, R., Baxter, P., Elliott, T. (2001). Routine intracranial pressure monitoring in acute coma. *Cochrane Database System Review*, **3**, CD002043.

Smith, M. (2008). Monitoring intracranial pressure in traumatic brain injury. *Anesthesia and Analgesia*, **106**, 240–48.

Stocchetti, N., Rossi, S., Buzzi, F., Mattioli, C., Paparella, A., Colombo, A. (1999). Intracranial hypertension in head injury: management and results. *Intensive Care Medicine*, **25**, 371–6.

☼ Severe head injury

Definition
Severe traumatic head injury—GCS ≤8 after resuscitation.

Presentation
- Unconscious patient following any trauma, clinically apparent head trauma, and obtunded conscious level.

Investigations
- Check FBC, U&Es, ABGs, and cross-match blood.
- Neurological examination prior to sedation/intubation—GCS (with eyes–verbal–motor scores) and localizing signs and secondary survey.
- Cranial CT scan is the investigation of choice, skull X-ray is of little value if CT easily accessible.

Risk factors
- Road traffic collision
- Assault
- Falls from significant height

Exclusions
- Alcohol or other drug intoxication
- Subarachnoid haemorrhage or other spontaneous intracranial haemorrhage
- Anoxic/hypoxic intracranial event

Paediatric implications
- The relatively large head size and weak neck muscles render the child's brain more susceptible to acceleration–deceleration injuries.
- In children under 2 years of age, brain swelling is accommodated by expansion of the skull and may be assessed by examination of the fontanelles (the anterior fontanelle closes between 7 and 19 months) and measurement of head circumference. Skull fractures are less common than in adults.
- Scalp lacerations and intracranial haematomas may result in hypotension because of the relatively large head size and small circulating blood volume.
- Surgically treatable intracranial haematomas occur less frequently than in adults (20–30% of paediatric head injuries compared to 50% in adults).
- Cerebral blood flow is higher in children than adults and this may offer some 'protection' against ischaemic damage.
- Neurological outcome is better for children than for adults with the same GCS after resuscitation.

Immediate management

☑ Oral endotracheal intubation under direct vision, with manual in-line immobilization of the cervical spine (association between cervical spine and head injury).

☑ IV induction agent to prevent rise in ICP secondary to laryngoscopy. Choice of agent not important, but appropriate dose should be chosen to avoid fluctuations in blood pressure. Propofol or ketamine with fentanyl or alfentanil is widely used.

☑ Rapid sequence induction using rocuronium (1mg/kg)—a full stomach or acute gastric dilatation must be assumed.

☑ Pass orogastric tube to decompress the stomach. Avoid nasal gastric tubes where there may be a base of skull fracture.

☑ Mechanical ventilation to maintain P_aO_2 >13.3 kPa (100 mmHg) and P_aCO_2 4.5–5.0 kPa (34–38 mmHg).

☑ Maintain sedation and paralysis with short-acting agents (e.g. propofol, fentanyl, atracurium) to allow ventilation and prevent coughing.

☑ Fluid resuscitation to maintain mean BP >90 mmHg—if ICP monitored, aim for CPP >60 mmHg. Choice of fluid not as important as volume administered, but glucose-containing fluids and hypotonic solutions should be avoided.

☑ Inotropes may also be required to maintain BP at adequate levels, particularly to offset the hypotensive effects of sedative agents. Noradrenaline is the agent of first choice.

☑ Mannitol 20% (0.5 g/kg) or hypertonic saline may be used to reduce ICP pending definitive treatment—seek advice from neurosurgical centre.

☑ Urgent CT scan for patients at high risk of intracranial haematoma or post-resuscitation GCS ≤8 (Table 7.1).

Subsequent management

☑ Detailed secondary survey and appropriate investigations to identify other injuries.

☑ Active bleeding and other life-threatening chest and abdominal injuries must be treated prior to definitive neurosurgical treatment, but it is sufficient to stabilize non-life-threatening injuries.

☑ Treat seizures with anticonvulsants—phenytoin 15 mg/kg loading dose.

☑ Discuss with neurosurgical unit (see p. 195).

Table 7.1 The Glasgow coma scale (GCS)

	Score
Eye-opening	
Spontaneous	4
To speech	3
To pain	2
None	1
Best verbal response	
Orientated	5
Confused	4
Inappropriate words	3
Incomprehensible sounds	2
None	1
Best motor response	
Obeying	6
Localizing to painful stimulus	5
Withdrawing from painful stimulus	4
Abnormal flexion to painful stimulus (decorticate)	3
Extension to painful stimulus (decerebrate)	2
No response	1

Reprinted from *The Lancet*, 304, 7872, Teasdale, G. & Jennett, B. Assessment of coma and impaired consciousness. A practical scale. pp. 81–4. Copyright © 1974 Published by Elsevier Ltd, with permission from Elsevier. doi:10.1016/S0140-6736(74)91639-0.

Indications for CT scanning after head injury

Indications for adult CT head scan within 1 h of risk factor being identified

- GCS less than 13 on initial assessment in the emergency department.
- GCS less than 15 at 2 h after the injury on assessment in the emergency department.
- Suspected open or depressed skull fracture.
- Any sign of basal skull fracture (haemotympanum, 'panda' eyes, cerebrospinal fluid leakage from the ear or nose, Battle's sign).
- Post-traumatic seizure.
- Focal neurological deficit.
- More than one episode of vomiting.

A provisional written radiology report should be made available within 1 h of the scan being performed.

Indications for adult CT head scan within 8 h
Any patient who has experienced loss of consciousness/amnesia with one or more of the following risk factors:
- 65 y or older.

- Any history of bleeding or clotting disorders/anticoagulation.
- Dangerous mechanism of injury (a pedestrian or cyclist struck by a motor vehicle, an occupant ejected from a motor vehicle or a fall from a height of greater than 1 metre or 5 stairs).
- More than 30 min retrograde amnesia of events immediately before the head injury.

A provisional written radiology report should be made available within 1 h of the scan being performed.

Reasons to discuss with a neurosurgical centre

- Persisting coma GCS 8 or less after initial resuscitation.
- Unexplained confusion which persists for more than 4 h.
- Deterioration in GCS score after admission.
- Progressive focal neurological signs.
- Seizure without full recovery.
- Definite or suspected penetrating head injury.
- CSF leak.

Transfer

➜ See also 'Transport of the critically ill', p. 502.

- 20% more patients are now surviving severe trauma since the introduction of Major Trauma Networks in 2010.
- Ensure adequate resuscitation and stabilization prior to transfer.
- Appropriate emergency and monitoring equipment, drugs, intravascular access, and infusion devices should be available for the journey (including backup equipment and power suppliers).
- Medical staff involved in transfer should have suitable training, skills, and experience in resuscitation and intensive care medicine, and accompanied by an appropriately trained assistant.
- Good communication between referring and receiving centre before and during transfer.
- Notes, prescription charts, observation charts, and CT scans should accompany the patient.

Further reading

Brain Trauma Foundation (2007). The American Association of Neurological Surgeons. Joint section of neurotrauma and critical care. *Journal of Neurotrauma*, **13**, 671–734.

Dinsmore, J. (2013). Traumatic brain injury: an evidence-based review of management. *CEACCP British Journal of Anaesthesia*, **13**(6), 189–95.

Stocchetti, N., Carbonara, M., Citerio, G., Ercole, A., Skrifvars, M. B., Smielewski, P., ... Menon, D. K. Severe traumatic brain injury: targeted management in the intensive care unit. *The Lancet Neurology*, 16(6), 452–464.

Ghajar, J. (2000). Traumatic brain injury. *Lancet*, **356**, 923–9.

Helmy, A., Vizcaychipi, M., Gupta, A. (2007). Traumatic brain injury: intensive care management. *British Journal of Anaesthesia*, **99**, 32–42.

Maas, A.I., Dearden, M., Servadei, F., Stocchetti, N., Unterberg, A. (2000). Current recommendations for neurotrauma. *Current Opinion in Critical Care*, **6**, 281–92.

Moppett, I. (2007). Traumatic brain injury: assessment, resuscitation and early management. *British Journal of Anaesthesia*, **99**, 18–31.

NICE (2014). *Head Injury: Assessment and Early Management: Clinical Guideline CG176*. Available at: https://www.nice.org.uk/CG176

Trauma Audit and Research Network (TARN) (2013). *National Audit*. Available at: https://www.tarn.ac.uk/

☼ Subarachnoid haemorrhage

Definition

Non-traumatic subarachnoid haemorrhage (SAH) is characterized by extravasation of blood into the CSF of the subarachnoid space. It occurs secondary to a ruptured intracranial aneurysm in 85% of cases.

Presentation

- Symptoms—sudden onset headache (often described as 'worst imaginable' or 'like a hammer blow'), nausea, vomiting, photophobia, and neck stiffness.
- Focal neurological signs, including third or sixth cranial nerve palsies, motor deficits, or obtunded conscious level.
- Seizures (in 6–8% at presentation).
- Neurogenic pulmonary oedema, dysrhythmias.
- Catastrophic SAH presents as sudden loss of consciousness.

Immediate management

☑ ABC—O_2.
☑ Maintain systemic blood pressure in 'high normal' range prior to control of the aneurysm (>120 mmHg) — maintains cerebral perfusion while minimizing risk of re-bleeding.
☑ Treat hypertension if systolic BP exceeds 160 mmHg in a previously normotensive patient.
☑ Treat hypotension with intravenous fluids followed by vasopressors.
☑ Oral endotracheal intubation and mechanical ventilation in unconscious patients or those with deteriorating conscious level:
☑ Maintain P_aO_2 >13.3 kPa (100 mmHg) and P_aCO_2 4.5–5.0 kPa (34–38 mmHg).
☑ Urgent CT scan.
☑ Regular neurological observations.
☑ Nimodipine 60 mg PO/NG 4-hourly.
☑ Transfer to neurosurgical unit.

Complications and Further management

- Re-bleeding:
  - occurs in 7%.
    ☑ prevented by early protection of the ruptured aneurysm.
    ☑ endovascular intervention is now the treatment of choice for the majority of aneurysms.
- Hydrocephalus:
  - occurs in approx. 25% patients.
    ☑ treated by surgically placement of external ventricular drainage.
- Vasospasm:
  - can result in delayed cerebral ischaemic neurological deficit.
  - most common cause of morbidity and mortality after re-bleeding.
  - peaks at 4–10 days after the event.
  - detected clinically by changes in conscious level or focal neurological deficits.

- confirmed by transcranial Doppler ultrasonography or cerebral angiography.
  - ☑ triple-H therapy (hypervolaemia, hypertension and haemodilution) is no longer used in the treatment of vasospasm. Hypertension alone is beneficial. Aim for euvolaemia and a Hb concentration between 80 and 100 g/L.
  - ☑ maintain systemic BP using vasopressors/inotropes.
  - ☑ balloon angioplasty and intra-arterial vasodilating agents may be applied in vasospasm resistant to hypertensing.
- Systemic complications:
  - ECG changes and 'stunned' myocardial syndrome common in poor grade SAH.
  - pulmonary oedema.
  - hyponatraemia often secondary to SIADH (syndrome of inappropriate antidiuretic hormone secretion) or cerebral salt wasting (CSW).
  - fever and hyperglycaemia.

Endovascular treatment of intracranial aneurysm

Procedures usually carried out in isolated areas of the hospital, at some distance from main theatre.

Complications include:
- Acute rupture of aneurysm, detected by:
  - visualization of extravasation of contrast media during angiography
  - abrupt rise in mean arterial pressure and change in heart rate
  - immediate management:
    - ☑ reduce systemic blood pressure with short-acting hypotensive agent (e.g. labetalol) or by deepening anaesthesia to allow radiologist to gain control of bleeding.
    - ☑ maintain P_aCO_2 4.5–5.0 kPa (34–38 mmHg).
    - ☑ consider reversal of heparin with protamine (1 mg for each 100 IU of heparin given).
    - ☑ consider mannitol (0.25–0.5 g/kg).
  - subsequent management:
    - ☑ urgent CT scan when bleeding controlled.
    - ☑ alert main theatre.
    - ☑ arrange transfer to an ICU post procedure.
  - risk factors for intraprocedural aneurysmal rupture:
    - ☑ prolonged or anatomically difficult coiling.
    - ☑ thin-walled aneurysm.
    - ☑ anticoagulant and/or antiplatelet therapies.
  - special considerations:
    - ☑ preferred treatment is packing of aneurysm with coils. Some patients may require emergency craniotomy to evacuate clot and clip the aneurysm.
- Thromboembolism:
  - ☑ consider administration of an antiplatelet agent such as abciximab (ReoPro®).

- Vasospasm:
  - ☑ consider intra-arterial administration of vasodilators such as glyceryl trinitrate (GTN) or nimodipine via the angiographic catheter.
  - ☑ hypertensing the patient using vasopressors post procedure to blood pressure parameters decided by the degrees of vasospasm and the neurological deficit.

Investigations

- Check FBC, U&Es, ABGs, clotting, and cross-match blood.
- Cranial CT scan demonstrates blood in the basal cisterns and throughout the CSF spaces.
- Lumbar puncture if CT-negative or equivocal. Typical findings include high CSF opening pressure, elevated red cell count, and xanthochromia after 12 h.
- Four-vessel cerebral angiography to identify aneurysm and delineate vascular anatomy.

Risk factors

- 85% of cases of non-traumatic SAH are caused by ruptured intracranial aneurysm.
- Female sex.
- Afro-Caribbean and Japanese races.
- Hypertension.
- Alcohol intake >2 units/day.
- First-degree relative with SAH.

Exclusions

- Ischaemic or haemorrhagic stroke
- Migraine
- Tension headache

Grades of SAH

Several grading scales quantify the severity of SAH but that described by the World Federation of Neurological Surgeons (WFNS) is widely used:

- Grade 1: GCS 15 and no motor deficit
- Grade 2: GCS 13–14 and no motor deficit
- Grade 3: GCS 13–14 with motor deficit
- Grade 4: GCS 7–12 with or without motor deficit
- Grade 5: GCS 3–6 with or without motor deficit

Further reading

Louma, A., Reddy, U. (2013). Acute management of aneurysmal subarachnoid haemorrhage. CEACCP *British Journal of Anaesthesia*, **13**(2), 52–8.

Smith, M. (2007). Intensive care management of patients with subarachnoid haemorrhage. *Current Opinion in Anaesthesiology*, **20**, 400–7.

Suarez, J., Tarr, R., Selman, W. (2006). Aneurysmal subarachnoid hemorrhage. *New England Journal of Medicine*, **354**, 387–96.

Varma, M., Price, K., Jayakrishnan, V., Manickam, B., Kessell, G. (2007). Anaesthetic considerations for interventional neuroradiology. *British Journal of Anaesthesia* **99**, 75–85.

Wartenberg K.E., Mayer S.A. (2006). Medical complications after subarachnoid hemorrhage: new strategies for prevention and management. *Current Opinion in Critical Care*, **12**, 78–84.

Wilson, S., Hirsch, N., Appleby, I. (2005). Management of subarachnoid haemorrhage in a non-neurosurgical centre. *Anaesthesia*, **60**, 470–85.

☼ Spontaneous intracerebral haemorrhage

Definition
Acute extravasation of blood into the brain parenchyma.

Presentation
- Rapid onset of focal neurological deficit, signs of raised ICP, decreased consciousness level.
- Acute hypertension (blood pressure >150/100 mmHg) occurs in >90% patients.
- Severe intracerebral haemorrhage results in immediate unconsciousness.

Investigations
- Check FBC, U&Es, ABGs, clotting, and cross-match blood.
- Cranial CT scan allows estimation of volume of haematoma and differentiates between haemorrhagic and ischaemic stroke.
- Angiography in young patients, those with no obvious risk factors for ICH or pattern of bleeding suggestive of underlying aneurysm/ arteriovenous malformation.
- MRI if underlying lesion suspected (e.g. amyloid angiopathy, neoplasm).

Risk factors
- Warfarin therapy (5–10-fold increase in risk of ICH).
- High dose aspirin in older people.
- Hypertension—especially untreated.
- High alcohol intake.
- Cocaine abuse.
- Cerebral amyloid angiopathy.
- Arteriovenous malformation.

Exclusions
- Ischaemic stroke.
- Subarachnoid haemorrhage— ⊃ see p. 196.

Immediate management
☑ ABC—O_2.
☑ Oral endotracheal intubation and mechanical ventilation in unconscious patients or those with deteriorating conscious level.
☑ Maintain P_aO_2 >13.3 kPa (100 mmHg) and P_aCO_2 4.5–5.0 kPa (34–38 mmHg).
☑ Maintain systemic blood pressure within tight limits around premorbid BP—balancing risk of perihaematoma ischaemia against risk of haematoma expansion.
☑ Do not treat hypertension unless >180/105 mmHg
☑ Always maintain systolic BP >100 mmHg.
☑ Consider mannitol (0.5 g/kg) or hypertonic saline if signs of raised ICP.
☑ Urgent CT scan.

Subsequent management

☑ Regular neurological observations.

☑ Reverse therapeutic anticoagulation: vitamin K or fresh frozen plasma until normal coagulation indices are restored.

rFVIIa is not indicated—it reduces haematoma volume but does not reduce mortality or improve outcome.

Treat hypertension—consensus guidance recommends treatment only when systolic BP >180 mmHg.

Recent evidence suggests that reduction of systolic BP to 140 mmHg is associated with reduced haematoma expansion and no increase in cerebral ischaemic events, but further studies are required to determine if this is associated with improved outcome

☑ Seek neurosurgical advice for large ICH or deterioration in clinical status.

Further management

- Surgery:
  - evacuation of haematoma is controversial.
  - cerebellar haemorrhage >3 cm should be evacuated because of risk of early deterioration.
  - younger patients with lobar haemorrhage causing significant mass effect may also derive benefit from surgery.
  - external ventricular drain for hydrocephalus.
- Fever and glycaemic control.
- Thromboembolic prophylaxis. TEDS and calf compression devices. LMWH only considered outside of the acute phase when no further surgery is anticipated and after prior discussion with the neurosurgeons.
- Seizures occur in 10% of patients and should be treated aggressively.
- Optimal time for resumption of anticoagulation therapy is unclear. Risks and benefits of withholding or restarting treatment should be assessed for each patient.

Further reading

Anderson, C., Heeley, E., Huang, Y. (2013). Rapid blood pressure lowering in patients with acute intracerebral haemorrhage. *New England Journal of Medicine*, **368**(25), 2355–65.

Anderson, C., Huang, Y., Wang, J., et al. (2008). Intensive blood pressure reduction in acute cerebral haemorrhage trial (INTERACT): a randomised pilot trial. *Lancet Neurology*, **7**, 391–9.

Mayer, S., Rincon, F. (2005). Treatment of intracerebral haemorrhage. *Lancet Neurology*, **4**, 662–72.

Rincon, F., Mayer, S. (2004). Novel therapies for intracerebral hemorrhage. *Current Opinion in Critical Care*, **10**, 94–100.

① Sodium disturbances after brain injury

Definition
Hyponatraemia: serum sodium <135 mmol/L (➲ see also p. 319)
Hypernatraemia: serum sodium >145 mmol/L (➲ see also p. 317)

Presentation
- **Hyponatraemia**—lethargy, irritability, nausea and vomiting, headache, and muscle cramps/weakness in moderate hyponatraemia. Severe hyponatraemia (<120 mmol/L) presents with drowsiness, seizures, and unconsciousness.
- **Hypernatraemia**—thirst, lethargy, and irritability in moderate hypernatraemia. Severe hypernatraemia (>165 mmol/L) results in seizures and coma.

Causes
- Hyponatraemia:
  - syndrome of inappropriate ADH secretion (SIADH).
  - cerebral salt-wasting syndrome (CSWS).
- Hypernatraemia:
  - cranial diabetes insipidus (DI).

Investigations
- Plasma sodium
- Plasma osmolality
- Urine sodium
- Urine osmolality
- Cranial CT scan

Risk factors
- Head injury (➲ see p. 192)
- Subarachnoid haemorrhage (➲ see p. 196)
- Iatrogenic
- Drugs:
  - diuretics
  - mannitol
- Water intoxication

Exclusions
- Inappropriate administration of hypotonic fluids.
- Inadequate water intake or excessive water loss.
- Hyperglycaemia.
- Adrenal insufficiency.
- Hypothyroidism.
- Renal failure.

Immediate management
☑ Expectant and supportive treatment in asymptomatic patients—brain-injury-related sodium disturbances are often transient and self-limiting.
☑ ABC—in patients with decreased consciousness or those in coma.

☑ Prompt treatment of acute sodium disturbance in acute symptomatic patients to minimize risk of neurological complications and death.

☑ Gradual correction of sodium deficit (0.5 mmol/L/h or 8–10 mmol/L/day) to minimize neurological sequelae.

☑ Target treatment to the alleviation of symptoms rather than arbitrary serum sodium values.

☑ Correct associated water deficits.

Diagnosis
- SIADH:
  - serum Na^+ <135 mmol/L and osmolality <280 mOsm/kg—i.e. hypotonic hyponatraemia.
  - urine osmolality > serum osmolality.
  - urinary Na^+ concentration >20mmol/L.
  - normal thyroid, adrenal, and renal function.
  - clinical euvolaemia.
- CSWS:
  - low serum Na^+ concentration in association with a low serum osmolality.
  - high urine osmolality with a high urinay sodium > 40mmol/L.
  - high haematocrit and urea.
  - biochemical criteria may be inconclusive—the key clinical diagnostic feature is the presence of volume depletion.
- DI:
  - polyuria, polydipsia, and thirst in awake patients.
  - high urine volume (>3ml/kg/hr for more than 3 hours with a low urine specific gravity < 1.01).
  - serum Na^+ >145 mmol/L.
  - serum osmolality >305 mOsm/kg.
  - abnormally low urine osmolality (<350 mOsm/kg).

Specific management
- SIADH:
  ☑ often self-limiting—treatment should be initiated if patient symptomatic or serum Na^+ significantly low or falling rapidly.

  ☑ fluid restriction (800–1000 mL/24 h).

  ☑ 1.8% saline in acute symptomatic hyponatraemia–discontinue when serum Na^+ approx. 125 mmol/L.

  ☑ pharmacological treatment if saline resuscitation fails and diagnosis certain—furosemide, demeclocycline (900–1200 mg/24 h; note this is higher than licensed dose) or ADH-receptor antagonists (e.g. conivaptan).

  ☑ in general, do not increase serum Na^+ by more than 0.5 mmol/L/h or 8–10 mmol/L/day–over-rapid correction can lead to central pontine myelinolysis (➔ see also p. 319).

- CSWS:
  - ☑ volume and sodium resuscitation—initially with 0.9% saline.
  - ☑ 1.8% saline 25-50mls/hr in acute symptomatic hyponatraemia—discontinue when serum Na⁺ approx. 125 mmol/L.
  - ☑ replace ongoing losses when normovolaemia and normonatraemia restored—0.9% saline IV and sodium tablets via NG tube.
  - ☑ fludrocortisone (100mcg PO/NG tds)in refractory CSWS.
  - ☑ as with SIADH, avoid over-rapid correction of serum Na concentration (➲ see also p. 319).

- DI:
  - ☑ key aims are replacement and retention of water and replacement of ADH.
  - ☑ conscious patients are often able to increase their own water intake—may be sufficient treatment in self-limiting disease.
  - ☑ 5% glucose IV or water via NG tube in unconscious patients.
  - ☑ Desmopressin (100–200 µg intranasally or incremental doses of 0.4 µg IV) if urine output >250 mL/h with a rapidly rising serum sodium
  - ☑ in general, do not reduce serum Na⁺ quicker than 10 mmol/L/day—over-rapid correction can result in pulmonary or cerebral oedema (➲ see also p. 317).

Further reading

Bradshaw, K., Smith, M. (2008). Disorders of sodium balance after brain injury. *CEACCP British Journal of Anaesthesia*, **8**(4), 129–33.

Diringer, M., Zazulia, A. (2006). Hyponatremia in neurologic patients: consequences and approaches to treatment. *Neurologist*, **12**, 117–26.

Lien, Y., Shapiro, J. (2007). Hyponatraemia: clinical diagnosis and management. *American Journal of Medicine*, **120**, 653–8.

Tisdall, M., Crocker, M., Watkiss, J., Smith, M. (2006). Disturbances of sodium in critically ill adult neurologic patients. *Journal of Neurosurgical Anesthesiology*, **18**, 57–63.

☠ Venous air embolism

Definition
Entry of air into the pulmonary arterial circulation through open veins or sinuses (➲ see also p. 77).

Presentation
- Immediate fall in $ETCO_2$, fall in S_pO_2.
- Rise in end-tidal nitrogen as air enters circulation. This is more specific than changes in $ETCO_2$ as it is not influenced by cardiovascular changes.
- Air entry noted by surgeon, detection of air bubbles with precordial ultrasonography or transoesophageal echocardiography.
- Tachyarrhythmias, hypotension, and shock with cardiovascular collapse if left untreated.
- Awake patients may complain of chest pain, dyspnoea, and wheeze.
- Auscultation may reveal the classic millwheel murmur in the right precordial area.

Investigation
- Clinical diagnosis and ultrasonography/echocardiogram.
- ABG.

Risk factors
- Presence of central venous catheters—particularly during insertion or removal.
- Surgery:
  - operative site above level of heart, creating negative hydrostatic pressure (e.g. posterior fossa surgery, ENT surgery).
  - surgery involving lung parenchyma.
  - cardiothoracic surgery.
  - iatrogenic introduction of air, CO_2, or other gases to systemic veins (e.g. laparoscopic, hysteroscopic, and arthroscopic surgery).
  - obstetric surgery.
- Blunt and penetrating chest trauma.
- Barotrauma:
  - IPPV, blast injuries.

Paediatric implications
- Cardiovascular instability may be more common in children as an equivalent air bubble would be larger relative to blood volume in children and, therefore, more likely to cause compromise.

Immediate management

☑ Inform surgeon.
☑ ABC—100% O_2.
☑ Stop nitrous oxide (N_2O) if in use.
☑ Flood open wounds with saline/cover wound with wet swabs.
☑ Raise venous pressure, elevate legs, compress neck veins (during cranial surgery), and occlude open ports on CVP lines.
☑ Attempt to aspirate air from CVP line.
☑ Arterial blood gas analysis.

Subsequent management

☑ Position patient in head-down, left lateral position to limit airflow to pulmonary circulation.
☑ Standard resuscitation if cardiovascular collapse ensues, initially with fluids, but with inotropes/vasopressors if necessary.
NB: Adrenaline may worsen arrhythmias precipitated by air embolism; therefore careful administration advisable.
☑ Echocardiography or ultrasonography if available.
☑ 8 mg dexamethasone IV followed by maintenance dosage may limit delayed cardiovascular and pulmonary sequelae, although clinical evidence for this is poor.
☑ Admit to critical care facility for observation.

Special considerations

• Prevent venous air embolism in high-risk procedures by elevating central venous pressure—volume loading, compression of the lower limbs with bandages, 'G-suit', or medical antishock trousers.
• Ensure patient is head down and venous catheters are flushed prior to insertion. Check lines are closed to air when not in use.
• Do not use nitrous oxide in high-risk procedures—causes expansion of air bubbles.
• Closed chest compressions may give additional benefit by dissipating emboli into the pulmonary arterial tree.

Further reading

Marek, A., Lele, A.V., Fitzsimmons, L., Toung, T.J. (2007). Diagnosis and treatment of vascular air embolism. *Anesthesiology*, **106**, 164–77.
Smith, M. (2004). Anaesthesia for posterior fossa surgery. In: Pollard, B. (ed). *Handbook of Clinical Anaesthesia*, pp. 299–302. Edinburgh, UK: Churchill Livingstone.

:O: **Acute spinal cord injury and spinal shock**

Definition
Traumatic injury, leading to interruption of both somatic and sympathetic pathways in the spinal cord.

Presentation
- Initial hypertension will be quickly replaced by profound hypotension and reduced systemic vascular resistance in the acute phase of spinal cord injury. Often bradycardia will be seen due to interruption of cardiac sympathetic denervation.
- Acute respiratory compromise if the lesion is above C4.
- Impaired systolic function may manifest as congestive cardiac failure, particularly with fluid loading.
- Bladder and bowel atony are frequently present.

Investigations
- FBC, U&E.
- ASIA (American spinal injuries association) assessment and score of sensory and motor function.
- Imaging; plain films/computerized tomography/MRI scan.
- ABGs.

Risk factors
- Trauma.
- 50% of spinal cord injuries are associated with another injury, traumatic brain injury and chest trauma being the most common.
- Spinal shock is most common in high thoracic or cervical cord injuries.

Exclusions
- Exclude haemorrhagic shock as a cause of hypotension. Associated bradycardia is more indicative of neurogenic (spinal) shock.
- Anaphylaxis.
- Vascular volume assessment with CVP/pulmonary artery catheter or oesophageal Doppler monitoring may be helpful.

Paediatric implications
- Paediatric spinal cord injury is very rare.
- Children with spinal cord injury often develop scoliosis in later life.

Immediate management

☑ ABC—100% O_2.
☑ Spinal immobilization with rigid cervical collar and spinal board.
☑ Early intubation with manual in-line stabilization of cervical spine. Consider awake fibreoptic intubation.
☑ Large-bore IV cannula.
☑ **Careful** IV fluid boluses.
☑ Atropine—up to 3 mg in 0.3–0.6 mg increments for bradycardia.
☑ Consider vasopressors (e.g. noradrenaline) if patient remains hypotensive despite above treatment.

Subsequent management

☑ Insertion of central venous and oesophageal Doppler to monitor responses in cardiac output and filling pressures to fluid challenges.
☑ Titration of vasopressors and inotropic agents to cardiac output and systemic vascular resistance.
☑ Nasogastric suctioning for gastric/bowel distension.
☑ Urinary catheterization for monitoring of fluid balance and bladder atony.
☑ Venothromboprophylaxis. TEDS and calf compression devices. LMWH only considered outside of the acute phase when no further surgery is anticipated and after prior discussion with the neurosurgeons.

Special considerations

Hypotension should be treated aggressively with volume expansion and vasopressor/inotropic therapy to optimize spinal cord perfusion, thereby reducing the risks of 2° spinal cord injury.

Suxamethonium should be avoided beyond 3 days post injury.

Steroids and acute spinal cord injury

• Methylprednisolone may be administered to patients with an acute spinal cord injury within 3 h of the injury. Dose is 30 mg/kg bolus dose over 15 min, followed 45 min later by an infusion at 5.4 mg/kg/h for 23 h.
• While administration of methylprednisolone may not treat spinal shock, there is some evidence to suggest that it may produce some neurological improvement in incomplete spinal cord injury, although the potential side effects of administration should also be considered.

Further reading

Stevens, R.D., Bhardwaj, Kirsch, J.R., Mirski, M.A. (2003). Critical care and perioperative management in traumatic spinal cord injury. *Journal of Neurosurgical Anesthesiology*, **15**, 215–29.

☼ Autonomic dysreflexia

Definition
Massive sympathetic discharge in patients with an SCI.

Presentation
- Condition characterized by massive autonomic discharge of the sympathetic chain, below the level of the spinal cord lesion, in response to certain stimuli.
- Severe hypertension (most common clinical feature), cardiac arrhythmias, headache, flushing, and sweating above the level of the lesion.
- Less common features—Horner's syndrome, nausea, anxiety.

Investigations
- Clinical diagnosis
- Thorough examination for the trigger
- Invasive pressure monitoring

Risk factors
- Occurs from 3 weeks to 12 y after SCI.
- Most commonly seen in high spinal cord lesions—occurs in up to 60% of patients with cervical lesions and 20% in those with thoracic lesions. Rarely a problem with lesions below T10.
- More common in complete lesions of the spinal cord.
- Usually related to provoking stimuli such as bladder distension, blocked urinary catheter, faecal impaction, uterine contractions/labour.

Exclusions
- Exclude other pathology—bone fractures, DVT/PE, phaeochromocytoma (rare).

Paediatric implications
- Autonomic dysreflexia is rarely seen in children.
- Should be treated as per adult management.

Immediate management
- ☑ ABC—100% O_2.
- ☑ Place patient in upright position to produce fall in blood pressure.
- ☑ Loosen all tight clothing and shoes.
- ☑ Treat/stop any obvious precipitating stimuli, including during general or local anaesthesia.
- ☑ Rapid-onset, short-acting vasodilators—nifedipine 10 mg capsule (contents) sublingually, glyceryl trinitrate (0.5–10 mg/h IV infusion, 0.3–1 mg sublingually prn, 5 mg in 24 h dermal patch), or phentolamine (2–10 mg IV prn).
- ☑ Consider early invasive blood pressure monitoring.

Subsequent management

☑ Continue antihypertensive of choice in incremental doses until blood pressure is controlled.

☑ Patient and carer education; regular catheter checks, bowel management, management of uterine contractions.

☑ Consider long-term pharmacological therapies:
- prazosin 1–20 mg PO daily.
- guanethidine 10–20 mg IM, repeated 3-hourly prn.
- calcium channel blockers, clonidine, and hydralazine have also been recommended.

Special considerations

- Episodes of autonomic dysreflexia may result in myocardial ischaemia, pulmonary oedema, cerebral haemorrhage, seizures, coma, and death. Severe hypertension should be treated promptly and these outcomes recognized, investigated, and treated as appropriate.
- Spinal anaesthesia obliterates autonomic dysreflexia, although numerous cases have been reported under general and epidural anaesthesia. In addition to short-acting antihypertensive therapy, increasing depth of anaesthesia may be effective in treating these cases.
- Obstetric patients are at high risk of autonomic dysreflexia therefore epidural anaesthesia should be continued for 48 h after delivery.

Further reading

Bycroft, J., Shergill, I.S., Chung, E.A., Arya, N., Shah, P.J. (2005). Autonomic dysreflexia, a medical emergency. *Postgraduate Medical Journal*, **81**, 232–5.

① Dystonic reactions

Definition
Severe, sustained muscular spasms or abnormal posturing.

Presentation
- Recent history of antipsychotic or antidepressant drug ingestion:
  - antipsychotics—phenothiazines (e.g. prochlorperazine), butyrophenones (e.g. haloperidol), thioxanthenes (e.g. flupentixol).
  - antiemetics—prochlorperazine, metoclopramide.
  - antidepressants—selective serotonin reuptake inhibitors.
  - in 90% of patients, onset is within 4 days of starting medication.
  - Should be considered in any patient exhibiting symptoms within 7 days of starting medications.
- Characteristic muscle spasms:
  - oculogyric crisis—blepharospasm, upward/lateral deviation of eyes.
  - torticollic crisis—spasm of neck muscles.
  - buccolingual crisis—spasm of facial muscles and tongue, dysphagia, dysarthria.
  - tortipelvic crisis—painful abdominal wall spasm.
  - vocal cord dystonia—stridor/laryngospasm.
- Cessation of symptoms within 5–15 min of antimuscarinic administration.

Investigations
- U&Es, magnesium, calcium

Risk factors
- Recent treatment with triggering agents (see earlier)
- Male sex, teenagers/young adults
- Previous history of acute dystonia
- Cocaine abuse

Exclusions
- Tetanus
- Seizures including temporal lobe epilepsy and status epilepticus
- Metabolic disturbances (e.g. hypocalcaemia, hypomagnesaemia)
- Cerebrovascular accident

Paediatric implications
- Antiemetics are the most common cause of dystonic reactions in children.
- Meningitis should be considered as a differential diagnosis.

Immediate management

- ☑ Assess and stabilize airway, consider 100% O$_2$.
- ☑ Reassure patient.
- ☑ IV access.
- ☑ Centrally acting antimuscarinic—procyclidine 5–10 mg IM, consider IV only in life-threatening emergency.
- ☑ Consider diazepam 5–10 mg IV in severe cases resistant to treatment with antimuscarinic agents.

Subsequent management

- ☑ If immediate management fails, consider another diagnosis.
- ☑ Discontinue trigger agent if possible.
- ☑ Consider longer term treatment with anticholinergic therapy:
  - procyclidine 5 mg PO tds or amantadine 100 mg od–tds.

Special considerations

- Life-threatening dystonias may occur rarely.
- Severe stridor due to laryngospasm has been reported.

Further reading

Dressler, D., Benecke, R. (2005). Diagnosis and management of acute movement disorders. *Journal of Neurology*, **252**, 1299–306.

Van Harten, P.N., Hoek, H.W., Kahn, R.S. (1999). Acute dystonia induced by drug treatment. *British Medical Journal*, **319**, 623–6.

☠ **Status epilepticus**

Definition
Continuous seizure activity lasting >30 min.
Intermittent seizure activity lasting >30 min during which consciousness is not regained.

Presentation
Loss of consciousness, tonic–clonic muscle activity, tongue biting, and urinary incontinence.
May be partial/absence seizures.

Investigations
- ABGs, FBC, and inflammatory markers, U&Es, blood glucose, anti-epileptic drug plasma levels
- EEG
- CT or MRI scan if intracranial lesion suspected

Risk factors
- Acute processes:
  - electrolyte imbalance (e.g. Na^+, Ca^{2+}, glucose)
  - stroke, cerebral anoxic/hypoxic damage
  - CNS infection (e.g. encephalitis, meningitis)
  - trauma
  - drug overdose/toxicity
  - sepsis syndrome
  - acute renal failure
- Chronic processes:
  - pre-existing epilepsy, poor compliance with therapy, or recent change of anti-epileptic medication
  - alcoholism
  - intracranial space-occupying lesion

Exclusions
- Rigors due to sepsis
- Myoclonic jerking
- Generalized dystonia
- Pseudostatus epilepticus, including seizures that are psychogenic in origin

Paediatric implications
- Fever or infection are the most common causes of Status Epilepticus in the paediatric population. Children should be given immediate antipyretics and cooled.
- Drug efficacy is similar to that in adults, although children may tolerate more rapid IV administration.
- Drug dose calculations are the same as for adult patients on a weight by weight basis, but the maximum dose of lorazepam should not exceed 4 mg/dose in children. Buccal midazolam (0.5 mg/kg) may also be considered.
- The adult treatment protocol is generally followed, although there is no evidence that this is applicable to children.

Immediate management

See Figure 7.1.

☑ ABC—100% O₂.
☑ Check blood sugar treat hypoglycaemia where necessary.
☑ Termination of seizures with IV lorazepam (0.1 mg/kg) as first line therapy. May be repeated once after 10–20 min if seizures not terminated.
☑ Second-line therapy if seizures not terminated within 10 min: phenytoin 15–18 mg/kg by slow IV infusion (rate <50 mg/min), or fosphenytoin 22.5 mg/kg (equivalent to phenytoin 15 mg/kg) at a rate of up to 225 mg/min (equivalent to phenytoin 150 mg/min).
☑ Intubation and ventilation to maintain PₐO₂ and PₐCO₂ within normal range.
☑ Fluid resuscitation to maintain adequate systemic blood pressure and CPP.
☑ Inotropes may also be required, particularly if general anaesthesia is needed to control seizures.

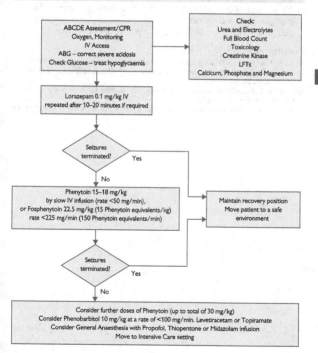

Figure 7.1 Algorithm for status epilepticus.

Subsequent management

☑ Search for cause of seizures and treat underlying problem:
- known epileptic ± recent change in anti-epileptic medication.
- alcohol withdrawal, drug overdose.
- CNS infection, intracranial pathology (e.g. stroke, subarachnoid haemorrhage).

☑ Start propofol or barbiturate anaesthesia (under EEG control) for refractory status epilepticus if seizures not controlled after 30 min with second-line therapy. Anaesthesia should be continued for 12–24 h after the last clinical or electrographic seizure.

☑ Ensure therapeutic levels of long-acting anticonvulsant drugs.

☑ Consider third-line therapy, e.g. phenobarbital 10 mg/kg by infusion (rate <100 mg/min; max 1 g) or one of the newer anti-epileptic drugs such as levetiracetam or topiramate. Levetiracetam is now available as an IV preparation and is being widely used in the ICU setting because of rapid titration and ease of transition to maintenance therapy. There are limited data on its efficacy in status epilepticus.

☑ Manage complications—hyperthermia, rhabdomyolysis (screen for myoglobinuria and measure creatinine kinase), cardiac arrhythmias, pulmonary aspiration, and neurogenic pulmonary oedema.

Further reading

Adapa, R., Absalom, A. (2009) Status epilepticus. *Anaesthesia and Intensive Care Medicine*, **10**, 137–40.

Costello, D., Cole, A. (2007). Treatment of acute seizures and status epilepticus. *Journal of Intensive Care Medicine*, **22**, 319–47.

NICE (2012). *Epilepsies: Diagnosis and Management. Clinical Guideline CG137.* Available at: https://www.nice.org.uk/guidance/cg137

Penas, J., Molins, A., Puig, J. (2007). Status epilepticus: evidence and controversies. *Neurologist*, **65**, S62–S73.

Thoracics

James Bennett and Gerard Gould

☼: Intrathoracic tracheal/bronchial obstruction

Definition
Partial or complete obstruction of the tracheobronchial tree.

Presentation
- **Symptoms**: dyspnoea, weak voice, wheeze, prefer to sit up (particularly to sleep).
- **Signs**: hypoxia, ↑work of breathing, stridor, talking in incomplete sentences, ineffective cough, see-saw abdominal movements.

Central airway obstruction can progress insidiously with symptoms and signs presenting with advanced lesions.

Immediate management
Management depends on:
1) Urgency of intervention
2) Level of obstruction
3) Condition of patient

General approach
☑ 100% O_2 via non-rebreathing facemask.
☑ Consider Heliox (can be useful in upper airway obstruction due to its low density as a temporary measure but delivers limited F_iO_2).
☑ Give dexamethasone 6.6 mg IV, then 3.3 mg 6–hourly.
☑ Antisialagogues (e.g. glycopyrrolate 200 µg can be beneficial in selected patients).
☑ Insert arterial catheter to monitor ABGs (check pH, P_aCO_2).
☑ Transfer to HDU/ITU environment.
☑ Make plans for rigid bronchoscopy +/− debulking of tumour +/− stenting.

Airway management
Clinical urgency often limits opportunities to optimize medical comorbidities:
☑ May need tracheal intubation—use small tube (5.0–6.0 mm).
☑ Ensure tube tip is below level of obstruction (use FOB).

Airway obstruction is likely to get worse during anaesthesia or airway manipulation due to loss of airway tone, airway reflexes, trauma, and bleeding.

Options
☑ Awake fibreoptic bronchoscopy (if situation not critical) to diagnose site and extent of problem and urgent radiotherapy to debulk malignancy.
☑ Awake fibreoptic intubation and maintenance of spontaneous respiration.
☑ Inhalational induction.
☑ RSI and rigid bronchoscopy (may be life-saving).
☑ Site of obstruction may not allow cricothyroidotomy or tracheostomy.

Subsequent management

Rigid bronchoscopy:
- ☑ TIVA with Sanders injector.
- ☑ Surgeon can manipulate bronchoscope through obstruction or into bronchus.

Tumour debulking:
- ☑ by grabbing with forceps.
- ☑ laser: can be possible through flexible bronchoscope without GA.

Stenting of narrowed airway:
- ☑ TIVA.
- ☑ X-ray screening with patient on X-ray lucent table,
- ☑ wire placed through obstruction into distal bronchus,
- ☑ stent advanced over wire into bronchus, trachea, or both.

Consider
- ☑ radiotherapy, chemotherapy, or surgical removal of mass.
- ☑ Inflammatory tracheal narrowing requires tracheostomy followed by immunosuppression.

Investigations

- The nature and extent of obstruction must be clearly defined.
- CXR.
- CT of airway (multislice).
- Echocardiography (excludes cardiac causes/pericardial effusions).
- Flow-volume loop (limited value in acute setting, can precipitate respiratory failure).

Risk factors/causes

Benign:
- Traumatic (e.g. postintubation).
- Inflammatory (e.g. Wegener's granulomatosis, amyloid).
- Infection (e.g. TB).
- Neoplastic (e.g. neurofibroma).
- Anastomotic (e.g. lung transplant, sleeve resection).

Malignant:
- Primary:
  - Intraluminal (e.g. bronchogenic, carcinoid).
  - Extraluminal (e.g. oesophageal, lymphoma, mediastinal—thymus, thyroid).
- Metastatic (e.g. breast, bronchogenic, colon).

Problems likely if trachea narrowed by >50% on CT.

Exclusions

- Asthma (⊕ see p. 70)
- Worsening of COPD
- Cardiac causes of wheeze (e.g. LVF)
- Foreign body aspiration (⊕ see p. 219)
- Anaphylaxis (⊕ see p. 272)
- Neurological weakness

Special considerations

- Cardiopulmonary bypass is sometimes necessary (e.g. pulmonary artery compression).
- Carinal obstruction is difficult to overcome—try intubating one bronchus and surviving on one lung temporarily.
- Tissue diagnosis may allow therapeutic intervention (e.g. antibiotics, steroids, chemotherapy, or radiotherapy).
- Mediastinal masses are one cause of unexpected failed ventilation and intubation after induction of general anaesthesia.

Subsequent management

Conacher, I.D. (2003). Anaesthesia and tracheobronchial stenting for central airway obstruction. *British Journal of Anaesthesia*, **90**, 367–74.

Hammer, G.B. (2004). Anaesthetic management for the child with a mediastinal mass. *Paediatric Anaesthesia*, **14**, 95–7.

Worrell, S.G., DeMeester, S.R. (2014). Thoracic emergencies. *Surgical Clinics of North America*, **94**, 183–91.

☼ Inhaled foreign body

Definition
Foreign body (FB) in the airway.

Presentation
Immediate
- 'Classical': choking, coughing, stridor, wheeze, and cyanosis. Only seen in a minority of patients.

Late
- Non-resolving collapse, consolidation, wheeze:
  - Adults: impaction is in distal airways.
  - Children: impaction is in main-stem bronchi (right > left).

Immediate management
- Back blows, chest thrusts, and abdominal thrusts all ↑ intrathoracic pressure and can expel foreign bodies from the airway.
- Assess after **each** intervention. Stop immediately after expulsion.

Adults
Assess severity:

Severe: ineffective cough
- patient conscious:
  - ☑ up to five back blows (heal of hand between shoulder blades), then
  - ☑ up to five abdominal thrusts, then
  - ☑ if no relief return to start of cycle (5 back blows and so on).
- patient unconscious:
  - ☑ initiate chest compressions even if pulse.
  - ☑ 100% O_2.
  - ☑ Assess airway—remove visible obstruction.
  - ☑ Protect airway:
    - FB occasionally seen at laryngoscopy
    - ET tube may push FB distally allowing ventilation.

Mild: effective cough
- no intervention required, observe only.

Child (>1 year old)

Severe, conscious
- ☑ 5 back blows, 5 chest thrusts, check airway, 5 back blows, 5 abdominal thrusts, check airway, then repeat if necessary.

Severe, unconscious
- ☑ Open airway, 5 rescue breaths, initiate chest compressions.

Mild
- ☑ Encourage coughing, continually re-assess.

Infant (<1 year old)

Ineffective cough, conscious
- ☑ Support infant in head-downwards position.

☑ Up to five back blows, reassessing after each blow.
☑ Up to five chest thrusts, reassessing after each thrust.
☑ Do not use abdominal thrust due to risk of internal organ damage.

Ineffective cough, unconscious
☑ Attempt five rescue breaths.
☑ If no response, proceed to chest compressions.

Surgical management
• Flexible bronchoscopy remains gold standard of diagnosis.
  ☑ Retrieval may be possible in adults by flexible bronchoscopy using topical anaesthesia, allowing spontaneous ventilation.
• Respiratory distress may require intubation and immediate transfer to theatre for rigid bronchoscopy.
  ☑ Typically a balloon catheter is placed beyond the object and is pulled proximally to the carina. FB then extracted via grasping forceps.
  ☑ Other tools include magnets, baskets, snares, cryotherapy probes, and laser.

Anaesthetic management
☑ IV access, atropine 600 μg IV (or 20 μg/kg for a child).
☑ Standard monitoring.
☑ Two anaesthetic options: gas induction or TIVA.
☑ **1. Gas induction**
  • with O_2/sevoflurane to maintain spontaneous ventilation.
  • consider switching to isoflurane (sevoflurane wears off rapidly).
  • ensure adequate depth of anaesthesia before airway instrumentation.
☑ **2. TIVA**
  • ensure muscle relaxation (especially when FB removal at vocal cords).
  • anaesthetic depth monitoring useful, e.g. bispectral index (BIS).
  • jet ventilation or HFJV.
☑ Tape and pad eyes.
☑ Dexamethasone 0.1 mg/kg IV to minimize laryngeal oedema.
☑ Insertion of rigid bronchoscope and connection to breathing system.
☑ Procedure may be prolonged: ensure patient warmth and appropriate fluid therapy.
☑ Consider intubation postprocedure and transfer to ITU.

Subsequent management
• Complications of foreign body aspiration depends on physical properties of FB (organic vs. inorganic, sharp vs. blunt edged), location, and duration of impaction.
• Organic material (especially oily nuts) can produce local inflammatory reactions that may cause tissue degranulation.
• Antibiotics only if clinically indicated.

Investigations
CXR (inspiratory/expiratory views). Only 11% of FB are radio-opaque therefore history and examination are important.

Risk factors

- Extremes of age (immature or obtunded swallowing or airway reflexes).
  Children: lack of adult supervision, availability of nuts, seeds, beads.
  Adults: dentures, senility, mental illness, intoxication.
- Neurological disorders, poor swallow.

Exclusions

- Chest infection
- Asthma
- Acute laryngotracheobronchitis
- Anaphylaxis
- Intrathoracic tumour

Paediatric implications

- Rigid bronchoscopy and GA commonest therapeutic intervention.
- Reduced airway diameter gives rise to greater risk of obstruction,
  asphyxiation, and gas trapping (ball-valve mechanism).
- 400 choking deaths/year in EU—food accounts for 85% choking deaths.

Special considerations

- Maintenance of spontaneous breathing allows:
  - fewer interruptions to surgery for ventilation
  - ↓ risk of distal dislodgement
  - ↓ risk of dynamic hyperinflation
- Maybe more than 1 FB.
- Organic FBs can fragment at removal.
- Prolonged impaction can cause atelectasis and bronchiectasis.
- Erosion and perforation can cause pneumothorax, haemoptysis, and
  pneumomediastinum.

Further reading

Fidkowski, C.W., Zheng, H., Firth, P.G. (2010). The anesthetic considerations of tracheobronchial foreign bodies in children: a literature review of 12,979 cases. *Anesthesia and Analgesia*, **4**, 1016–25.

Pinzoni, F., Boniotti, C., Molinaro, S.M., Baraldi, A., Berlucchi, M. (2007). Inhaled foreign bodies in pediatric patients: review of personal experience. *International Journal of Pediatric Otorhinolaryngology*, **71**, 1897–903.

UK Resuscitation Council. *BLS Guidelines*. Available at: https://www.resus.org.uk

☼ Tracheal injury or laceration

Definition
Loss of structural integrity of tracheobronchial tree.

Presentation
Laryngotracheal trauma
- Presentation rare as majority die out of hospital.
- Injury rare as mandible and sternum offer bony protection.

Blunt injury:
- Involves both larynx and trachea.
- Injury at cricotracheal junction can cause airway transection:
  - air dissects through oesophageal submucosa.
  - high mortality.
- Associated with head, maxillofacial, and cervical spine injury.

Penetrating injury:
- Trachea at greater risk of injury than larynx.
- Associated with oesophageal and cervicothoracic vascular injury.
- **Symptoms**: stridor, hoarseness, cough, neck pain, dysphagia, preferring to sit forward.
- **Signs**: haemoptysis, neck swelling, subcutaneous emphysema, sucking chest wound.
- >25% of patients with laryngotracheal injury have no symptoms or signs until 24–48 h following injury.

Tracheobronchial trauma
- Seen in up to 2% of blunt chest trauma.

Blunt injury:
- Low tracheal tears more common.

Penetrating injury:
- High tracheal tears.

Associated injuries:
- Oesophageal, cardiac, aortic, great vessel injury.
- Cervical spine trauma.
- **Signs**: respiratory distress, cyanosis, vocal cord palsy, simple, tension, or open pneumothorax, haemothorax, flail chest, superficial bruising, subcutaneous emphysema, bubbly or frothy blood in airway, pulmonary contusion, lung collapse.

Immediate management
- ☑ Manage as per ATLS guidelines (i.e. identify and treat immediate threats using an ABC approach).
- ☑ 100% O_2 with cervical spine precautions.
- ☑ Maintain spontaneous respiration whenever possible:
  - massive air leak may occur with IPPV.
  - anaesthetic induction, muscle relaxation, and direct laryngoscopy are all potentially hazardous.

☑ Continuous airway re-assessment:
- >50% of patients require emergency airway intervention.
- partially obstructed airway can rapidly obstruct.

☑ Multidisciplinary planning of care (anaesthetics, ENT, and thoracic surgeons).

Anaesthetic management

☑ Large-bore access essential, arterial line is useful.

☑ Airway protection:
- intubation by direct laryngoscopy may fail to intubate distal trachea if there is laryngeal or tracheal disruption.
- may be possible to pass tracheal tube directly into trachea through penetrating injury of cervical trachea.

☑ Tracheostomy under LA (or directly into exposed trachea) may be required:
- particularly with blunt laryngeal trauma.
- likely to be technically difficult.

☑ Awake fibreoptic intubation in theatre if injuries not immediately life-threatening:
- load a cuffed tube on intubating fibrescope.
- use uncut small tube (6.0–7.0 mm) in case intubation of one bronchus required.
- inspection of airway fibre-optically using stack system allows surgeons to view airway also, allowing collective strategy of care.
- view impaired by blood, oedema, and laryngotracheal disruption.
- attempt to pass scope and tube beyond any trauma, even down to intubation of an unaffected bronchus.

☑ Avoid IPPV until airway below tear has been isolated with cuffed tube.

Subsequent management

☑ If fibreoptic assessment of airway demonstrates normal or minor findings, can be observed in critical care environment.

☑ Find and treat any associated injuries.

Investigations

- Bloods: FBC, coagulation, cross-match 4 units, regular ABGs
- Radiology:
  - C-spine: fractures, dislocations.
  - CXR: pneumomediastinum, pneumothorax, haemothorax.
  - Pelvic: disruption.
  - CT chest and neck: airway calibre.
- Flexible nasendoscopy:
  - laryngeal oedema, haematoma, vocal cord paralysis, cartilage disruption.

Risk factors

- Blunt injuries:
  - Direct impact (e.g. steering wheel).
  - Crush injury (e.g. strangulation).

- Penetrating injuries:
  - Iatrogenic (e.g. difficult intubations, double lumen tube insertions).
  - Knife injuries and gunshots.
- Thermal injury.

Special considerations
- Direct trauma to airway is rare (<1%).
- 70–80% of patients with airway injury die before reaching hospital.
- Blunt thoracic trauma has higher mortality than penetrating trauma.
- 80% tears in blunt thoracic trauma are within 2.5 cm of carina.
- Repair of low tracheal tears may require mediastinal sternotomy or thoracotomy.
- Cricoid cartilage injury associated in 15% of airway trauma:
  - 25% have recurrent laryngeal nerve palsy.
- Air embolism:
  - Pulmonary vein laceration may lead to left-sided (systemic) air embolism.
  - Systemic embolism may present with haemoptysis, coronary and cerebral dysfunction, air in retinal vessels and in arterial sample.

Further reading

Karmy-Jones, R., Wood, D.E. (2007). Traumatic injury to the trachea and bronchus. *Thoracic Surgical Clinics*, **17**, 35–46.

Schneider, T., Storz, K., Dienemann, H., Hoffmann, H. (2007). *Annals of Thoracic Surgery*, **6**, 1960–4.

Welter, S. (2014). Repair of trachea-bronchial injuries. *Thoracic Surgery Clinics*, **1**, 41–50.

⊙ Bronchopleural fistula (BPF)

Definition

Abnormal communication between bronchial tree and pleural cavity.

Presentation

Diagnosis usually made clinically:
- **Symptoms**: dyspnoea, cough, fever +/− haemoptysis.
- **Signs**: subcutaneous emphysema, contralateral deviation of the trachea, large air leak through intercostal drain, tension pneumothorax.
- Severity of symptoms relates to the size of the fistula.

Immediate management

☑ Oxygen by mask.
☑ Antibiotics to treat infection secondary to soiling of lung.
☑ Insert chest drain (prior to induction) to drain any pus.

Anaesthetic management

☑ Prevent soiling of unaffected lung:
  - Position patient head up.
  - Semi-sitting.
  - Lateral tilt (good lung uppermost).
☑ Control distribution of ventilation:
  - IPPV can cause large air leaks that contribute to the development of tension pneumothorax, ↑ pulmonary shunt and impaired face mask/alveolar ventilation.
  - Minimize airway pressures during IPPV using pressure-controlled ventilation.
☑ Isolate the unaffected lung (➋ see 'Special considerations', p. 226):
  - insertion of a DLT under FOB guidance.
  - DLT intubates the healthy bronchus.
  - Clamp side of BPF.
  - Suction frequently down tracheal lumen to remove pus.

Surgical management

- BPFs are associated with significant morbidity and mortality and almost always require surgical intervention, especially large leaks.
- Small leaks (<5 mm) can be managed by various endoscopic treatments including fibrin glue, endobronchial valves, or bronchial stents.

Subsequent management

☑ Attempt to extubate as soon as possible postprocedure.
☑ If postoperative ventilation required, minimize airway pressures and PEEP.
☑ Transfer to critical care environment as patients commonly have preoperative comorbidities and have associated significant postoperative mortality.

Investigations
- Bloods: Hb, ABG, cross-match 2 units (usually minimal blood loss but can be high).
- CXR: shows falling fluid level in postpneumonectomy space.
- Bronchoscopic examination.
- Sinograms: contrast used to identify and map pathway of fistula.
- Methylene blue: injected into pleural space, positive finding if retrieved in sputum.

Risk factors
- Most frequent following lung resection, greatest incidence following pneumonectomy (stump dehiscence).
- Postpneumonectomy BPF is more common with preoperative infection and postchemotherapy.
- Erosion of bronchus by carcinoma or chronic inflammation.
- Rupture of lung abscess, bronchus, bulla, cyst into pleural space.

Exclusions
Bronchopneumonia: cough, fever, dyspnoea, hypoxia, ± haemoptysis.

Paediatric implications
- Smallest DLT available is 28 Fr, not suitable for children <30 kg.
- Single lumen ETT with 'built in' bronchial blocker available from 5.5 mm ID.
- Using a small paediatric fibreoptic bronchoscope (3.4 mm), the smallest bronchial blocker (5 Fr) can fit through a 4.5 mm ID ETT.

Special considerations
- Isolation and prevention of soiling of the unaffected lung is central to the anaesthetic management and can be achieved in a number of ways:
- ☑ Awake fibreoptic intubation with a SLT or DLT or BB
  - induction of GA once lung isolation complete.
- ☑ Rapid IV induction
  - FOB guided endobronchial intubation with DLT, or
  - SLT placed endobronchially (if postpneumonectomy).
- ☑ Inhalational induction
  - maintains spontaneous ventilation.
  - avoids IPPV until lung isolation has occurred.
  - difficult to carry out safely.
- ☑ BB should be considered if unable to pass DLT.

If DLT insertion unsuccessful or problematic in the presence of a **major** air leak, then consider the following:
- ☑ Isolate and ventilate 'good lung' using uncut SLT (6 mm) over FOB
  - control air leak by passing 'Arndt' bronchial blocker (guided by FOB) or Fogarty embolectomy catheter into the fistula.
  - this will only act as a holding measure.

Further reading

Gothard, J.W.W. (2008). Principles and practice of thoracic anaesthesia. *Anaesthesia and Intensive Care Medicine*, **12**, 545–9.

Hammer, G., Fitzmaurice, B., Brodsky, J. (1999). Methods for single lung ventilation in pediatric patients. *Anesthesia and Analgesia*, **89**, 1426–9.

Kozian, A., Schilling, T., Strang, C., Hachenberg, T. (2006). Anesthetic considerations in patients with previous thoracic surgery. *Current Opinions in Anaesthesiology*, **19**, 26–33.

☼ Hypoxia during one-lung ventilation (OLV)

Definition
Oxygen saturation <90% during OLV.

Presentation
- Usually gradual decrease in S_pO_2 following change from two-lung ventilation to one lung.
- Usually develops over 3–10 min, then gradually improves.

Immediate management
- ☑ Increase F_iO_2 to 100%.
- ☑ Check DLT patency and position—both clinically and with fibrescope.
- ☑ Adjust tidal volume to 7–8 mL/kg or inflation pressure to 30 cmH₂O.
- ☑ Suction to the dependent lung to remove mucus, blood, or pus.
- ☑ Manual inflation of the dependent lung to assess compliance and to expand areas of collapse.
- ☑ Auscultate lower lung for added sounds.
- ☑ Ensure adequate cardiac output (for a given shunt fraction, a fall in cardiac output leads to lower arterial oxygen partial pressures).
- ☑ Insufflation of 1–2 L/min oxygen through catheter in tracheal limb.
- ☑ CPAP of 5–10 cmH₂O with 100% oxygen to the non-dependent lung is highly effective and may be acceptable to the surgeon.
- ☑ Try PEEP 5 cmH₂O to the dependent lung, but may be ineffective or worsen situation (by increasing PVR).
- ☑ Re-inflate operative, non-dependent lung with 100% oxygen following discussion with the surgeon (particularly if saturations sustained at <85–90%).
- ☑ Clamping the pulmonary artery will eliminate the shunt to the operative lung (consider during pneumonectomy).
- ☑ May need to revert to two-lung ventilation if hypoxia persists.

Subsequent management
- ☑ Surgery may need to continue with intermittent two-lung ventilation.
- ☑ Switching from inhalational to intravenous anaesthesia may help to preserve hypoxic pulmonary vasoconstriction—consider when all else fails, but beware of falling cardiac output during changeover.
  - IV almitrine (4–12 µg/kg/min), a pulmonary vasoconstrictor, has been effective in small studies but is not available in the uk.
  - Nitric oxide to the lower lung has usually little or no beneficial effect.

Investigations
ABGs, fibreoptic bronchoscopy

Risk factors

- Arterial oxygen tension always dips following institution of OLV, but O_2 saturation <90% occurs in only 5–10% patients.
- Young may be more susceptible than elderly.
- Best predictor is P_aO_2 when ventilating both lungs.

Exclusions/Causes

- Malposition of DLT, malfunction of DLT or the bronchial cuff (cuff herniation).
- Soiling of the dependent lung with sputum, mucus, or blood.
- Breathing circuit dysfunction:
  - kinks in the circuit.
  - incorrect application of clamp to 'Y' connector.
  - obstruction within the breathing circuit.
- Bronchospasm, anaphylaxis.

Re-inflating the non-dependent lung

☑ Use 100% oxygen.
☑ Suction using catheter provided with the DLT to remove any blood or secretions before re-inflation.
☑ Re-inflate using high sustained CPAP (35–40 cmH_2O) to expand areas of atelectasis under direct surgical vision.
☑ May return to original two-lung ventilation settings (care if extensive lung resection).
☑ Maintain normocapnia.
☑ May need to return to OLV if complications occur (e.g. large air leak from operative lung).

Further reading

Eastwood, J., Mahajan, R. (2002). One-lung anaesthesia. *British Journal of Anaesthesia CEPD Reviews*, **2**, 83–7.
Karzai, W., Schwarzkopf, K. (2009). Hypoxia during OLV: prediction, prevention and treatment. *Anesthesiology*, **110**, 1402–11.

⚙ Sudden high airway pressure during OLV

Definition
Peak airway pressure >30 cmH$_2$O on OLV with tidal volumes of 7–8 mL/kg.

Presentation
Airway pressure >30 cmH$_2$O during OLV with volume-controlled ventilation.

Immediate management
☑ 100% O$_2$ if S$_a$O$_2$ <90%.
☑ Check delivered tidal volume only 7–8 mL/kg.
☑ Switch to manual ventilation to assess compliance and to exclude dynamic hyperinflation (➲ see p. 234).
☑ Auscultate dependent lung for wheeze.
☑ Treat bronchospasm appropriately (➲ see p. 70).
☑ Inspect DLT and connector for obvious kinks or obstruction to gas flow and ensure the DLT is at an appropriate distance at the teeth (➲ see p. 242).
☑ Check positioning of DLT with fibrescope, particularly in relation to RUL, and rule out cuff herniation.
☑ Ensure the clamp is applied to the appropriate limb of the 'Y' connector and the correct lumen is open to the atmosphere.
☑ Suction, using catheter provided with DLT, to remove particulate matter within the DLT. Ask the surgeon to evaluate the dependent lung space under direct vision.
☑ If the problem is serious, consider going to two-lung ventilation to regain control.
☑ Surgery may need to continue on two-lung ventilation (discuss with surgeon).

Subsequent management
☑ Continue high F$_I$O$_2$ as required.
☑ Treat pneumothorax (➲ p. 66), bronchospasm (➲ p. 70), and suspected anaphylaxis (➲ p. 272) appropriately.
☑ Always check position of DLT with fibrescope following any change in patient position or ventilatory dynamics.
☑ Pulmonary oedema may be treated with postoperative IPPV, diuretics, nitrates, inotropes (➲ p. 68). Consider CVP/PAP monitoring.

Investigations
Fibreoptic bronchoscopy.

Risk factors

- The severity of underlying disease in the dependent lung will affect the peak airway pressure following institution of OLV.
- Surgical handling may displace tube.

Exclusions

- Malposition of DLT (especially right DLT).
- Obstruction within the DLT by sputum, blood.
- Clamp incorrectly applied to 'Y' connector.
- Dynamic hyperinflation (➔ p. 234).
- Pneumothorax of the dependent lung (➔ p. 232).
- Bronchospasm in dependent lung (➔ p. 70).
- Anaphylaxis (➔ p. 272).
- Cardiogenic pulmonary oedema (➔ p. 68).
- FB (➔ p. 219).

Special considerations

- Consider the use of pressure-controlled ventilation during one-lung anaesthesia to prevent exposure to high peak airway pressures.
- Airway pressures above 40 cmH$_2$O have been associated with postpneumonectomy pulmonary oedema.
- In ARDS, consider ventilation strategies to limit tidal volume and accept hypercapnia.

Further reading

Klein, U., Karzai, W., Bloos, F., et al. (1998). Role of fibreoptic bronchoscopy in conjunction with the use of double-lumen tubes for thoracic anesthesia. *Anesthesiology*, **88**, 346–50.

Moloney, E.D., Griffiths, M.J.D. (2004). Protective ventilation of patients with acute respiratory distress syndrome. *British Journal of Anaesthesia*, **92**, 261–70.

☹ Pneumothorax of dependent lung during OLV

Definition
Pneumothorax of ventilated 'good lung' during OLV.

Presentation
- Decreased S_aO_2, BP, ETCO$_2$, increased P_{aw}, cyanosis, bradycardia.
- Decreased breath sounds on auscultation.

Immediate management
☑ Stop N_2O if used and increase F_iO_2 to 100%.
☑ Ventilate both lungs gently to assess compliance and improve oxygenation.
☑ If during thoracotomy, ask surgeon to evaluate dependent pleural space and decompress tension pneumothorax without having to return patient supine.
☑ If during VATS, consider rapid needle decompression (second intercostal space mid-clavicular line).
☑ If tension:
  • turn patient supine.
  • place chest drain.

Subsequent management
☑ Formal chest drain insertion.
☑ CXR on table or in recovery/HDU.
☑ Insert arterial line if not *in situ*—check ABGs.
☑ Consider HDU post-op.
☑ Aim to return to spontaneous ventilation as soon as possible post-op.

Investigations
Clinical diagnosis, consider on-table CXR.

Risk factors
- High ventilatory pressures.
- Connective tissue disorders.
- Long procedures.
- Incidence unknown, but risk is greater if bullous disease of non-operative side.

Exclusions
- Dynamic hyperinflation (➲ p. 234).
- Bronchospasm, anaphylaxis (➲ p 70, 272).
- Obstruction to expiratory gas flow.

Special considerations
Consider advisability of continuing with planned surgery (particularly major lung resection) if a critical stage not yet reached.

☉ Dynamic hyperinflation (DHI)

Definition
Pulmonary gas trapping can occur in patients with lungs that have ↓ elastic recoil combined with expiratory flow limitation (e.g. COPD).
IPPV can exacerbate pulmonary gas trapping when expiratory flow time is longer than time allowed for exhalation; producing DHI.

Presentation
- Awake patients with hyperinflation complain of dyspnoea, limited exercise tolerance, and a reduction in functional and physical abilities.
- DHI under anaesthesia can present as ↑P_{aw}, ↑JVP/CVP, ↓BP and ↓S_pO_2, pulsus paradoxus, and a slow rising capnography trace.

Immediate management
☑ Increase F_iO_2 to 100%.
☑ **Disconnect patient from ventilator and breathing circuit**.
  - Clinical improvement (i.e. ↑S_pO_2, ↑BP, and ↓HR) following disconnection is pathognomonic of DHI (or tension pneumothorax).
  - Improvement is rapid.
☑ Vaso-active medication to support circulation.
☑ Listen to the end of disconnected ET tube (long expiration time).
☑ Discontinue N_2O if in use.
☑ Limit tidal volumes V_t to 7–8 mL/kg.
☑ Accept hypercarbia (≤8.5 kPa [64 mmHg]).
☑ Limit inspiratory pressure to ≤20 cmH_2O. Consider pressure control mode.
☑ ↑Expiratory phase (I:E ratio 1:4).
☑ Optimize bronchodilator therapy.

Subsequent management
- Arterial line, monitor ABGs (especially P_aCO_2).
- Aim to return to spontaneous ventilation ASAP.
- Consider HDU post-op.

Investigations
Audible prolonged expiration at open end of ET tube.

Risk factors
- Parenchymal pathology causing ↓elastic recoil.
- Dysfunctional airways with expiratory flow limitation.
- Inappropriate mechanical ventilation settings (↑↑Vt, ↑↑ inflation pressures).

Exclusions
- Bronchospasm (Ð p. 70).
- Tension pneumothorax of dependent lung (Ð p. 232).
- Distension of bulla in dependent lung.
- Malposition of DLT (Ð p. 242).

Special considerations

- The use of PEEP in mechanically ventilated patients with COPD should be avoided:
  - risk of air-trapping.
  - correct expiratory PEEP target difficult to define.
  - limited evidence of benefit.

Further reading

Conacher, I.D. (1998). Dynamic hyperinflation—the anaesthetist applying a tourniquet to the right side of the heart. *British Journal of Anaesthesia*, **81**, 116–17.

Gagnon, P., Guenette, J.A., Langer, D., et al. (2014). Pathogenesis of hyperinflation in chronic obstructive pulmonary disease. *International Journal of Chronic Obstructive Pulmonary Disease*, **9**, 187–201.

:☼: Cardiac herniation postpneumonectomy

Definition
- A rare complication of intrapericardial pneumonectomy.
- Herniation of the heart occurs typically when surgically created pericardial defect is not closed.

Presentation
- Symptoms and signs depend on side of herniation.
- 75% present in immediate postoperative period and all within 24 h.
- Right-sided herniations occur more often.
- Usually dramatic symptoms/signs, but may occur with little initial disturbance:

Right-sided
- **'Superior vena cava syndrome'**—distension of neck veins due to kinking of SVC.
- ↓ right ventricular filling causing ↓BP, ↑HR and shock.

Left-sided
- **'Strangulation of left ventricle'**—arrhythmias, cardiac ischaemia.
- Impaired left ventricular performance with profound hypotension.

Immediate management
- ☑ 100% oxygen by facemask.
- ☑ Turn patient so that non-operative lung is dependent.
- ☑ Alert surgeons.
- ☑ Keep chest drain (if present) clamped.
- ☑ Insert arterial line (if not present).
- ☑ Vasoactive medication immediately available.
- ☑ Intubate if patient collapsed.
- ☑ Organize immediate transfer to theatre.

Anaesthetic management
- ☑ Continue spontaneous ventilation for as long as possible.
- ☑ Consider CVP line (if not present).
- ☑ Induction in semi-lateral position, non-operative side dependent.
- ☑ Single lumen tube.
- ☑ Arterial monitoring during induction.
- ☑ Pressure-controlled ventilation to limit pressure on bronchial stump.
- ☑ Start inotropes as required.

Surgical management
- ☑ Treatment for cardiac herniation is surgical:
  - repositioning of heart.
  - placement of patch over defect.

Subsequent management

☑ Extubate as soon as safe to do so.
☑ LV dysfunction due to ischaemia, oedema, or infarction may persist.
☑ May require postop IPPV ± inotropes in critical care environment.
☑ Surgical repair of defect should prevent recurrence.

Investigations

- CXR: distorted cardiac shadow.
- ECG: findings non-specific.
- Echo: to exclude other cardiac causes of sudden postop shock.
- CT: impractical in emergency setting.

Risk factors

- Pneumonectomy:
  - when intrapericardial ligation of great vessels required, leaving pericardial defect.
  - heart can herniate through breakdown of pericardial patch.
- Other contributing factors:
  - ↑ intrathoracic pressure (e.g. coughing).
  - positive pressure ventilation.
  - rapid lung re-expansion.
  - suction on chest drain.
  - patient position change (operative side becomes dependent).

Exclusions

- Bleeding (haemorrhage, cardiac tamponade) (➔ pp. 38, 418).
- Myocardial ischaemia/infarction (➔ p. 35).
- Primary arrhythmia (➔ p. 25, 27).
- Acute mediastinal shift.
- PE (➔ p. 41).

Paediatric implications

- Cardiac herniation can occur spontaneously through congenital pericardial defects.

Special considerations

- 100% mortality if unrecognized.
- 50% mortality when recognized and treated promptly.

Further reading

Chambers, N., Walton, S., Pearce, A. (2005). Cardiac herniation following pneumonectomy—an old complication revisited. *Anaesthesia and Intensive Care*, **33**, 403–9.

Kawamukai, K., Antonacci, F., Di Saverioa, S., Boaron, M. (2011). Acute postoperative cardiac herniation. *Interactive Cardiovascular and Thoracic Surgery*, **12**, 73–4.

Ponten, J.E.H., Elenbaas, T.W.O., Woorst, J.F.T., Korsten, E.H.M., Van der Borne, B.E.E.M., Van Strath, A.H.M. (2012). Cardiac herniation after operative management of lung cancer. A rare and dangerous complication. *General Thoracic and Cardiovascular Surgery*, **60**, 668–72.

☠ Major airway bleeding

Definition
Haemorrhage from tracheobronchial tree.
- **Massive haemoptysis**: >600 mL in 24 h.
- **Exsanguinating haemoptysis**: >1000 mL or bleeding rate >150 mL/h.
- **Catastrophic haemoptysis**: major bleed from airway causing immediate threat to life requiring immediate surgery.

Presentation
- Acute haemoptysis.
- Bleeding at bronchoscopy.
- Cough, hypoxia, tachypnoea, cardiovascular instability.

Mortality due to haemoptysis is related to rate of bleeding.

Immediate management
☑ 100% O_2.
☑ Turn patient good lung up.

Anaesthetic management
☑ Tracheal intubation and suction to remove blood and clots.
☑ Insert arterial line, ensure large-bore IV access.
☑ Proceed to rigid bronchoscopy in theatre.

Surgical management
If catastrophic bleeding occurs at bronchoscopy:
☑ Do not remove rigid bronchoscope.
☑ Advance and wedge bronchoscope into bleeding bronchus to partially tamponade.
☑ Suction under direct vision.
☑ Pass balloon tip vascular catheter/bronchial blocker beyond bleeding focus.
☑ Withdraw bronchoscope and balloon slowly until bleeding source seen.
☑ Inflate balloon—assess extent of bleeding with suctioning.

Subsequent management
☑ Following initial resuscitation, individuals should be re-assessed for:
  - rate of bleeding.
  - detection and correction of any clotting derangement (e.g. FFP, platelets, or cryoprecipitate).
  - comorbidities.
  - lung function.
☑ Bleeding cavitating lesions (such as aspergillomas) will need pulmonary resection and possibly pneumonectomy.
  - External radiation, bronchial artery embolization and laser (YAG) application are unsuitable in catastrophic haemoptysis.

- Bronchial irrigation with iced saline, vasoconstrictors, or coagulants not suitable with heavy bleeding due to dilution.
- Gauze packed in the airway can become mobile and cause bronchial obstruction.

Investigations

- Bloods: Hb, serial haematocrit, cross-match 4–6 units.
- CXR.
- Bronchoscopy.

Risk factors

- Biopsy at bronchoscopy.
- Tracheobronchial tumour/trauma.
- Bleeding disorder.
- Aspergilloma.

Special considerations

- Consider double lumen tube if:
  - known unilateral disease.
  - unilateral trauma.
  - thoracotomy required.
- Double lumen tube placement as an initial life-saving measure may worsen clinical situation:
  - difficulties in correct placement.
  - lumens blocked by blood.
  - risk of displacement.
  - loss of lung isolation.
- Mortality following massive haemoptysis predominantly caused by asphyxiation rather than exsanguination—blood floods the alveoli leading to irreversible hypoxia.

Further reading

Maguire, M.F., Berry, C.B., Gellett, L., Berrisford, R.G. (2004). Catastrophic haemoptysis during rigid bronchoscopy: a discussion of treatment options to salvage patients during catastrophic haemoptysis at rigid bronchoscopy. *Interactive Cardiovascular and Thoracic Surgery*, **3**, 222–5.

:Ο: **Bleeding during mediastinoscopy**

Definition
- Haemorrhage during mediastinoscopy.
- Mediastinoscopy is the passage of an endoscope into the mediastinum through an incision above the sternal notch. The procedure allows inspection and biopsies of mediastinal masses and lymph nodes.

Presentation
- Large mediastinal vessels—arterial or venous—may be damaged during procedure leading to torrential haemorrhage (e.g. brachiocephalic artery tear).
- Major venous bleeding associated with superior vena cava obstruction.

Immediate management
- ☑ Monitor heart rate and measure BP every 2.5 min.
- ☑ Non-invasive BP should be taken in both arms.
- ☑ Obtain large-bore access in **lower limb** (fluids given through IV line in the arm may enter the mediastinum through tear in large mediastinal vessel).
- ☑ Cross-match 4 units.
- ☑ Consider activating Major Haemorrhage protocol.
- ☑ Prepare rapid infuser/fluid warmer.
- ☑ Consider cell salvage.
- ☑ Site arterial line in **left radial artery**, as endoscope may compress innominate artery—giving false low readings in right radial artery.

Surgical management
- ☑ Pack wound and wait 10 min (consider digital compression).
- ☑ An emergency thoracotomy or median sternotomy may be required to control bleeding.

Anaesthetic management
- ☑ Keep single lumen tube in place.
- ☑ Position patient appropriately.
- ☑ If OLV preferable: use bronchial blocker or advance tube into bronchus with fibrescope.

Subsequent management
Airway can become compromised by external tracheal compression.
- ☑ Consider continued intubation post-op and transfer to ITU.

Investigations
- FBC, coagulation, cross-match 4 units.
- CXR: all patients in the immediate postoperative period.

Risk factors
- Aberrant blood vessel in front of trachea.
- Grossly abnormal mediastinal anatomy.
- SVC obstruction.

Special considerations

- Haemorrhage associated with 0.73% of mediastinoscopies.
- Carotid artery perfusion may be compromised by vascular compression or damage by endoscope leading to impaired cerebral blood flow.
- Mediastinoscopy morbidity rate 1.5–3.0%, mortality 0.09%.
- Profound, persistent bleeding may need cardiopulmonary bypass (rare).

Further reading

Minowa, M., Chida, M., Eba, S., Matsumura, Y. (2011). Pulmonary artery injury during mediastinoscopy controlled without gauze packing. *Journal of Cardiothoracic Surgery*, 6, 15–17.

Park, B.J., Flores, R., Downey, R.J., Bains, M.S., Rusch, V.W. (2003). Management of major hemorrhage during mediastinoscopy. *Journal of Thoracic and Cardiovascular Surgery*, **126**, 726–31.

⑦ Double-lumen tubes (DLT)

Indications for DLT
- Pulmonary surgery.
- Avoid contamination of lung secondary to infection, haemorrhage, bronchopulmonary lavage.
- Control distribution of ventilation if large air leaks or unilateral lung disease (e.g. giant bullae, lung cysts).

DLT
- Broncho Cath single-use PVC:
  - 28–41 Fr, low-pressure, high-volume cuff.
  - transparent with coloured endobronchial cuff for fibreoptic recognition.
  - right-sided tubes have a slot for ventilation of RUL.
- Robertshaw:
  - small, medium, or large, red-rubber, reusable.
  - high-pressure, low-volume cuff.

Pre-insertion checks
- What size?
  - ☑ Use largest DLT that passes without difficulty through the glottis.
  - ☑ 39–41 Fr Broncho Cath for males (large or medium Robertshaw).
  - ☑ 35–37 Fr for females (medium or small Robertshaw).
- Which side?
  - ☑ Left-sided DLT usually used. Easier to place and avoids problems with right upper lobe orifice (2.5 cm from carina).
  - ☑ Will need right-sided DLT if surgery on left main-stem bronchus.
- Cuffs and connectors:
  - ☑ Check both bronchial and tracheal cuffs and connectors prior to insertion.

Insertion of DLT
- ☑ Insert DLT initially with concavity facing anteriorly.
- ☑ Once tip is past the glottis, withdraw the stylet and rotate tube through 90° in direction of the bronchus to be intubated.
- ☑ To aid endobronchial intubation, rotate the patient's head to the side opposite the bronchus to be intubated.
- ☑ Advance the tube gently.
- ☑ Height determines depth of insertion. Usually 29 cm at the teeth in men, 27 cm in women.
  - Depth increases or decreases by 1 cm for each 10 cm in height above or below 170 cm.
- ☑ Inflate the tracheal cuff and confirm ventilation of the lungs.
- ☑ Inflate bronchial cuff slowly (usually <3–4 mL air).

Checking position of DLT

Clinical confirmation

☑ Inflate tracheal cuff.
☑ Check ventilation via bronchial lumen.
☑ Clamp flow to tracheal lumen and open tracheal lumen to air.
☑ Inspect for correct unilateral chest movement (be aware of pre-op pathology) and confirm air entry to all lobes by auscultation.
☑ Check for leaks around the bronchial cuff.
☑ Inflate bronchial cuff slowly to abolish leak. If >4 mL air required, then DLT position incorrect, or incorrect size for the patient (care with cuff volume, bronchial rupture reported).
☑ Check ventilation of contralateral lung by reconnecting tracheal limb and switching clamp to bronchial limb. Open bronchial lumen, and check selective ventilation by inspection and auscultation.

Fibreoptic confirmation

('Gold standard' for checking placement of DLT.)

☑ Pass scope via tracheal lumen, visualize carina, and open main bronchus.
☑ Superior surface of the bronchial cuff should be visible at the carina.
☑ Ensure no bronchial cuff herniation into lower trachea.
☑ Pass scope down endobronchial limb of right-sided DLT to check correct positioning of 'slit' opposite RUL orifice.
☑ Scope can also be used to 'railroad' the DLT into the appropriate main bronchus if placement is difficult.

Paediatric implications

- Smallest available DLT is 28 Fr and is unsuitable for patients under 30 kg.
- BB are available that pass through 3.5 mm ID ETT.
- Single lumen ETT with 'built in' bronchial blocker available from 5.5 mm ID.

Special considerations

- Position of DLT should always be checked following repositioning of patient or if difficulty with ventilation and oxygenation.
- Recommendations to avoid DLT-induced tracheobronchial injury are to inflate cuffs slowly, limit intracuff pressure to <30 cmH2O, avoid N_2O, deflate endobronchial cuff when not needed, on turning patient, and repositioning the DLT.
- Olympus LF-DP fibrescope (external diameter 3.1 mm) goes down all DLTs. Standard intubating fibrescope (ED 4.0 mm) is a tight fit down 37 Fr and may not fit down 35 Fr.

Further reading

Campos, J.H. (2007). Which device should be considered the best for lung isolation: double-lumen tube versus bronchial blockers. *Current Opinion in Anaesthesiology*, **20**, 27–31.

⑦ Bronchial blockers (BB)

Definition
Balloon-tipped luminal catheters that occlude the operative side bronchus.

Indications for use
Inability to place DLT, distorted anatomy, difficult intubation, tracheostomy, patient <30 kg, limited mouth opening, ITU patient already intubated, planned postoperative ventilation.

Function
Block main-stem bronchus or segmental bronchi to facilitate single lung ventilation or selective lobar blockade.

Types
• Wire-guided bronchial blocker (Arndt).
• Single lumen ETT with enclosed bronchial blocker (Univent).
• Fogarty embolectomy catheter.

'Arndt' wire-guided endobronchial blocker
• 7 Fr (use 7.0 mm ETT) or 9 Fr catheter (use at least 8.0 mm ETT).
• 65 or 78 cm in length.
• Inner lumen 1.4 mm diameter.
• Inner lumen contains flexible nylon wire, exits as a small flexible wire loop.
• Advantages:
  • passes through nasotracheal tube.
  • use if tracheostomy *in situ*.
  • can be used as selective lobar blocker.
  • allows CPAP through inner channel.
  • useful if anticipated or actual difficult intubation with DLT.
  • guided directly into position with fibrescope.
  • high-volume, low-pressure cuff.
• Disadvantages:
  • difficult to pass if ETT <7.0 mm internal diameter.
  • wire cannot be re-inserted once removed (repositioning difficult).
  • small suction channel (increased time to lung collapse when compared with DLT).
  • takes longer to place than DLT.
• Placement:
  • passes through single lumen ETT.
  • attach 'Arndt multiport' adaptor and maintain ventilation.
  • lubricate the distal part of the blocker.
  • fully deflate balloon to prevent damage.
  • insert blocker through port.
  • insert FOB through port and place FOB through loop on the blocker.
  • pass FOB into appropriate bronchus.
  • slide blocker down over FOB into bronchus.
  • advance far enough so that deflated cuff is within bronchus.
  • withdraw FOB into trachea and check blocker position.

- inflate balloon (5–8 mL air for bronchial blockade).
- once position confirmed with FOB, remove wire loop.
- Complications:
  - malposition (reported as more frequent than with Univent).
  - prone to dislodgement when moving to lateral position.
  - balloon shearing has been reported when withdrawn through multiport. Withdraw blocker along with multiport connector and not through unlocked blocker port.

'Univent' endobronchial blocker

- Single lumen tube, sizes from 3.5 to 9.0 mm ID.
- Tube incorporates a channel enclosing a moveable bronchial blocker.
- Advantages:
  - can block right, left, or any specific secondary bronchi.
  - non-latex, small lumen for suctioning and oxygenation.
- Disadvantages:
  - bronchial rupture reported, high-pressure, low-volume cuff.
- Placement:
  - lubricate bronchial blocker.
  - retract blocker into standard lumen of ETT.
  - place tube in trachea and insert FOB.
  - advance BB into appropriate bronchus under FOB vision.
  - inflate cuff of blocker and listen for leaks.
  - outer surface of cuff should be just below carina.
  - end of Univent tube should be at least 1–2 cm above tracheal carina.
- Complications:
  - failure to achieve lung separation (no seal, abnormal anatomy).
  - inclusion of blocker in stapling line (communication with surgeon!)
  - prolonged suctioning to facilitate lung collapse can cause pulmonary oedema (use low pressure for just a few seconds).
  - lung rupture has been reported (blind insertion).
  - malposition and displacement when turning patient.

Fogarty embolectomy catheter

- Least commonly used, minimal literature to support use.
- 80 cm length, 0.5–10 mL air to achieve occlusion of bronchus.
- Passed down ETT or as a separate device external to ETT.
- Positioned in appropriate bronchus under vision with FOB or via rigid bronchoscope.
- Ideal position is with superior surface of cuff 10 mm distal to carina.
- Advantages:
  - can be passed through single lumen ETT.
  - used for selective lobar blockade.
  - can be used with tracheostomy.
  - can be used nasally.
- Disadvantages:
  - high-pressure, low-volume cuff.
  - vascular device, not designed for bronchial blockade.
  - made of natural rubber latex.
  - cannot suction or oxygenate.
  - cannot be coupled with FOB placement.

- Complications:
  - minimal use, so no complications reported, risk of airway rupture, but very soft catheter.
  - inclusion in stapling line if used for selective lobar blockade.

Further reading

Campos, J.H. (2003). An update on bronchial blockers during lung separation techniques in adults. *Anesthesia and Analgesia*, **97**, 1266–74.

Hammer, B., Fitzmaurice, B.G., Brodsky, J.B. (1999). Methods for single lung ventilation in pediatric patients. *Anesthesia and Analgesia*, **89**, 1426–9.

Regional anaesthesia

Owen Davies

☼ Local anaesthetic toxicity

Definition
Toxicity due to excessive local anaesthetic blood levels.

Presentation
- CNS symptoms are often subtle or absent. Cardiovascular collapse may be the first sign toxicity has occurred.
- Light headedness, dizziness, drowsiness. Tingling around lips, fingers, or generalized. Metallic taste, tinnitus, blurred vision.
- Confusion, restlessness, incoherent speech, tremors, or twitching, leading to full-blown convulsions with loss of consciousness and coma.
- Bradycardia, hypotension, cardiovascular collapse, and respiratory arrest.
- ECG changes (prolongation of QRS and PR interval, AV block, and/or changes in T-wave amplitude).

Immediate management
- ☑ Discontinue injection.
- ☑ Immediately re-inflate tourniquet, if performing intravenous regional anaesthesia, to minimize LA entering circulation.
- ☑ ABC—100% O_2.
- ☑ Treat convulsions with IV midazolam (3–10 mg), diazepam (5–15 mg), lorazepam (0.1 mg/kg) or thiopental (50–150 mg). Titrate against patient response. Avoid propofol if cardiovascularly unstable.
- ☑ Intubate and ventilate if required to prevent hypoxic cardiovascular collapse. Hyperventilation may help by increasing pH in the presence of metabolic acidosis.
- ☑ CPR if pulseless—commence ALS protocol (⊙ see p. 13).
- ☑ Commence lipid emulsion therapy. Initial bolus of 1.5 mL/kg of 20% Intralipid® over 1 min. Then commence infusion.
- ☑ Consider cardiopulmonary bypass if available.

Lipid emulsion therapy
- ☑ Give an intravenous bolus injection of Intralipid® 20% 1.5 mL/kg over 1 min (100 mL for a 70 kg patient).
- ☑ Start an intravenous infusion of Intralipid® 20% at 15 mL/kg/h (1000 mL/h for a 70 kg patient).
- ☑ Repeat initial bolus twice at 5 min intervals if an adequate circulation has not been restored.
- ☑ Up to three boluses including initial bolus dose may be given.
- ☑ After 5 min, double the infusion rate if an adequate circulation has not been restored.
- ☑ Do not exceed a maximum of 12 mL/kg cumulative dose.

☑ Continue CPR and infusion until a stable adequate circulation has been restored.
☑ Recovery from local anaesthetic induced cardiovascular arrest may take >1 h.
☑ Propofol is NOT a suitable alternative to Intralipid® 20% and should be avoided if cardiovascular instability is suspected.

Subsequent management

☑ Simple, short-lived toxicity—observe and then consider if surgery can proceed.
☑ Treat hypotension with small doses of vasopressors— ephedrine, phenylephrine, noradrenaline, or adrenaline.
☑ Admit to ITU if cardiac arrest or complicated reaction has occurred.
☑ Document procedure, event, and management in detail.
☑ Explanation to patient and relatives at the appropriate time.
☑ Exclude pancreatitis by daily clinical review and monitoring amylase, lipase levels for 48 h.
☑ Report findings to National Patient Safety Agency (℘ http://www.npsa.nhs.uk) and to ℘ http://www.lipidrescue.org.

Investigations

• Heparin or EDTA plasma sample for local anaesthetic blood levels.
• If Intralipid® used, also collect blood in plain tube to measure plasma triglyceride concentrations.

Risk factors

• Large volumes/high concentrations of local anaesthetics.
• Location of local anaesthetic injection (e.g. lumbar plexus/intercostal blocks higher risk).
• Failure to aspirate before and during injection.
• Use of agent with narrow therapeutic window, e.g. bupivacaine vs. prilocaine.
• Intravenous regional anaesthesia (IVRA):
  • Premature release of tourniquet during intravenous regional anaesthesia, releasing large dose of local anaesthetic into the circulation. A double-cuff tourniquet should be used.
  • Inappropriate or faulty equipment including gas supply.
  • Swapping cuff inflation to diminish tourniquet pain.
  • Obese patient with large arm, very muscular arm, hypertensive patient.

Exclusions

• Fainting—vasovagal episodes are common. If cerebral anoxia occurs, convulsions may result.
• 'Acute anxiety' reaction sometimes associated with adrenaline-containing solutions.
• Epilepsy.
• Allergic reaction to LA (rare) or other drugs administered.
• Anaphylaxis.

Paediatric implications

- Since most regional blocks are carried out in anaesthetized children, many of the early warning signs of toxicity are masked. CVS collapse may be the first sign.
- Ensure dose and concentration are appropriate for size.
- Small children are more prone to methaemoglobinaemia than adults.

Special considerations

- All clinical areas where local and regional anaesthetic blockade is practised should have equipment and protocols for treating systemic toxicity from local anaesthetic drugs.
- Incidence of significant local anaesthetic toxicity is between 10–20/10 000 for peripheral nerve blocks and 4/10 000 for epidurals.
- Table 9.1 lists the maximum doses of some LAs.
- Bupivacaine binds to myocardial ion channels and may result in prolonged cardiac arrest.
- Allergic reactions to local anaesthetics are extremely rare. The ester groups are more prone to exhibit allergic reactions than amides because they are metabolized to para-aminobenzoic acid (PABA), which acts as a hapten. There is also a cross-sensitivity of ester LAs with sulphonamides. Allergic reactions range from simple local irritation, rash, or urticaria, to laryngeal oedema or anaphylaxis.
- Some guidelines now advocate the use of low-dose adrenaline boluses (<1 µg/kg) as part of their resuscitation guidelines for systemic local anaesthetic toxicity.

Avoiding toxicity

- Maximum dose varies depending on site to be anaesthetized, vascularity of the tissues, individual tolerance, and anaesthetic technique.
  - ☑ Use smallest dose for required effect.
  - ☑ Consider dose reduction in elderly and those with poor cardiac function.
  - ☑ Inject slowly with regular gentle aspirations, as the side-wall of a small blood vessel is easily sucked on to the needle/catheter.

Table 9.1 Maximum local anaesthetic drug doses

Drug	Max. dose for infiltration (mg/kg)	Max. dose for plexus anaesthesia (mg/kg)
Lidocaine	4	5
Lidocaine with adrenaline	7	7
Bupivacaine	2	2
Bupivacaine with adrenaline	3	
Prilocaine	6	7
Prilocaine with adrenaline/ octapressin	8	8
Ropivacaine	3	3

- Epidurals:
  - ☑ Use a test dose. When giving large volumes, give incrementally and aspirate or allow the catheter to hang below patient level for a few moments (observing for blood or clear fluid).
  - ☑ Inadvertent intrathecal injection of 3 mL 0.5% bupivacaine or lidocaine will be quickly apparent clinically (paraesthesia and decreased sensation in lower limbs and buttocks, depression, or absence of knee jerk reflexes in sedated patients).
  - ☑ Use of adrenaline in the test dose may help to identify an intravascular injection. 3 mL of 1:200 000 (15 µg) adrenaline injected intravenously will cause an increase in heart rate of 20 bpm and systolic blood pressure of 15 mmHg. However, these changes are short-lived and can be missed unless ECG and frequent BP monitoring is employed.
  - ☑ Risk associated with subsequent 'top-ups': the incidence of catheter migration is estimated to be 1 in 255.
- Levobupivacaine and ropivacaine are less toxic than bupivacaine. The higher toxicity of bupivacaine is related to the R-enantiomer which binds more firmly and is released more slowly from the myocardium. Although ropivacaine is less toxic than bupivacaine, in clinical practice, a higher concentration of ropivacaine is required.
- Toxicity from prilocaine is less likely because of its rapid metabolism (primarily by the liver). Methaemoglobinaemia may occur with high doses (>600 mg in an adult) and should be treated with methylthioninium chloride (methylene blue) (1–2 mg/kg).
- Intravenous regional anaesthesia:
  - ☑ Always site a second cannula in contralateral limb before starting the procedure.
  - ☑ Do not remove tourniquet for at least 20 min after injection of local anaesthetic.
  - ☑ Monitor patients undergoing IVRA by talking to them.
  - ☑ Never use bupivacaine for IVRA.

Further reading

American Society of Regional Anesthesia and Pain Medicine (2012). *Checklist for Treatment of Local Anesthetic Systemic Toxicity*. Available at: https://www.asra.com

Association of Anaesthetists of Great Britain and Ireland (2010). *Guidelines for the Management of Severe Local Anaesthetic Toxicity*. Available at: https://anaesthetists.org/Home/Resources-publications/Guidelines

Toledo, P. (2011) The role of lipid emulsion during advanced cardiac life support for local anesthetic toxicity. *International Journal of Obstetric Anaesthesia*, **20**, 60–3.

Weinberg, G.L. (2012). Lipid emulsion infusion. Resuscitation for local anesthetic and other drug overdoses. *Anesthesiology*, **117**, 180–7.

ⓘ Epidural abscess

Definition
Abscess formation in the extradural space.

Presentation
- Classical presentation is of back pain and fever with progressive neurological deficit.
- Four progressive phases of neurological symptoms —spinal ache, root pain with or without paraesthesia, weakness, and bladder/bowel dysfunction, and finally paralysis at or below relevant nerve roots.
- Pyrexia, general feeling of malaise, headache, neck stiffness or meningism, leading to full-blown meningitis.
- Possible evidence of skin infection with localized tenderness and swelling at site of recent needle puncture. However haematogenous spread rather than tracking infection is often the cause.

Immediate management
- ☑ Bloods for culture, FBC, C-reactive protein, ESR, coagulation screen.
- ☑ Document findings of a full neurological examination.
- ☑ Organize an urgent MRI scan and liaise with neurosurgical team.
- ☑ Monitor neurological function regularly to assess deterioration.
- ☑ Discuss timing of antibiotics with surgical team and liaise with local microbiology services.

Subsequent management
- ☑ Neurosurgical opinion, exploration, and decompression combined with prolonged high-dose antibiotic therapy.
- ☑ Surgical decompression via laminectomy is the usual treatment of choice for patients with neurological deficit.
- ☑ Patients with early diagnosis without neurological deficit have been managed with IV antibiotics alone but early multidisciplinary assessment with neurosurgical input is paramount.
- ☑ If surgery can be offered immediately antibiotics may be withheld until after intraoperative culture to maximize the likelihood of isolating the causative organism.
- ☑ Preoperative antibiotics should be commenced in the following circumstances; a significant surgical delay cannot be avoided, a critically ill or septic patient, paralysis, a poor surgical candidate.
- ☑ Carefully documented review of neurological loss/recovery.
- ☑ Outcome worsened by delays in diagnosis and surgery. Adversely affected by the use of steroids.

Investigations
- Frequent neurological observations to assess trend.
- FBC, serial C-reactive protein, ESR, coagulation screen, and blood cultures.
- MRI scan.

Risk factors

- Recent epidural or spinal.
- Time epidural catheter *in situ* (40% increased risk per day).
- Poor sterility. Re-connection of separated filters and frequency of syringe/infusion changes.
- Traumatic procedure with multiple attempts and needle passes.
- General abdominal and thoracic surgery.
- Compromised immunity including diabetes mellitus (20–50% of cases), steroid therapy, malignancy, systemic and localized infection, HIV infection, pregnancy, alcoholism, and cirrhosis.
- Intravenous drug abuse (10–40% of cases) and patients with indwelling vascular catheters.
- Antithrombotic therapy (LMWH or NSAIDs).
- Sources of bloodborne infection include; skin, infected indwelling catheters, respiratory tract, urinary tract, dental abscess, bacterial endocarditis, bacteraemia, or septicaemia.
- Combined factors increase risk considerably.

Exclusions

- Profound but reversible blockade due to excessive LA dose or concentration.
- Epidural haematoma—➔ see p. 255 (epidural abscess has a slower onset, 24–48 h vs. ≤24 h, and is associated with pyrexia and signs of sepsis).
- Malignancy usually has a much slower, insidious onset.

Special considerations

- Maintain vigilant sterility during procedures.
- The use of epidural catheters should be kept to the shortest time required with daily review of necessity.
- The quoted incidence accompanying central neuro-axial block has been reported as 1:47 000 (1:150 000 for the obstetric population).
- High clinical suspicion is required especially as presenting symptoms vary.
- Contrast-enhanced MRI is the gold-standard investigation for confirming a clinical diagnosis of epidural abscess. Epidural abscesses that contain no gas are difficult to diagnose on MRI without contrast enhancement as pus gives a similar image to cerebrospinal fluid. Gadolinium–diethylenetriamine penta-acetic acid (Gd–DTPA) enhances actively inflamed tissue, delineating the abscess cavity more clearly.
- *Staphylococcus aureus* is consistently the most commonly isolated causative organism (50–90% of cases). MRSA is an increasingly prevalent organism.
- TB and Gram-negative organisms may be the causative organism in the immunocompromised, those with a history of intravenous drug use or recent genitourinary tract procedures.
- Permanent neurological damage is likely if surgery is delayed for more than 12 h.
- Often slow neurological recovery, despite surgical decompression of abscess, suggests that local pressure is not the only mechanism.

Ischaemia due to leptomeningeal vessel thrombosis or spinal artery compression is also a major contributing factor.

- Likely outcomes—complete recovery (39%), residual neurological deficit (48%), death (13%). Poor outcome associated with increasing age (risk doubles with every decade of life), degree of thecal sac compression and duration of symptoms.

Further reading

Grewal, S., Hocking, G., Wildsmith, J.A.W. (2006). Epidural abscesses. *British Journal of Anaesthesia*, **96**(3), 292–302.

Shaha, N.H., Roosb, K.L. (2013). Epidural abscess and paralytic mechanisms. *Current Opinion in Neurology*, **26**, 314–17.

The Royal College of Anaesthetists (2009). *National Audit of Major Complications of Central Neuraxial Block in the United Kingdom*. Available at: https://www.rcoa.ac.uk/system/files/CSQ-NAP3-Full_1.pdf

Thompkins, M., Panuncialman, I., Lucas, P., Palumbo, M. (2010). Spinal epidural abscess. *Journal of Emergency Medicine*, **39**, 384–90.

ⓘ Epidural haematoma

Definition
Haematoma in the extradural space.

Presentation
- Unexpected neurological deficit following epidural and severe localized pain at the level of the haematoma.
- Sensory/motor block at or below relevant nerve root distribution. Unilateral or bilateral.
- Spinal cord compression at the level of the epidural haematoma may produce urinary retention or incontinence, faecal incontinence, hemiplegia, or paraplegia.

Immediate management
☑ Discontinue infusion of local anaesthetic.
☑ Optimize systemic blood pressure, avoid hypotension.
☑ Document findings of an immediate, full neurological examination.
☑ Monitor neurological function regularly to assess any deterioration.
☑ Organize an urgent MRI scan and liaise with neurosurgical team.
☑ Restore normal coagulation.
☑ Surgical evacuation of the haematoma. For optimal results surgery should take place within 8 h of diagnosis. Surgery beyond this time has a worse outcome but neurological improvements can still be expected.

Subsequent management
- Neurosurgical monitoring—meticulous documentation is important.

Investigations
- Frequent neurological observations to assess trend.
- FBC, C-reactive protein, ESR, coagulation screen, blood cultures.
- Arrange urgent MRI. If MRI is not available, CT myelography or conventional myelography may reveal a mass.

Risk factors
- Rarely, can occur spontaneously (incidence <1:150 000 people each year).
- Female, old age, history of gastrointestinal bleeding.
- Bleeding disorders or altered bleeding state, including haemophilia, platelet deficiency, pre-eclampsia, sepsis, and syndrome of haemolysis, elevated liver enzymes, and low platelets (HELLP).
- Anticoagulation (e.g. warfarin, LMWH, heparin, dabigatran, and others). Risk enhanced with renal failure for drugs eliminated via this route.
- Thrombolytic therapy—risks may exist for up to 10 days following the use of epidurals if a vessel was damaged during insertion or removal of the catheter.
- Removal or accidental displacement of extradural catheter shortly after VTE prophylaxis dose.
- Epidural catheter insertion > spinal anaesthetic block.
- Traumatic epidural or spinal technique.
- Spinal surgery.

Exclusions
- Epidural abscess—slower onset and associated with pyrexia and signs of sepsis (⮑ see p. 252).
- Malignancy has a much slower, insidious onset.

Special considerations
- Incidence 0.85:100 000 with central neuro-axial block (CNB) although higher risk with epidural catheter placement.
- Use of minimal concentration of local anaesthetics reduces the incidence of unintended motor blockade and may allow earlier detection of neurological deficit.
- Concurrent use of several preparations (e.g. NSAIDs, clopidogrel, warfarin, LMWH) may increase the risk of haematoma without influencing clotting/platelet test results.
- Review local and national guidelines on the use of anticoagulants and CNB. Table 9.2 gives recommendations for central neuraxial blockade and anticoagulation.
- Appropriate postoperative monitoring for all neuro-axial blocks especially with catheter insertion.

Further reading
Association of Anaesthetists of Great Britain and Ireland (2013). *Regional Anaesthesia and Patients with Abnormalities of Coagulation*. Available at: https://www.aagbi.org

Royal College of Anaesthetists (2009). *National Audit of Major Complications of Central Neuraxial Block in the United Kingdom*. Available at: https://www.rcoa.ac.uk/system/files/CSQ-NAP3-Full_1.pdf

SreeHarsha, C.K., Rajasekaran, S., Dhanasekararaja, P. (2006). Spontaneous complete recovery of paraplegia caused by epidural hematoma complicating epidural anesthesia: a case report and review of literature. *Spinal Cord*, **44**, 514–17.

Table 9.2 Recommendations for central neuraxial blockade and anticoagulation

Drug	Type	Recommendations	Notes
Thrombolytic therapy	rt-PA, streptokinase, etc.	Avoid administration for 10 days following block. Avoid block after thrombolysis for minimum 10 days	Very high risk. Fibrinogen level **may** be useful indicator
Unfractionated heparin	Prophylactic SC	Normal APTR. No contraindication to neuraxial block. If possible, delay next dose until 1 h after block	Check platelet count after 4 days' therapy
	Treatment IV	Normal APTR. Give heparin >4 h after block. Do not remove catheter until 4 h after dosage	If bloody/traumatic tap, discuss need for heparin with surgeon
LMWH	Prophylactic	Block more than 12 h after last dose	Allow 4 h after block before next dose
	Treatment	Block more than 24 h after last dose	Allow 4 h after block before next dose
Warfarin	Long term	Stop 4–5 days pre-op. INR <1.4 for block	Recommence drug after catheter removed
Antiplatelets	NSAIDs	No additional precautions	
	Aspirin	No additional precautions	
	Dipyridamole	No additional precautions before procedure	Allow 6 h before recommencing drug
	Clopidogrel	Stop for 7 days pre-block	Allow 6 h before recommencing drug
	Ticlopidine	Stop for 14 days pre-block	Allow 6 h before recommencing drug
	Abciximab	Stop for 48 h pre-block	Allow 6 h before recommencing drug
	Eptifibatide, tirofiban	Stop for 8 h pre-block	Allow 6 h before recommencing drug
Synthetic penta-saccharide	Fondaparinux (Arixtra®) 2.5 mg od SC	Allow 36 h after last dose for block	12 h before next dose after block or catheter removal
Direct thrombin inhibitors	Dabigatran CrCl >80 mL/min CrCl 50–80 CrCl 30–50	Acceptable time 48 h 72 h 96 h	Allow 6 h before recommencing drug

Adapted with permission from Harrop-Griffiths, W. et al. (2013). Regional anaesthesia and patients with abnormalities of coagulation. *Anaesthesia*, 68(9), 966–72. © Association of Anaesthetists.

☼ Total spinal

(➔ See also 'Total spinal—obstetrics', p. 171.)

Definition
Blockade of all spinal nerves including CNS.

Presentation
- Profound onset of regional block within seconds to minutes following administration of local anaesthetic into the spinal, subdural, or epidural space.
- Tingling in fingers or hands warns of block to T1. Nauseated or faint due to severe fall in BP and/or bradycardia. Dilated pupils late sign when the brainstem becomes involved.
- Initial difficulty in breathing due to intercostal paralysis (T1–T12) may progress to gasping and respiratory arrest due to diaphragmatic paralysis (C3–C5). Inability to cough or difficulty in speaking or whispering suggests onset of phrenic nerve block.
- Initial tachycardia (from hypotension) followed by bradycardia (cardiac accelerator fibres T1–T4 or activation of the Bezold–Jarisch reflex). Other cardiac arrhythmias may occur.

Immediate management
- ☑ ABC—100% oxygen. Reassure conscious patient that they are safe.
- ☑ Secure airway with ETT and ventilate as necessary. Unconscious patient will not need a GA. Conscious patient will need a GA or sedation as dictated by blood pressure.
- ☑ Raise legs to increase venous return (pillows/Trendelenburg).
- ☑ Monitor S_pO_2, ECG, and BP.
- ☑ Establish large-bore intravenous infusion—infuse colloids or crystalloids 1000 mL stat. Repeat as necessary.
- ☑ Treat bradycardia with atropine 0.6–1 mg IV up to 3 mg.
- ☑ Treat hypotension with IV vasopressors:
  - ephedrine 6–9 mg boluses
  - metaraminol 1–2 mg boluses
- ☑ Adrenaline 100 µg IV boluses—if not responding or imminent cardiac arrest.

Subsequent management
- ☑ If cardiovascular stability achieved, it is possible to proceed with urgent surgery.
- ☑ Patient may require ventilation for 2–4 h and block will regress from cranial to spinal. Sedation (propofol infusion ideal) when consciousness starts to return.
- ☑ Transfer to ICU post-op.
- ☑ Document incident in detail, since there is the possibility of medico-legal claim.

☑ Offer explanation and reassurance to the relatives and patient upon recovery.
☑ Write to GP with copy of letter to patient so details are understood.
☑ A total spinal during labour is not necessarily an indication for a CS—unless fetal distress occurs. After recovery, an assisted forceps delivery may be indicated. Hypotension should be managed appropriately.

Investigations
• Clinical diagnosis.

Risk factors
• 'Large' dose spinal anaesthesia—particularly in parturients, short, or obese patients.
• Epidural anaesthesia without effective test dose or following dural tap.
• Subdural catheter placement (may present with an unexpectedly high block, often with sacral sparing).
• Combined epidural/spinal anaesthesia.
• Multiple attempts at siting epidural.
• Caudal block.
• Retrobulbar, interscalene, stellate ganglion block.

Exclusions
• Vasovagal.
• IV injection of LA may present as sudden loss of consciousness with or without convulsions and cardiovascular collapse.
• Anaphylaxis.
• Hyperventilation may cause tingling in fingers in an anxious patient.
• Sensation of breathing difficulties occurs in spinals due to intercostal blockade.

Paediatric implications
• Same basic principles as in adults—although fluids may be more useful than vasopressors.
• Use appropriate needle size while doing caudal. Avoid cephalad advancement of needle further than absolutely necessary into caudal epidural space.

Special considerations
• Vasopressors are more effective than fluids to reverse hypotension, but both are required.
• There should be no permanent sequelae if handled correctly. Total spinal was previously used as anaesthetic to reduce blood loss.
• There are case reports of successful, short term, non-invasive ventilation (BiPAP) of patients with high spinal block suffering from respiratory failure without haemodynamic instability.

Further reading
Guterres, A.P, Newman, M.J. (2010). Total spinal following labour epidural analgesia managed with non-invasive ventilation. *Anaesthesia and Intensive Care*, **38**, 373–5.

ⓘ Injection of adrenaline-containing local anaesthetic around digit

Definition
Inadvertent injection of adrenaline-containing solutions around end-arteries (e.g. digit, penis).

Presentation
- Error discovered on checking syringes.
- Pallor, blanching in affected digit, possibly pain and paraesthesia.

Immediate management
- ☑ Assess blood flow to the digit using pulse oximeter, Doppler ultrasound, capillary return, or blanching.
- ☑ Usually the effect is temporary, so observe over 30 min.
- ☑ Massage may help to disperse the solution.
- ☑ Injecting papaverine (40 mg in 20 mL saline; unlicensed use) into the affected area may relieve arterial spasm. Alternatively, use of 1 mL lidocaine 2% with 0.15 mg phentolamine has been described.
- ☑ Consider warming the affected area—it may hasten digit ischaemia, but may also relieve arterial spasm.
- ☑ Consider use of regional block technique (e.g. brachial plexus block) to increase blood flow.
- ☑ Do nothing (see next).

Subsequent management
- ☑ If ischaemia remains severe after 30 min, refer for urgent vascular surgical review.

Investigations
- Pulse oximetry of affected digit.
- Doppler ultrasonography.

Risk factors increasing the likelihood of harm
- Concentration of adrenaline injected.
- Large volume injection.
- Concurrent infection.
- Peripheral vascular disease or other underlying vascular compromise.
- Use of mechanical tourniquets.

Exclusions
- Using a high volume of local anaesthetic for ring blocks can stop arterial blood flow due to a pressure effect. Massaging the area is usually effective.

Special considerations

- The established tradition of avoiding adrenaline for extremity blocks is weakly supported by limited numbers of case reports involving unknown concentrations of adrenaline and other confounding variables (e.g. infection). No case reports of digital gangrene exist following the use of commercial lidocaine with adrenaline preparations, despite a number of case series and randomized controlled trials supporting its routine use. As always, a balance of risk should be struck between the use of adrenaline in local anaesthetics and the potential advantages it may bring through the avoidance of mechanical tourniquets and prolonged analgesia.
- The current literature suggest that in the absence of risk factors local anaesthetic with adrenaline 1:200 000 is safe to use in digital ring blocks.

Further reading

Mohan, P.P. (2007). *Epinephrine in Digital Nerve Block. BestBets.* Available at: https://bestbets.org/bets/bet.php?id=1212

Thomson, C.J., Lalonde, D.H. (2006). Randomized double-blind comparison of duration of anaesthesia among three commonly used agents in digital nerve block. *Plastic and Reconstructive Surgery,* **118**, 429–32.

Wilhelmi, B.J., Blackwell, S.J., Miller, J.H., et al. (2001). Do not use epinephrine in digital blocks: myth or truth? *Plastic and Reconstructive Surgery,* **107**, 393–7.

⚠ Retrobulbar haemorrhage

Definition
Bleeding behind the globe from puncture of vessels in the orbital cone usually following retrobulbar or peribulbar block.

Presentation
- Rapid onset of proptosis with a taut, immovable eye. Increase in intraocular pressure—may be high enough to be palpable (>26 mmHg).
- Pain, decreased visual acuity, and ophthalmoplegia.
- Blood may be visible in the subconjuctival space and eyelid.

Immediate management
- ☑ Withdraw needle.
- ☑ Main danger is retinal/optic nerve ischaemia due to retrobulbar pressure preventing blood flow through the central retinal artery.
- ☑ Degree of haemorrhage is usually assessed clinically. A severe haemorrhage is indicated by:
  - globe that feels stony hard (compare with normal eye).
  - immobile globe due to severe proptosis.
  - inability to close eyelid.
  - pain.
  - decreased blood flow in central retinal artery on fundoscopy (pale/white optic disc, white blood vessels).
- ☑ If haemorrhage is mild, then gentle external pressure for 20–30 min in sitting position may reduce bleeding. However, excessive pressure in the presence of raised intraocular pressure may further disrupt retinal artery circulation and worsen ischaemia.
- ☑ If haemorrhage is severe—discuss further management immediately with ophthalmic surgeon.
- ☑ If circulatory compromise is suspected, a lateral canthotomy is performed as a temporary measure to relieve pressure by increasing retrobulbar volume.

Subsequent management
- ☑ Formal decompression is carried out as an emergency under GA. Surgery within 2 h has an improved outcome.
- ☑ Acetazolamide (250–500 mg IV) or mannitol (0.5 g/kg IV) can be used to reduce intraocular pressure. Steroids may reduce inflammation and stabilize cell membranes against ischaemic damage.

Investigations
- Measure intraocular pressure using a tonometer (normal 10–21 mmHg).
- Record keeping is essential and all observations must be recorded.

Risk factors
- Use of sharp vs. blunt needles (sub-Tenon's block).
- Retrobulbar block/retrobulbar needle placement.
- Long needles (>25 mm).
- Patients on warfarin (INR >2.0), dabigatran or antiplatelet drugs.
- Bleeding disorders (e.g. haemophilia, thrombocytopenia).
- Severe hypertension.

Exclusions
- Accidental intraocular injection of local anaesthetic following inadvertent globe perforation—presents as severe, acute rise in intraocular pressure, associated with severe pain (➜ see 'Globe perforation', p. 264).
- Proptosis due to large volume of local anaesthetic agent.
- Allergic reaction to local anaesthetic.

Special considerations
- Dabigatran accumulates in reduced creatinine clearance Consider stopping 5 days prior to surgery.
- Sub-Tenons injection considered safer option for patients on anticoagulant or antiplatelet medication.

Further reading
Kumar, N., Jivan, S., Thomas, P., McLure, H. (2006). Sub-Tenon's anesthesia with aspirin, warfarin and clopidogrel. *Journal of Cataract and Refractive Surgery*, **32**, 1022–5.

⚠ **Globe perforation**

Definition

Accidental perforation of the globe during administration of a local anaesthetic eye block.

Presentation

- Operator may feel sudden loss of resistance as the needle perforates globe, or notices marked globe deviation followed by sudden return to neutral gaze. If in doubt, ask patient to look right then left with needle *in situ*. May be single perforation (entry) or double perforation (entry and exit).
- Patient may experience sudden severe intraocular pain or sudden loss of vision.
- Poor red reflex (vitreous haemorrhage).
- 50% of cases of globe perforations go unrecognized at the time of their occurrence.

Immediate management

- ☑ Refer to surgeon for indirect ophthalmoscopy. Will look for puncture sites, retinal detachment, and vitreous haemorrhage.
- ☑ Surgery should be postponed.

Subsequent management

- ☑ Management may be conservative.
- ☑ Consider cryopexy/laser retinopexy if vitreous haemorrhage, vitreous contraction, or retinal detachment occur.

Investigations

- Urgent indirect ophthalmoscopy. 'B' scan (ultrasound) if dense cataract.

Risk factors

- Abnormally shaped globe: long eye (myopic >26 mm axial length), enophthalmos, staphyloma.
- Previous extraocular surgery (e.g. for strabismus).
- Sharp needles vs. blunt needles. Sharp needles are more likely to perforate sclera but blunt needles that do perforate are likely to cause more intraocular trauma.
- Elevated, adducted gaze in an inferotemporal needle insertion increases the risk of optic nerve and macular damage.

Exclusions

- Intraneural injection (optic nerve).

Special considerations

• There should be a careful risk discussion and consenting process prior to any periocular injections including the risks and benefits of general anaesthesia.
• Patients with highly myopic eyes (>26 mm axial length) need to be informed their risk of globe perforation may be increased up to 10 to 30 times.

Further reading

Schrader, W.F., Schargus, M., Schneider, E., Josifova, T. (2010). Risks and sequalae of scleral perforation during retrobulbar anaesthesia. *Journal of Cataract and Refractive Surgery*, **36**, 885–9.

Thind, G.S., Rubin, A.P. (2001). Local anaesthesia for eye surgery—no room for complacency. *British Journal of Anaesthesia*, **86**, 473–6.

ⓘ **Neurological injury after regional anaesthetic block**

Definition

A new sensory and/or motor deficit following regional anaesthesia that is consistent with a peripheral nerve or plexus area of distribution and has no other identifiable cause.

Presentation

- New onset of abnormal sensation in a previously blocked anatomical area that extends beyond the reasonable duration of local anaesthetic effect (this may not become apparent until after removal of a regional catheter days after the initial procedure).
- Sensation may be reduced or abnormal (paraesthesia/dysaesthesia) or both.
- Abnormal sensation may be accompanied by motor deficit.
- Motor deficit is uncommon but concerning and should prompt immediate review.

Immediate management

- ☑ Detailed history and full examination of the affected limb.
- ☑ Identify other possible causes of perioperative nerve injury including swelling, compartment syndrome, infection, or haematoma at surgical or block site.
- ☑ Check coagulation status and INR for deep peripheral nerve blocks.
- ☑ Immediate referral to neurologist or neurosurgical team for complete (sensory and motor) or progressive deficits.
- ☑ Consider early neurophysiological testing (nerve conduction studies or electromyography).
- ☑ MRI or CT for deep nerve blocks may help to rule out compressive lesions.
- ☑ Reassure patient, most postoperative neuropraxias will resolve over a few days and the exact cause may never be known.

Subsequent management

- ☑ Minor nerve lesions including paraesthesia and dysaesthesia require ongoing follow-up.
- ☑ Minor nerve lesions that fail to resolve in in 2–3 months should prompt neurophysiological studies and neurology referral.
- ☑ Early liaison with chronic pain specialists for exacerbations of pain or allodynia caused by peripheral nerve blocks (PNB).
- ☑ Figure 9.1 shows an example strategy for follow-up and referral of minor nerve lesions.

Investigations

- Serial neurological examination as determined by degree of nerve injury and progression of symptoms.

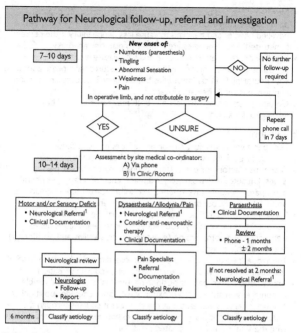

Figure 9.1 Pathway for neurological follow-up, referral, and investigation of minor nerve lesions.

Reprinted with permission from IRORA (International Registry of Regional Anaesthesia).

- Electrophysiology. Abnormalities detected on nerve conduction studies and electromyography are most marked at 3–5 weeks. Earlier testing may be useful to rule out pre-existing neuropathy or establish a baseline for repeat testing.
- Measurements include nerve conduction velocity, compound muscle action potentials, and F waves (which allow testing of proximal segment of the motor nerve). Although useful for diagnosing nerve pathology, electrophysiology does not indicate the cause of the lesion.
- MRI or CT for deep nerve blocks if compressive lesions are suspected.

Risk factors

- Intraneural, intrafascicular injection exposes nerves to direct toxicity of local anaesthetics (concentration and time dependent). There is currently insufficient evidence that nerve localizing techniques including ultrasound-guided nerve blocks or nerve stimulation techniques avoid intraneural injection or reduce the incidence of neurological injury following PNB.

- Needle calibre and bevel. Smaller calibre and shorter (40 degree) bevelled needles recommended over larger and longer (14 degree) bevelled needles and believed to cause less neural injury if the nerve is penetrated. Touhy needles are difficult to place intraneurally.
- Injection pressure effect on nerve and vasculature is thought to contribute to nerve injury. High injectate pressures have been associated with neural injury in canine studies but the benefit of pressure monitors in practice is yet to be established.
- Co-administration of adrenaline in PNB may reduce neural blood flow leading to ischaemia.

Exclusions

- Perioperative nerve injury can originate from multiple causes with patient, surgical, and anaesthetic factors all contributing.
- Patient risk factors for pre-existing neuropathy or chronic pain issues. Diabetes mellitus, vascular disease, chemotherapy, peripheral neuropathy, preoperative trauma, alcoholism, carpal tunnel syndrome, proximal nerve root compression, or spinal stenosis.
- Surgical causes: orthopaedic procedures carry the highest risk of perioperative nerve injury. Tourniquet induced neuropathy, nerve transection and compression (dressings, casts, swelling and positioning) are all possible causes.
- Tourniquet neuropathy features: motor loss, diminished touch, vibration, and position sense with preserved heat, cold, and pain sensation.
- Anaesthetic causes: patient positioning. Brachial plexus is vulnerable to compression and stretch proximally with poor shoulder positioning. The ulnar nerve is vulnerable at the elbow as it courses through the superficial postcondylar groove. Compression and injury are more likely with the arm in a flexed pronated position.

Special considerations

- Postoperative neurological symptoms following PNB are not uncommon (maybe up to 10%) but most resolve.
- The incidence of serious neurologic complications directly related to PNB are rare and stated at 1.5 to 4 in 10 000.
- Perioperative nerve injury is a common cause of medical litigation (15% of closed claims) with brachial plexus injury being the most common. A fully documented account of the risk discussion and consent process is required for all patients undergoing PNB.
- Documentation of pre-existing neurological deficits.
- Regional anaesthesia often puts high-risk patients at risk of neurological injury with patient, surgical, and anaesthetic factors all contributing to the disease process and outcome.
- Differentiating a true PNB-related nerve injury from other causes of perioperative nerve injury is challenging but it should be noted that postoperative neuropathy is 10 times more likely to have a cause unrelated to PNB. It is often a diagnosis of exclusion.
- It is useful for any department with a significant regional anaesthesia practice to develop clear referral pathways with local neurology colleagues who may be called on to assist with postoperative patient assessment.

Avoiding nerve injury

- Adequate supervision and training in regional anaesthesia techniques including the use of nerve localizing adjuncts (ultrasound and nerve stimulation) and a knowledge regional anatomy is essential for safe and successful practice of PNB.
- Avoid sharp, long bevelled needles.
- Consider volume and dose reduction in older and at-risk patients.
- Co-administration of adrenaline with local anaesthetic reduces neural blood flow. Consider avoiding in high-risk patients.
- Limit tourniquet time and pressure to the minimum required.
- Careful patient positioning with attention to neck flexion, shoulder, and elbow position.

Further reading

Barrington, M.J., Watts, S.A., Gledhill, S.R., et al. (2009). Preliminary results of the Australasian Regional Anaesthesia Collaboration: a prospective audit of more than 7000 peripheral nerve and plexus blocks for neurologic and other complications. *Regional Anesthesia and Pain Med*, **34**, 534–41.

Jeng, C.L, Torillo, T.M., Rosenblatt, M.A. (2010). Complications of peripheral nerve blocks. *British Journal of Anaesthesia*, **105**(S1), i97–i107.

Neal, J.M., Barrington, M.J., Brull, R., et al. (2015). The second ASRA practice advisory on neurological complications associated with regional anaesthesia and pain medicine: executive summary. *Regional Anesthesia and Pain Medicine*, **40**(5), 401–30.

Neal, J.M., Brull, R., Chan, V.W., et al. (2010). The ASRA evidence-based medicine assessment of ultrasound-guided regional anesthesia and pain medicine. *Regional Anaesthesia and Pain Medicine*, **35 (2)** S1–9.

Steinfeldt, T., Nimphius, W., Werner, T., et al. (2010). Nerve injury by needle nerve perforation in regional anaesthesia: does size matter? *British Journal of Anaesthesia*, **104**(2), 245–53.

Metabolic and endocrine

Hannah Blanshard

:☠: Anaphylaxis

(● See also 'Paediatric anaphylaxis', p. 141.)

Definition

Anaphylaxis is a severe, life-threatening, generalized, or systemic hypersensitivity reaction.

Presentation

- Clinical manifestations are wide ranging and inconsistent. Have a high index of suspicion.
- Most common presentations include cardiovascular collapse (88%), erythema (48%), bronchospasm (40%), angioedema (24%), cutaneous rash (13%), and urticaria (8%).
- Recognition of anaphylaxis during anaesthesia is often delayed because the key features of hypotension and bronchospasm more commonly have a different cause.

Immediate management of anaphylaxis during anaesthesia

☑ Stop any likely trigger agents including IV colloids, latex, and chlorhexidine. Maintain anaesthesia if necessary with an inhalational agent.
☑ Call for help and note the time.
☑ Maintain airway and give 100% oxygen.
☑ Exclude airway/breathing system obstruction (● see p. 91). Intubate if necessary and ventilate with oxygen.
☑ If the patient is hypotensive, elevate the legs, or tip the operating table head-down.
☑ If appropriate, start CPR immediately according to ALS guidelines (● see p. 13).
☑ Give adrenaline intravenously. An initial dose of 50 µg (0.5 mL of 1:10 000) is appropriate. Several doses may be required if there is hypotension or bronchospasm.
☑ If several doses of adrenaline are required, consider starting an adrenaline infusion IV. CVS instability may last several hours and 5% of cases relapse.
☑ Start rapid IV infusion with crystalloid. Adult patients may require 2–4 L.

Subsequent management

☑ Give antihistamines (chlorphenamine 10 mg by slow IV injection).
☑ Give corticosteroids (200 mg hydrocortisone IV 6-hourly).
☑ Consider adding metaraminol (or other vasopressors) if BP does not recover despite an adrenaline infusion.

☑ Give bronchodilators for persistent bronchospasm:
- Salbutamol 250 µg IV or 2.5–5 mg by nebulizer (may be given back to back).
- Aminophylline 250 mg by slow IV injection (up to 5 mg/kg)—not if taking theophylline.
- Consider giving magnesium sulphate 2 g in 5% glucose or 0.9% saline IV over 15 min (may worsen hypotension).

☑ Refer to ITU.

☑ Check for airway oedema by letting the cuff down prior to extubation and ensuring there is a leak.

☑ Report suspected anaphylactic reactions associated with anaesthesia to the MHRA using the 'Yellow Card' scheme (https://yellowcard.mhra.gov.uk).

Investigations

☑ Take three blood tests for mast cell-released tryptase, each 5–10 mL clotted blood:
- as soon as feasible after resuscitation has started—do not delay resuscitation to take the sample.
- 1–2 h after the reaction.
- 24 h after the reaction or in convalescence. This is a measure of baseline tryptase levels.

☑ Store sample at –20°C until it can be sent for measurement of serum tryptase.
- Elevated serum tryptase indicates the reaction was associated with mast cell degranulation, and rises after both anaphylactic and anaphylactoid reactions. A negative test does not completely exclude anaphylaxis.
- Plasma histamine rises during the first several minutes of a reaction and generally stays up briefly; measurement is impractical because it requires special collection and handling techniques.

☑ Refer the patient to a regional allergy centre. With the referral send:
- photocopies of anaesthetic chart, drug chart, and recovery documentation.
- description of reaction and time of onset in relation to drug administration.
- a note of tests sent and their time.
- a standard referral form can be found on the AAGBI website under 'Safety/Allergies and anaphylaxis' and 'Suspected anaphylactic reactions associated with anaesthesia'.
- The allergist will perform skin-prick tests to GA drugs 4–6 weeks after the reaction. Specific IgE antibodies in the serum can be measured for suxamethonium.

Risk factors

- Previous allergic reaction to the agent.

- No other valid predictor of anaphylaxis—history of previous exposure not necessary.
- Factors which increase severity include asthma, β-adrenoceptor blockade, hypovolaemia, and neuraxial anaesthesia. These are associated with a reduced endogenous catecholamine response.

Exclusions

- Breathing circuit obstruction (→ see p. 413):
  - filter or catheter mount obstruction.
  - kinked ETT.
  - cuff herniation.
  - endobronchial intubation/tube migration.
- Check breathing system not at fault—disconnect breathing circuit distal to all connections/filters and ventilate directly with a self-inflating bag. If inflation pressure still feels high, the problem is due to airway/ETT obstruction or reduced compliance.
- Foreign body in the airway (→ see p. 219).
- Air embolus (→ see p. 77).
- Tension pneumothorax (→ see p. 66):
  - history of CVP line insertion or trauma.
  - trachea not central.
- Severe bronchospasm (→ see p. 70).
- Type IV allergy—localized cutaneous reaction to a substance. This is T-cell mediated and is not life-threatening. It occurs 6–48 h after exposure. In the medical context, it is generally an allergy to chemical accelerators used in the manufacture of both latex and synthetic gloves.

Paediatric implications

Anaphylaxis in children is covered on → p. 141.

Special considerations

- UK Resuscitation Guidelines recommend the IM route for adrenaline administration (500 µg adrenaline, 0.5 mL 1 in 1000) as the best compromise between safety and speed of onset for most healthcare workers. IV adrenaline should only be given in specialist settings by those familiar with its use (e.g. anaesthetists), and if the patient is monitored and IV access is already available. It should not be given without continuous ECG monitoring because of the risk of precipitating dysrhythmias, especially in the presence of hypoxia and acidosis. SC adrenaline should be avoided because absorption time is extremely erratic.
- Latex anaphylaxis during anaesthesia presents in an atypical fashion. Most cases present 30–60 min after induction. This coincides with either a delayed airborne exposure or with mucous membrane exposure at the beginning of the surgical procedure. Minimize risks by using a breathing circuit filter, and non-latex gloves. Most antibiotic bottles and IV-giving sets are now latex-free.
- 'Diprivan' TCI propofol syringes are also latex-free.

Further reading

Hepner, D.L., Castells, M.C. (2003). Anaphylaxis during the perioperative period. *Anesthesia and Analgesia*, **97**, 1381–95.

National Institute for Health and Care Excellence (NICE) (2011). *Anaphylaxis: Assessment and Referral After Emergency Treatment*. Available at: https://www.nice.org.uk/guidance/cg134/chapter/1-recommendations

Resuscitation Council UK (2015). *UK Resuscitation Guidelines*. Available at: https://www.resus.org.uk/pages/reaction.pdf

The Association of Anaesthetists of Great Britain and Ireland and British Society for Allergy and Clinical Immunology (2008). *Suspected Anaphylactic Reactions Associated with Anaesthesia*. Available at: https://www.aagbi.org

:O: Diabetic ketoacidosis

Definition

Acute, severe, uncontrolled diabetes characterized by hyperglycaemia, ketonaemia, and acidosis.

Presentation

- 2–3-day history of gradual deterioration, associated with polydipsia, polyuria, abdominal pain, nausea and vomiting, dehydration, and drowsiness.
- Triad of:
  - hyperglycaemia (blood glucose >11 mmol/L).
  - ketonaemia >3 mmol/L (ketonuria—urinary ketones ≥3+).
  - acidaemia (bicarbonate below 15 mmol/L and/or venous pH <7.3).

Investigations

- To diagnose DKA—blood glucose, blood ketones, venous or arterial blood gases (to look at bicarbonate, pH, and potassium), dipstick urine.
- To assess cause—FBC, U&Es, CRP, troponin, cultures, MSU, ECG, and CXR.

Delivery of care

- The diabetes specialist team should be involved as soon as possible.
- Patients should be nursed in areas where staff are experienced in the management of ketoacidosis.

Immediate management—0–60 min

1. Intravenous access and initial investigations

☑ Rapid ABC and conscious level. Consider nasogastric tube and airway protection if patient obtunded.

☑ Full clinical assessment.

☑ Consider precipitating causes and treat appropriately.

☑ The presence of one or more of the following may indicate severe DKA requiring admission to a high dependency area, insertion of a central line and immediate senior review:
- blood ketones >6 mmol/L
- bicarbonate <5 mmol/L
- venous/arterial pH <7.1
- K^+ <3.5 mmol/L on admission
- GCS <12
- oxygen saturation <92% on air
- systolic blood pressure (SBP) <90 mmHg
- pulse >100 or <60 bpm
- anion gap >16. Anion gap = $(Na^+ + K^+)—(Cl^- + HCO_3^-)$

2. Restoration of circulating volume

☑ Assess severity of dehydration using pulse and BP.

☑ If hypotensive on admission, (SBP <90mmHg), likely to be due to low circulating volume, but consider other causes such as heart failure and sepsis. Give 500 mL 0.9% sodium chloride over 10–15 min. If SBP remains below 90 mmHg, consider repeating.

☑ Once SBP >90 mmHg give the average 70 kg patient fluid replacement of 0.9% sodium chloride, 1 L over the first hour, then 1 L over 2 h, 1 L over next 2 h, 1 L over 4 h, 1 L over 4 h, 1 L over 6 h, and then 8 hourly fluids.

3. Potassium replacement

• Serum potassium is often high on admission, but falls quickly on treatment with insulin.

☑ If K+ over 5.5 mmol/L do not give K+ but check level every 2 h.

☑ If K+ 3.5–5.5 mmol/L give 40 mmol in each litre of fluid.

☑ If K+ below 3.5 mmol/L withhold insulin and give 40 mmol K+ over 1 h until K+ >3.5 mmol/L.

4. Commence a fixed rate intravenous insulin infusion (IVII)

☑ Infuse insulin at a fixed rate of 0.1 unit/kg/h.

☑ If the patient normally takes insulin Lantus® or Levemir® subcutaneously continue this at the usual dose and usual time.

Subsequent management—60 min to 6 h

☑ Aim to clear the blood of ketones and suppress ketogenesis.

☑ Achieve a rate of fall of ketones of at least 0.5 mmol/L/h. If not increase insulin infusion rate by 1 unit/h. Continue fixed rate IVII until blood ketones <0.3 mmol/L, venous pH >7.3 and /or venous bicarbonate >18 mmol/L.

☑ If ketone measurement not available, bicarbonate should rise by 3 mmol/L/h and blood glucose should fall by 3 mmol/L/h.

☑ Monitor urine output and aim for >0.5 mL/kg/h.

☑ Regular observations and Early Warning Score charting.

☑ If blood glucose falls below 14 mmol/L commence 10% glucose at 125 mL/h alongside the 0.9% sodium chloride solution.

☑ Measure glucose hourly.

☑ Investigate cause of diabetic ketoacidosis.

☑ Consider venous thromboembolic prophylaxis according to NICE guidelines.

Subsequent management—6–12 h

☑ Continue intravenous fluids and insulin.

☑ Assess for complications of treatment (e.g. fluid overload or cerebral oedema).

☑ Avoid hypoglycaemia.

Resolution of DKA

• Defined as ketones <0.3 mmol/L and venous pH >7.3.

• Do not used bicarbonate at this stage (➲ see 'Special considerations', p. 278). Patients may demonstrate a hyperchloraemic acidosis secondary to high volumes of 0.9% sodium chloride.

• Resolution should be by 24 h.

Risk factors
- Usually occurs with type I diabetes, but may occur with type II.
- Caused by infection, omission of/or inadequate insulin, medical illness (i.e. MI), or initial presentation of diabetes mellitus.

Exclusions
Severe metabolic acidosis in the absence of hyperglycaemia due to:
- Sepsis
- Renal failure
- Salicylate overdose
- Inborn errors of metabolism
- Alcoholic ketoacidosis
- Hyperosmolar non-ketotic coma (marked hyperglycaemia but no detectable ketoacidosis)

Paediatric implications
- See guidelines prepared for the British Society of Paediatric Endocrinology and Diabetes (web address in Further reading).
- Involve paediatricians early.

Special considerations
- The likelihood of intraoperative cardiac arrhythmias and hypotension is much reduced if the metabolic decompensation can be at least partially reversed prior to surgery. However, delaying surgery where the underlying condition will continue to exacerbate ketoacidosis is futile.
- Resuscitation should be continued perioperatively.
- If surgery necessary, hyperventilate to maintain respiratory compensation for metabolic acidosis—insert arterial line and check ABGs.
- Sodium bicarbonate is virtually never indicated. A small percentage of patients who have diabetic ketoacidosis present with metabolic acidosis and a normal anion gap. Therefore, they have fewer ketones available for the regeneration of bicarbonate during insulin administration. Consider bicarbonate in this subset of patients or if pH <7.0 and compromised.

Hyperglycaemic, hyperosmolar, non-ketotic coma (HONK)
- Only occurs in type 2 diabetes.
- Patient is often old and presenting for the first time.
- Presents with a long history and often marked dehydration.
Characteristic features include:
- Hypovolaemia
- Marked hyperglycaemia (>30 mmol/L) without significant hyperketonaemia (<3 mmol/L) or acidosis (pH >7.3, bicarbonate >15 mmol/L)
- Osmolality usually >320 mosmol/kg.
- There is sufficient insulin to prevent lipolysis and ketogenesis, so no acidosis.
- A mixed picture of HONK and DKA may occur.

- HONK has a higher mortality than DKA and may be complicated by vascular complications such as myocardial infarction, stroke, or peripheral arterial thrombosis, also seizures, cerebral oedema, and central pontine myelinolysis.

Management of HONK

☑ Measure osmolality (using osmometer) or calculate osmolarity ($2Na^+$ + glucose + urea [all in mmol/L]) frequently to monitor the response to treatment. Normal osmolality of plasma is 285–295 mosmol/kg. (Osmolarity, expressed as mosmol/L, is usually within 1–2% of the osmolality unless significant ethanol/methanol, etc. has been ingested.)

☑ Use 0.9% sodium chloride to restore volume and reverse dehydration. Only switch to 0.45% sodium chloride solution if the osmolality is not declining despite adequate positive fluid balance. An initial rise in sodium is expected and is not itself an indication for hypotonic fluids. The rate of fall of plasma sodium should not exceed 10 mmol/L in 24 h.

☑ The fall in blood glucose should be no more than 5 mmol/L/h. Low-dose IV insulin (0.05 units/kg/h) should only be commenced once the blood glucose is no longer falling with IV fluids alone OR immediately if there is significant ketonaemia (>1 mmol/L or urine ketones greater than 2+).

☑ Intravenous fluid replacement aims to achieve a positive balance of 3–6 L by 12 h and the remaining replacement of estimated fluid losses within next 12 h though complete normalization of biochemistry may take up to 72 h.

☑ Patients with HONK have an increased risk of arterial and venous thromboembolism. The risk of venous thromboembolism is greater than in DKA. All patients should receive prophylactic LMWH for the full duration of admission unless contraindicated. Full anticoagulation should only be considered in patients with suspected thrombosis or acute coronary syndrome. Consider extending prophylaxis for 3 months in high-risk patients.

Further reading

BSPED (2015). *BSPED Recommended DKA Guidelines*. Available at: https://www.bsped.org.uk/clinical-resources/guidelines/

Joint British Diabetes Societies Inpatient Care Group (2013). *The Management of Diabetic Ketoacidosis in Adults*. Available at: http://www.diabetes.org.uk/About_us/What-we-say/Improving-diabetes-healthcare/The-Management-of-Diabetic-Ketoacidosis-in-Adults/

Joint British Diabetes Societies Inpatient Care Group (2012). *The Management of the Hyperosmolar Hyperglycaemic State (HHS) in Adults with Diabetes*. Available at: http://www.diabetologists-abcd.org.uk/JBDS/JBDS_IP_HHS_Adults.pdf

☠ Malignant hyperthermia

Definition
Inherited disorder of skeletal muscle that can be triggered pharmacologically to produce a potentially fatal combination of hypermetabolism, muscle rigidity, and muscle breakdown.

Trigger agents
- All inhalational agents.
- Succinylcholine.

Presentation
Early signs
- Earliest indication is masseter muscle spasm following suxamethonium— defined as excess and prolonged jaw rigidity (2–4 min). NB Only 30% with masseter spasm as the sole sign go on to develop MH.
- Tachypnoea in the spontaneously breathing patient, or a rise in end-tidal CO_2 if mechanically ventilated.
- Unexplained tachycardia.
- Generalized muscle rigidity.
- Progressing to hypoxaemia due to increased oxygen consumption.

Later signs
- Rise in body temperature.
- Raised plasma CK and myoglobin.
- Dark-coloured urine due to myoglobinuria occurs even later.
- At this stage, hyperkalaemia, cardiac arrhythmias, and DIC are likely to develop.

Immediate management
☑ Stop all trigger agents and give 100% oxygen.
☑ Call for help.
☑ Hyperventilate with high fresh gas flows and new breathing circuit that does not allow rebreathing.
☑ Expedite surgery and maintain anaesthesia with intravenous drugs (e.g. propofol and opioid). Avoid suxamethonium if intubation is needed.
☑ Give dantrolene 2.5 mg/kg immediate IV bolus. Repeat 1 mg/kg boluses to max 10 mg/kg until the tachycardia, rise in CO_2 production, and pyrexia start to subside. The average dose is 3 mg/kg. Warm solution to increase solubility and give through a blood administration set or bolus using syringes.

Subsequent management
☑ Commence active cooling by infusing cold IV solutions, applying ice to the axilla/groins, applying a cooling blanket. Avoid peripheral vasoconstriction which will prevent heat loss.
☑ Consider inserting an arterial line, central line, and urinary catheter.

☑ Take regular blood gas and electrolyte measurements.
☑ Give sodium bicarbonate IV if pH <7.2 and hyperventilate to normocapnia.
☑ Treat hyperkalaemia with 250 mL 10% dextrose with 10 units actrapid (adult dose) and 10% $CaCl_2$ 0.1–0.2 mL/kg (max 10 mL). ➲ See also p. 313.
☑ Measure clotting and CK (peaks at 12–24 h after episode).
☑ Limit renal tubular damage from myoglobin by maintaining a diuresis of at least 2 mL/kg/h preferably with alkalinized urine (0.5–1 g/kg mannitol ± 1 mL/kg 8.4% sodium bicarbonate when P_aCO_2 is within normal limits) and furosemide 0.5–1 mg/kg.
☑ Treat coagulopathies and arrhythmias as usual. Do not use calcium channel blocking drugs, which in combination with dantrolene can produce marked cardiac depression.
☑ Transfer to ITU for monitoring.
☑ Repeat dantrolene 1 mg/kg as necessary.
☑ Prior to discharge, warn patient and family of potential implications of MH.

Investigations

• ABGs, U&Es, CK, FBC, and clotting.
• Muscle biopsy for *in vitro* contracture testing (➲ see 'Special considerations', p. 282).

Risk factors

• Family history.
• May occur despite previously uneventful anaesthetics.
• History of unexpected death of relative during anaesthetic (50% risk of being MH).
• 1:10 000–1:15 000 patients.

Exclusions

• Inadequate anaesthesia/analgesia.
• Infection/sepsis—sepsis may present with tachycardia and pyrexia, with a metabolic acidosis which requires respiratory compensation; whereas MH presents with tachycardia, hypertension, and a mixed respiratory and metabolic acidosis. Both may cause a reduction in P_aO_2 and subsequently S_aO_2.
• Tourniquet ischaemia can cause tachycardia, hypertension, and in children in particular, a rise in core temperature. End-tidal CO_2 will rise briefly when tourniquet is released, but then symptoms settle.
• Anaphylaxis. Check blood pressure—usually decreased in anaphylaxis.
• Phaeochromocytoma.
• Thyroid storm.
• Ecstasy or other dangerous recreational drugs.

Paediatric implications

In children <20 kg, give dantrolene in doses of 1 mg/kg up to 10 mg/kg as required.

Special considerations

Confirmation of diagnosis

- The only MH centre in the United Kingdom is in Leeds. Tel 0113 2065274, hotline 07947 609601 for medical emergencies only.
- MH is confirmed by *in vitro* contracture testing (IVCT) using a muscle biopsy from the vastus medialis taken under ultrasound-guided femoral nerve block. The tissue is exposed to halothane and caffeine and the tension measured.
- MH is an inherited disorder so once a case is confirmed, further family members are investigated. DNA analysis can aid diagnosis but cannot be used in isolation.

Obstetric patients

- Baby has 50% chance of being affected if one parent is MH susceptible, so treat as potentially MH.

Mother MH susceptible

☑ Use regional technique if at all possible.
☑ If GA, use MH safe technique. Use rocuronium instead of suxamethonium and maintain anaesthesia with propofol.

Father MH susceptible

☑ Avoid inhalational agents until after delivery of the baby.
☑ Suxamethonium is highly charged so does not cross the placenta to any great extent and so can be used.

Anaesthesia for susceptible patients

☑ Avoid trigger agents (see Table 10.1, trigger, and safe agents in MH).
☑ Use regional anaesthesia where appropriate.

Table 10.1 Trigger and safe agents in MH

Trigger agents for MH	Safe agents to use in MH
Suxamethonium	Nitrous oxide
All volatile agents	IV anaesthetic agents including ketamine
	Benzodiazepines
	Non-depolarizing neuromuscular blocking drugs
	Local anaesthetics
	Opioids
	Neostigmine
	Atropine
	Glycopyrronium
	Metoclopramide
	Droperidol

☑ For general anaesthesia, prepare the anaesthetic machine by removing vaporizers and flushing the machine and ventilator with 100% oxygen at maximum flows for 20–30 min. Use a new breathing circuit. Prophylactic dantrolene is not needed. It has side effects of nausea and vomiting, muscle weakness, and prolongation of non-depolarizing muscle relaxants.

☑ Monitor closely for signs of MH.

☑ Can be discharged 4 h after surgery if no problems.

Further reading

Association of Anaesthetists (2011). *Malignant Hyperthermia Crisis AAGBI Safety Guideline.* Available at: http://www.aagbi.org/publications/publications-guidelines/M/R

Glahn K.P.E., Ellis, F.R., Halsall, P.J., et al. (2010). Recognizing and managing a malignant hyperthermia crisis: guidelines from the European Malignant Hyperthermia Group. *British Journal of Anaesthesia,* **105**(4), 417–20.

Halsall, P.J. (2011). Malignant hyperthermia. In: Allman, K.G., Wilson, I.H. (eds). *Oxford Handbook of Anaesthesia,* **3rd** edition, pp. 270–5. Oxford, UK: Oxford University Press.

Gupta P.K., Hopkins P.M., (2017) Diagnosis and management of malignant hyperthermia. *BJA education* **17** (7) 249-254.

! Porphyric crisis

Definition
The porphyrias are a group of inherited or acquired enzymatic defects of haem synthesis.
- Acute porphyric crises typically cause rapid onset potentially life-threatening nervous system symptoms

Presentation
- Autonomic neuropathy—acute abdominal pain (lasts days), vomiting, constipation, hypertension, tachycardia, fever, and postural hypotension.
- CNS changes—confusion, hysteria, depression, convulsions. Peripheral neuropathy: motor > sensory.
- Red/purple urine—Hyponatraemia secondary to inappropriate secretion of ADH.

Immediate management
- ☑ Remove possible precipitants.
- ☑ Rehydrate with IV fluid.
- ☑ Aim is to decrease haem synthesis and the production of porphyrin precursors. Fasting will trigger continued production of porphyrins, so if possible give carbohydrate loading orally or via nasogastric tract. If not, give 2 L of 10% dextrose over 24 h. This will give 200 g of glucose per day. Watch for hyponatraemia.
- ☑ Give propranolol for hypertension and tachycardia.

Subsequent management
- ☑ Treat any underlying infection.
- ☑ Treat pain with any opioid apart from oxycodone or pentazocine.
- ☑ Treat nausea with prochlorperazine or ondansetron. Avoid metoclopramide.
- ☑ Treat seizures with diazepam, propofol, or magnesium sulphate. Avoid barbiturates and phenytoin.
- ☑ For severe attacks, particularly those with neurological symptoms, treat with haem arginate (3 mg/kg IV to a maximum of 250 mg once daily for 4 days). This provides negative feedback to the haem synthetic pathway and shuts down production of porphyrins and precursors. It can lead to intense thrombophlebitis so should be given through a central line.
- ☑ Refer to ITU.

Investigations
- U&Es, urinary porphobilinogen, and 5-aminolaevulinic acid.
- A raised urine porphobilinogen is pathognomic of the acute attack.

Risk factors

- Precipitating factors for a crisis may be drugs, dehydration, fasting, stress, infection, fluctuations in hormone levels during menstruation/pregnancy, alcohol.
- Maintain a high index of suspicion in first-degree relatives of those with porphyria presenting with the features described earlier.
- Only acute porphyrias can precipitate a crisis. These include acute intermittent porphyria, variegate porphyria, hereditary coproporphyria, and plumboporphyria (very rare).
- Patients are at greatest risk on first presentation since an abdominal emergency may be simulated.

Exclusions

- Acute abdomen—appendicitis, diverticulitis, biliary problems, pyelonephritis.
- Acute neurology, predominantly motor, can mimic Guillain–Barré syndrome.
- Manic–depressive illness.

Paediatric implications

Acute crises usually occur from puberty to 40 years of age, but porphyrinogenic drugs should be avoided in all children with a family history.

Special considerations

Anaesthetic drugs considered safe to use in a porphyric crisis

- Provided appropriate precautions are taken, most patients with acute porphyria can tolerate surgery and GA.
- It is difficult to be precise about which drugs definitely cause a porphyric crisis, since crises can also be triggered by infection or stress, but current advice is given in Table 10.2.
- For further details on safe drugs to use in a porphyric crisis, see the Further reading list for website of the Norwegian Porphyria Centre.
- In certain cases, regional anaesthesia may be preferred to general anaesthesia, in which case bupivacaine is the LA of choice. In the presence of any peripheral neuropathy, detailed preoperative examination and documentation are essential.
- Remember, the onset of a porphyric crisis may be delayed for 5 days after exposure to a porphyrinogenic drug.

Further reading

Findley, H., Philips, A., Cole, D., Nair, A. (2012). Porphyrias: implications for anaesthesia, critical care and pain medicine. *Continuing Education in Anaesthesia, Critical Care and Pain*, **12**(3), 105–9.
James, M.F.M., Hift, R.J. (2000). Porphyrias. *British Journal of Anaesthesia*, **85**, 143–53.
The Norwegian Porphyria Centre (NAPOS). The Drug Database for Acute Porphyria. Available at: http://www.drugs-porphyria.org

Table 10.2 Safety of drugs in porphyria

	Definitely unsafe	Probably safe	Controversial
Induction agents	barbiturates etomidate	propofol	ketamine sevoflurane
Inhalational agents		desflurane isoflurane nitrous oxide	halothane sevoflurane
Neuromuscular blocking agents	alcuronium	suxamethonium, vecuronium atracurium rocuronium mivacurium	pancuronium
Antimuscarinics		atropine glycopyrronium	
Neuromuscular reversal agents		neostigmine	
Analgesics	pentazocine	alfentanil aspirin buprenorphine codeine fentanyl ibuprofen morphine naloxone paracetamol pethidine tramadol	diclofenac, ketorolac, oxycodone sufentanil mefenamic acid
Local anaesthetics	mepivacaine ropivacaine	bupivacaine lidocaine prilocaine procaine	cocaine levobupivacaine
Sedatives	chlordiazepoxide nitrazepam	chloral hydrate chlorpromazine lorazepam midazolam, temazepam,	diazepam
Antiemetics and H_2-antagonists	metoclopramide	cyclizine droperidol phenothiazines ondansetron cimetidine	ranitidine

Table 10.2 (Contd.)

	Definitely unsafe	Probably safe	Controversial
CVS drugs	hydralazine, nifedipine, phenoxybenzamine	adrenaline α-agonists β-agonists β-blockers magnesium phentolamine, procainamide noradrenaline milrinone phenylephrine	diltiazem sodium nitroprusside verapamil
Antibiotics	rifampicin erythromycin	co-amoxiclav gentamicin penicillins tazocin vancomycin	
Others	phenytoin sulfonamides	carboprost syntocinon	aminophylline steroids

☼ Thyrotoxic storm

Definition
Life-threatening exacerbation of hyperthyroid state with evidence of de-compensation in one or more organ system. Mortality 20–30%.

Presentation
Usually 6–24 h after surgery.
Four main symptoms:
- Hyperpyrexia—temperature ≥41°C, sweating.
- CNS dysfunction including agitation, delirium, and coma.
- CVS signs:
  - sinus tachycardia >140 bpm
  - atrial fibrillation or ventricular arrhythmias
  - hyper- then hypotension
  - congestive cardiac failure (25%)
- GI symptoms:
  - nausea and vomiting
  - diarrhoea
  - hepatocellular dysfunction with jaundice

May present as renal failure secondary to rhabdomyolysis.

Immediate management
☑ ABC—100% oxygen.
☑ Rehydrate with IV saline and glucose, due to large insensible losses and depletion of hepatic glycogen stores. Heart failure may occur, particularly in older people.
☑ Treat hyperpyrexia with tepid sponging and paracetamol. Do not use NSAIDs or aspirin as these displace thyroid hormone from serum binding sites.
☑ To treat hyperadrenergic state give propranolol (1 mg increments IV up to 10 mg) with CVS monitoring (may precipitate CCF). Aim to decrease pulse rate to <90 bpm. Or give esmolol (loading dose 250–500 µg/kg IV followed by continuous infusion of 50–100 µg/kg per min). Alternatively, use the antiadrenergic agent reserpine intramuscularly 2.5–5.0 mg qds (unlicensed).
☑ Give hydrocortisone (200 mg IV qds) to treat adrenal insufficiency and to decrease T_4 release and conversion to T_3 at very high levels.
☑ Dantrolene has been used with effect in treating thyroid crisis. High circulating T_4 has an effect on calcium flux across the sarcoplasmic reticulum and dantrolene may inhibit this pathological mechanism.

Subsequent management

☑ Give propylthiouracil (1 g loading dose via NG tube followed by 200–300 mg qds). This inhibits thyroid hormone release and also decreases the peripheral conversion of T_4 to T_3.

☑ At least 1 h following blockade with propylthiouracil, give sodium iodide (500 mg tds IV), or potassium iodide (5 drops qds via NG) or Aqueous Iodine Oral Solution (Lugol's iodine) (5–10 drops qds via nasogastric). Iodine can exacerbate release of thyroid hormone if given without prior propylthiouracil.

☑ Treat underlying precipitating event.

☑ Transfer to ITU.

Investigations

- T_3, free T_4, and TSH (but levels correlate poorly with severity)
- U&Es—hypercalcaemia, hypokalaemia (50%), and hypermagnesaemia

Risk factors

- Precipitating factors include intercurrent illness (especially infection), trauma, surgery, uncontrolled DM, labour, and pre-eclampsia/eclampsia.
- A crisis is precipitated intraoperatively due to excessive palpation of the gland, incomplete preparation, and inadequate doses of β-blockers preoperatively.

Exclusions

- Malignant hyperthermia—do not get mixed metabolic and respiratory acidosis in thyrotoxic storm and no raised CK.
- Phaeochromocytoma—would not expect pyrexia in phaeochromocytoma.
- Infection, sepsis.

Special considerations

- It is important to establish an adequate depth of anaesthesia to avoid exaggerated sympathetic nervous system responses.
- Reversal of muscle relaxants should include glycopyrronium instead of atropine.
- Treat any intraoperative hypotension with a direct-acting vasopressor, such as phenylephrine.
- Non-cardioselective β-blockers are more effective (e.g. propranolol). $β_1$-adrenergic blockade treats the symptoms of tachycardia, but $β_2$-adrenergic blockade prevents peripheral conversion of T_4 to T_3.

Further reading

Farling, P.A. (2000). Thyroid disease. *British Journal of Anaesthesia*, **85**, 15–28.

Migneco, A., Ojetti, V., Testa, A., De Lorenzo, A., Gentiloni Silveri, N. (2005). Management of thyrotoxic crisis. *European Review for Medical and Pharmacological Sciences*, **9**, 69–74.

Tay, S., Khoo, E., Tancharoen, C., Lee, I. (2013). Beta-blockers and the thyrotoxic patient for thyroid and non-thyroid surgery: a clinical review. *OA Anaesthetics*, **1** (1), 5.

Ross D.S. et al. (2016) American Thyroid Association Guidelines for diagnosis and management of hyperthyroidism and other causes of thyrotoxicosis. *Thyroid* **26** (10)

☼ Undiagnosed phaeochromocytoma

Definition
A functionally active catecholamine tumour of chromaffin cells typically found in the adrenal medulla (90%).

Presentation
- Sustained or paroxysmal hypertension, arrhythmias, MI.
- Most likely to occur during induction of anaesthesia/endotracheal intubation, or tumour manipulation.
- History of severe headache, anxiety, palpitations, tremor, weakness, chest pain, faintness, paraesthesia, drenching perspiration, facial pallor, anxiety, and tremor.

Immediate management
☑ Stop all noxious stimuli immediately, administer opioids, and deepen inhalational anaesthesia to at least 2 MAC.

☑ Give phentolamine (1–2 mg increments IV up to 20 mg) to control hypertension. Titrate according to blood pressure. This is a competitive α_1- and α_2-blocker with a half-life of 10–15 min.

☑ Alternatively/additionally, give magnesium sulphate, which inhibits catecholamine release, exerts a direct vasodilator effect, and reduces alpha-receptor sensitivity. Give 5 g (20 mmol) IV loading dose then 2 g/h (8 mmol/h) to achieve a therapeutic level of 1.5 mmol/L. Beware of giving further muscle relaxation after magnesium.

☑ Establish arterial line monitoring while establishing BP control.

☑ If HR >100 bpm or >1:4 VEs after alpha-blockade, give labetalol—predominantly β-blocker (5–10 mg increments IV).

☑ Abandon surgery, but expedite if already commenced. Do not attempt to remove phaeochromocytoma at this stage.

☑ Consider sodium nitroprusside. Initial infusion 0.5–1.5 µg/kg per min. Titrate to BP with mean dose of 3–5 µg/kg/min.

☑ Control further tachyarrhythmias with esmolol (1.5 mg/kg bolus IV).

Subsequent management
- Transfer to ITU. Continue infusion of magnesium (2 g/h), or sodium nitroprusside, until established on phenoxybenzamine or doxazosin orally.
- 24-h urine collection for free catecholamines.
- Do not rebook for theatre until patient is stabilized with alpha-blockers (phenoxybenzamine up to 30 mg twice daily or doxazosin up to 16 mg daily).

Investigations
- 24-h collection for urinary catecholamines, vanillylmandelic acid, and metanephrine.
- Serial ECGs, CK-MB, troponin, and echocardiogram for evidence of acute and chronic heart damage.

Risk factors

Can be associated with other syndromes:
- MEN type-2 syndrome (phaeochromocytoma, medullary thyroid carcinoma, hyperparathyroidism).
- MEN type-3 syndrome (phaeochromocytoma, medullary thyroid carcinoma, mucosal ganglioneuromas, Marfanoid habitus).
- Von Hippel–Lindau disease (phaeochromocytoma, retinal angiomas, hemangioblastoma of CNS, renal and pancreatic cysts, renal cell carcinoma).
- Neurofibromatosis.

Exclusions

- Inadequate anaesthesia/analgesia.
- Uncontrolled hypertensive disease during stimulating surgery or when in pain postoperatively.
- Pre-eclampsia.
- Raised intracranial pressure.
- Cocaine/amphetamine abuse.
- Thyroid storm—fever sweating, and tachycardia dominate.
- Malignant hyperthermia—get mixed respiratory and metabolic acidosis.

Paediatric implications

- Phaeochromocytomas are more often multifocal and extra-adrenal in children when compared to adults.

Special considerations

- Perioperative undiagnosed phaeochromocytoma carries a 50% mortality.
- Excess catecholamine secretion results in vascular contraction and a relatively low intravascular volume. α-Blockers cause a fall in peripheral resistance, mainly by a reduction in arteriolar tone. β-Blockers can then be used to counteract the resulting tachycardia. β-Blockade should never be instituted until α-blockade is fully established, as unopposed α–stimulation may lead to severe hypertension and fulminant congestive cardiac failure. Labetalol is not suitable as a solo therapy despite being both an α- and β-blocker. When given IV it is seven times more potent at β-adrenoceptors than α-adrenoceptors; following oral administration the relative potencies are 3 to 1.

Further reading

Naranjo J., Dodd S., Martin Y.N. (2017) Perioperative management of Pheochromocytoma. *J Cardiothorac Vasc Anesth* **31** (4)

Prys-Roberts, C. (2000). Phaeochromocytoma—recent progress in its management. *British Journal of Anaesthesia*, **85**, 44–57.

☼ Addisonian crisis

Definition
A collection of symptoms that indicates severe adrenal insufficiency. It is due to either stress in patients with chronic adrenal insufficiency without adequate steroid replacement, or due to acute adrenal haemorrhage or pituitary apoplexy (i.e. infarction or haemorrhage).

Presentation
- Severe hypotension or hypovolaemic shock, usually refractory to fluids and vasopressors.
- Acute abdominal pain, vomiting, and hyper- or hypothermia. May be misdiagnosed as having an acute abdomen.
- Mild hyponatraemia, hyperkalaemia, hypoglycaemia, and mildly elevated urea may be present.
- Addison's disease is typified by weakness, fatigue, and excess pigmentation.
- In patients with type I diabetes, deterioration of glycaemic control with recurrent hypoglycaemia can be the presenting sign of adrenal insufficiency.

Immediate management
☑ ABC—100% oxygen.
☑ IV fluids—saline 0.9% to replace Na⁺ deficit and glucose for hypoglycaemia.
☑ Hydrocortisone 100 mg IV or IM stat followed by 100 mg qds. Baseline cortisol and ACTH prior to administration of hydrocortisone. Dexamethasone (4 mg IV) can be used if the diagnosis has not been confirmed, since this does not interfere with measurement of cortisol and ACTH stimulation testing.
☑ Inotropes/vasopressors as required. May be resistant in the absence of cortisol replacement.

Subsequent management
☑ Treat primary cause or precipitating factor.
☑ Give antibiotics as clinically indicated.
☑ Refer to ITU.

Investigations
- U&Es and glucose.
- Baseline cortisol and ACTH.
- Short tetracosactide (Synacthen®) test—no response.
- Take blood, urine, and sputum for culture.
- ECG and troponin to exclude MI.

Risk factors

- Usually occurs in someone with Addison's disease, or one who is on long-term steroids but has forgotten to take their medication. Precipitating factors include:
  - surgery
  - trauma
  - cessation of steroid therapy
  - sepsis
  - coagulopathy
  - acute illness
  - burns
- In autoimmune polyendocrine syndrome type 2, onset of autoimmune hyperthyroidism can precipitate adrenal crisis due to enhanced cortisol clearance.
- Can also occur after bilateral adrenal haemorrhage.

Exclusions

- Acute abdomen.
- Septic shock.
- Myocardial infarction and cardiogenic shock.

Paediatric implications

- In children, acute adrenal insufficiency often presents as hypoglycaemic seizures.
- Give hydrocortisone initially 2 mg/kg IV. Often given as an infusion for the young child to prevent troughs in between boluses.

Further reading

Annane, D., Bellissant, E., Bollaert, P.E., Briegel, J., Keh, D., Kupfer, Y. (2004). Corticosteroids for severe sepsis and septic shock: a systemic review and *meta-analysis*. *British Medical Journal*, **329**, 480–4.

Bornstein S.R. et al. (2016). Diagnosis and treatment of primary adrenal insufficiency: An Endocrine Society Clinical Practice Guideline. *The Journal of Clinical Endocrinology and Metabolism* **101** (2), 364–89.

Chakera, A.J., Vaidya, B. (2010). Addison's disease in adults: diagnosis and management. *American Journal of Medicine*, **123**(5), 409–13.

☼ Disseminated intravascular coagulation (DIC)

Definition
DIC is a syndrome characterized by systemic activation of coagulation pathways leading to the formation of fibrin clots that may cause organ failure with concomitant consumption of platelets and coagulation factors that may result in clinical bleeding.

Presentation
- Presents with symptoms relating to underlying disease process.
- DIC can also present with bleeding (64%) or symptoms related to thrombotic complications, i.e. renal dysfunction (25%), hepatic dysfunction (19%), respiratory dysfunction (dyspnoea and cough), shock, and altered consciousness (2%).

Immediate management
- ☑ Treat underlying disease.
- ☑ Give platelets if platelet count <50 × 10^9/L and active bleeding or an invasive procedure is planned.
- ☑ In non-bleeding patients, assess bleeding risk but accept a lower count before giving platelets (i.e. if count falls below 10–20 × 10^9/L).
- ☑ Give fresh frozen plasma (FFP) at an initial dose of 15 mL/kg in actively bleeding patients with DIC or those requiring an invasive procedure, and prolonged PT and activated partial thromboplastin time (APTT).
- ☑ Give prothrombin complex concentrate if transfusion of FFP not possible due to fluid overload (Note this will only partially correct the deficiency.)
- ☑ Give fibrinogen concentrate 3 g or 2 pools cryoprecipitate if severe hypofibrinogenaemia (<1 g/L) that persists despite FFP replacement. (This should increase fibrinogen by 1 g/L.)

Subsequent management
- ☑ Consult a haematologist.
- ☑ Give further blood products guided by viscoelastometric point-of-care testing devices (ROTEM/TEG).

Anticoagulants
- ☑ In DIC where thrombosis predominates with arterial or venous thromboembolism, consider therapeutic doses of heparin.
- ☑ In non-bleeding patients with DIC, prophylaxis for venous thromboembolism with prophylactic doses of heparin or LMWH is recommended.

Other agents

The use of other anticoagulants in the treatment of DIC remains controversial:

- Antithrombin has been used in patients with sepsis and DIC. However, the beneficial effect is not conclusive.
- Activated protein C (APC) concentrates have been found to improve survival over that of heparin in the treatment of DIC due to severe sepsis. However, it should not be given if the patient is at high risk of bleeding.
- Recombinant factor VIIa (rFVIIa) may be used in patients with severe bleeding unresponsive to other treatment options.

Investigations

- Diagnosis made from the clinical picture and coagulation tests.
- Check platelet count, fibrin-related markers (D-dimer and fibrin degradation products), fibrinogen, PT, and APTT.
- The International Society on Thrombosis and Haemostasis developed a simple scoring system (Table 10.3). A score of 5 or more indicates overt DIC; a score of less than 5 does not rule out DIC but may indicate non-overt DIC.

Risk factors

DIC can be caused by:

- Infections (Gram-positive and -negative bacteria, viruses, fungi, and protozoa)
- Malignancy (acute myelocytic leukaemias)
- Obstetrics conditions (placental abruption, amniotic fluid embolism, acute fatty liver of pregnancy, eclampsia, retained dead fetus syndrome)
- Trauma
- Burns
- Snake envenomation
- Blood transfusion
- Acute hepatic failure

Table 10.3 Scoring system for DIC

Score	0	1	2	3
Platelet count	>100	<100	<50	
Elevated fibrin marker	No elevation		Moderate increase	Strong increase
Prolongation of PT (s)	<3	3–6	>6	
Fibrinogen level (g/L)	>1	<1		

Reproduced with permission from Taylor, F. B. Jr. et al. (2001). Towards definition, clinical and laboratory criteria, and a scoring system for disseminated intravascular coagulation. *Thromb Haemost.* 2001;86:1327–30. Copyright © 2001, Rights Managed by Georg Thieme Verlag KG Stuttgart • New York. doi: 10.1055/s-0037-1616068.

Exclusions
- Consumptive coagulopathies (e.g. trauma and major surgery).
- Severe liver disease may result in markedly reduced production of coagulation factors and inhibitors.
- Thrombotic thrombocytopenic purpura.
- Idiopathic thrombocytopenic purpura and heparin-induced thrombocytopenia are both also associated with low platelets with thrombus formation, but do not have the consumptive coagulopathy of DIC which causes APTT and PT to be elevated.

Paediatric implications
- 10–15 mL/kg FFP will increase coagulation factors by 10–20% in ongoing consumption.

Further reading
Franchini, M., Lippi, G., Manzato, F. (2006). Recent acquisitions in the pathophysiology, diagnosis and treatment of disseminated intravascular coagulation. *Thrombosis Journal*, **4**, 4.

Levi, M., Toh, C.H., Thachil, J., Watson, H.G. (2009) Guidelines for the diagnosis and management of disseminated intravascular coagulation. British Committee for Standards in Haematology. *British Journal of Haematology*, **145**, 24–33.

Wada, H., Matsumoto, T., Yamashita, Y. (2014). Diagnosis and treatment of disseminated intravascular coagulation (DIC) according to four DIC guidelines. *Journal of Intensive Care*, **20**(1), 15.

☼ Hypoglycaemia

Definition
- A lower level than normal blood glucose.
- A blood glucose <4.0 mmol/L should be treated.

Presentation
- Early:
  - shaking
  - pins and needles
  - palpitations
  - slurred speech, headache, double vision
  - hunger
- Intermediate to late:
  - altered behaviour, poor concentration
  - restlessness, sweating
  - fits
  - coma

Immediate management

Adults who are conscious and able to swallow
☑ Give four glucose tablets, dextrose gel (e.g. Glucogel/Hypostop™), any high-sugar drink or three spoonfuls of sugar in warm water.
☑ Check blood sugar after 10 min, if clinical symptoms remain repeat.
☑ Once symptoms have resolved, a high-fibre snack or carbohydrate meal should be eaten if the next meal is not due within the hour.
☑ Continue with normal regimen, but insulin review may be required.

Adults who are unconscious, aggressive, or having seizures
☑ Check airway (and give oxygen).
☑ Breathing.
☑ Circulation and gain IV access.
☑ Disability (including GCS and blood glucose).
☑ Exposure (including temperature).
☑ If patient has an insulin infusion running, stop immediately.
☑ Give 100 mL 20% dextrose or 200 mL 10% dextrose IV over 15 min. Repeat blood glucose measurement 10 min later.
☑ If IV access not available give glucagon 1 mg IM. This may take up to 15 min to take effect.

Subsequent management

☑ Once blood glucose >4.0 mmol/L, give longer acting carbohydrate or glucose infusion if blood sugar remains unstable.
☑ Liaise with diabetic team to improve blood sugar control.
☑ Monitor blood sugars closely for 24 h, rebound hypo-/hyperglycaemia may occur.
☑ Investigate cause if not obvious (e.g. incorrect insulin dosage).

Investigations

Blood glucose.

Risk factors

- Insulin or oral hypoglycaemic overdose—generally accidental.
- Insufficient oral intake—delayed meals, excess activity.
- Medical conditions—insulinoma, hypopituitarism, acute liver failure.
- Postoperative—pancreatectomy, gastric surgery.
- Extremes of age.
- Pregnancy.
- Alcohol excess.
- Severe sepsis, quinine therapy.

Exclusions

Any patient with an altered conscious level or CVS instability should have their blood sugar checked, as many conditions can mimic hypoglycaemia:

- excess alcohol intake
- drug overdose
- epilepsy and cerebral irritation of any cause
- sepsis
- cardiogenic shock

Paediatric implications

- Different age groups present differently.
- Children can develop nocturnal hypoglycaemia despite good diabetic control, therefore consider hypoglycaemia in children found collapsed in bed.
- Infants <1 y can develop hypoglycaemia with fasting.
- Neonates:
  - brisk reflexes, lethargy, coma
  - poor feeding
  - hypothermia
  - apnoeas/respiratory distress
  - bradycardia
- Infants/children:
  - sweating
  - hunger/poor appetite
  - anxiety/confusion/bad behaviour/seizures/coma
  - respiratory distress
  - cardiovascular instability

- Treatment:
  - If awake, encourage oral intake of simple carbohydrates (e.g. sugary drinks, milk).
  - If reduced conscious level:
    - 2.5 mL/kg of glucose 10% IV
    - repeat as necessary and infuse to maintain blood sugar >4 mmol/L
    - glucagon 500 µg IM/SC/IV if <12 y (1 mg if >12 y)

Special considerations

- Severe and prolonged hypoglycaemia may result in cerebral oedema. Intensive care and organ support may be required.
- 50% glucose can be highly irritant to blood vessels; therefore, if it is used instead of more dilute glucose preparations, care should be taken at time of injection. Avoid use in children due to small vessel size.
- Glucagon is relatively ineffective in liver failure, in those who are chronically malnourished (e.g. alcoholics) and after acute alcohol ingestion.
- Ongoing hypoglycaemia in the presence of liver disease may be a marker of acute liver failure.
- Hypoglycaemic attacks in previously well-controlled, insulin-dependent diabetics may indicate secondary pathology, e.g. Addison's disease (➐ see p. 292) or coeliac disease.
- Patient information and follow-up are vital. Liaise with local diabetic services.
- If the patient is not a known diabetic, investigate other causes.
- In cases of a hypoglycaemic agent overdose, rebound hypoglycaemia can occur after initial treatment, therefore consider transfer to HDU and initiate treatment with 10% glucose.
- NB: Blood glucose range on ABGs may be lower than recorded on BM stix.

Further reading

ABCD (2013). *The Hospital Management of Hypoglycaemia in Adults with Diabetes Mellitus*. Available at: http://www.diabetologists-abcd.org.uk/JBDS/JBDS.htm

Ly, T.T., Maahs, D.M., Rewers, A., Dunger, D., Oduwole, A., Jones, T.W. (2014) International Society of Pediatric and Adolescent Diabetes clinical practice consensus guidelines—hypoglycemia: assessment and management of hypoglycemia in children and adolescents with diabetes. *Pediatric Diabetes*, **15** (Suppl. 20), 180–92.

☼ Acute liver failure

Definition

- Encephalopathy, coagulopathy, and jaundice (often in individuals with no pre-existing liver disease). Defined according to the speed of onset of encephalopathy:
  - hyperacute: <7 days
  - acute: 7– 28 days
  - subacute: >28 days to 12 weeks.

Presentation

- Depends on the underlying cause:
  - non-specific symptoms; nausea, vomiting, abdominal pain
  - jaundice.
- Bleeding—deranged INR.
- Cardiovascular instability—patients usually have a high cardiac output with vasodilatation.
- Encephalopathy—grading is essential for management:
  - Grade I—Slow mental function, rousable, altered mood
  - Grade II—Inappropriate behaviour, drowsy but able to talk
  - Grade III—Drowsy, can be agitated or aggressive
  - Grade IV—Coma, may respond to painful stimulus.

Immediate management

- ☑ Assess ABC. Treatment is usually supportive initially, i.e. fluids, antibiotics (if indicated— ➔ see 'Special considerations', p. 302), monitor urine output.
- ☑ Grade III/IV encephalopathic patients should be transferred to ITU. Intubation, ventilation, and renal support (haemodialysis) nearly always required.
- ☑ Do not correct INR unless bleeding as this is used as a marker of hepatic impairment.
- ☑ Determine the cause of ALF to guide further management decisions.
- ☑ In those with paracetamol overdose or where there is a possibility of paracetamol overdose, give activated charcoal followed by acetylcysteine. Acetylcysteine should be given at a loading dose of 150 mg/kg followed by an infusion (➔ see pp. 375–377 and BNF).

Subsequent management

- ☑ Refer all patients with encephalopathy to a specialist liver unit.
- ☑ CVS—many patients require large volumes of fluid and should have CVP monitored. ALF results in a high cardiac output, vasodilated state, hence inotropes and vasoconstrictors are often required. Maintain mean arterial pressure ≥ 75 mmHg and cerebral perfusion pressure 60–80 mmHg.

☑ RS— intubate and ventilate patients with Grade III/IV encephalopathy to ensure airway protection and control of carbon dioxide in the presence of raised ICP.

☑ CNS—ICP is elevated in those with encephalopathy. Signs of raised ICP are late and as such ICP monitoring can be useful– ICP monitoring devices should be placed with caution due to concurrent coagulopathy. To reduce ICP consider head-up position, avoid tight ETT ties and practise minimal intervention care. If ICP remains high (>25 mmHg for >10 min) consider mannitol (0.5–1.0 g/kg). Maintain a higher serum sodium (145–155 mmol/L) with 1–2 mL/kg 5% saline to help reduce cerebral oedema.

☑ Metabolic—renal failure is common especially in those with hyperacute liver failure. If renal support is required, use a continuous mode rather than an intermittent mode to improve cardiovascular stability. Use lactate-free buffer solutions. Hypocalcaemia and hypoglycaemia can occur. Where hypoglycaemia is a problem an infusion of 10% glucose should be administered centrally and titrated according to blood glucose.

☑ Coagulation—patients should be cross-matched due to the risk of spontaneous haemorrhage. However, FFP should not be used to correct the INR unless bleeding occurs. The INR is used as a measure of hepatic synthetic function and as such reflects severity of disease. Thrombocytopenia also occurs.

Investigations

- To diagnose the cause and assess ongoing status:
  - viral serology
  - FBC, U&Es, LFTs (bilirubin, AST, ALT)
  - clotting—INR
  - monitor blood glucose
  - ABG and lactate
  - Autoantibodies
  - image hepatic vasculature (ultrasound)
  - send for immunology, microbiology (urine, sputum, blood for MC&S) and toxicology—including paracetamol levels
  - pregnancy test (females)
  - Consider ceruloplasmin if no obvious explanation for ALF (Looking for Wilson's disease).

Risk factors

- A thorough history is vital as the cause has implications for management, severity, and outcome.
- Infection—ask about recent travel and social history (sexual partners, recreational drug usage, recent tattoos).
- Drugs, e.g. paracetamol overdose (still the commonest cause in the United Kingdom), MAOIs, carbamazepine, isoniazid, ecstasy, phenytoin.
- Toxins—mycose phyllodes (mushrooms), herbal remedies.
- Vascular anomalies—Budd–Chiari syndrome, ischaemic hepatitis.
- Other—viral hepatitis, acute fatty liver of pregnancy, lymphoma, Wilson's disease.

Box 10.1 Criteria for consideration for liver transplantation in acute liver failure

Paracetamol overdose
- Arterial pH <7.3 (or 7.25 if NAC given)
  or
- PT >100 secs (INR >6.5) and
- Creatinine >300 µmol/L and
- Grade III/IV encephalopathy

Non–paracetamol
- PT >100 secs (INR >6.5)
  or three of the following:
  - Age <10 or >40 y
  - Jaundice >7 days prior to encephalopathy
  - PT >50 secs
  - Bilirubin >300 µmol/L
  - Aetiology—non-A non-B hepatitis, drug-induced hepatitis

Special considerations
- All ALF patients are at risk for bacterial or fungal infection or sepsis, therefore culture regularly. Prophylactic antibiotics and antifungals have not been shown to improve overall outcomes.
- Give histamine-2 blocking agents or proton pump inhibitors for acid-related gastrointestinal bleeding associated with stress.
- Early involvement of a specialist liver unit is important for advice and decision making with regard to transplantation (see criteria in Box 10.1).
- Despite advances in managing these patients, there is still a high mortality and morbidity associated with ALF. Those with subacute liver failure tend to have the worst prognosis.

Further reading

Lai, W.K., Murphy, N. (2004). Management of acute liver failure. Continuing education in anaesthesia. *Critical Care & Pain (CEACCP)*, **4**(2), 40–3.

Lee, W.M., Larson, A.M., Stravitz, R.T. (2011). *American Association for the Study of Liver Diseases Position Paper: The Acute Management of Acute Liver Failure: Update 2011*. Available at: https://www.aasld.org

Maclure, P., Salman, B. (2012) *Management of Acute Liver Failure in Critical Care. Anaesthesia Tutorial of the Week 251*. Available at: https://www.frca.co.uk/Documents/251%20Acute%20Liver%20Failure%20in%20Critical%20Care.pdf

☼ Sickle cell crisis

Definition

Acute, painful, and life-threatening occlusion of blood vessels by sickle cells. Often accompanied by haemolysis.

Presentation

- Signs of tissue infarction due to reduced blood flow and poor tissue oxygenation. Occlusion of vessels can occur at any site in the body:
  - RS—'acute chest syndrome'—hypoxia, dyspnoea, haemoptysis, chest pain. Long-term respiratory failure with pulmonary hypertension.
  - CNS—CVA, blindness, subarachnoid haemorrhages.
  - haematological—acute drop in haemoglobin levels, bone marrow failure resulting in neutropenia. Sequestration of cells in the spleen causes thrombocytopenia and increased sickling in the presence of a crisis.
  - skeletal and soft tissue—bone pain; disruption of growth plates, leading to gross limb deformities; osteomyelitis and cutaneous ulceration due to skin infarcts.
  - abdominal—renal impairment, priapism, haematuria, ileus, jaundice, gallstones, ascending cholangitis/empyema of gallbladder, liver failure.
- Evidence of multiorgan involvement due to recurrent episodes of vaso-occlusion.

Immediate management

- ☑ Aim to break the cycle of sickling.
- ☑ IV access and rehydrate.
- ☑ Admit to specialist ward, give oxygen if saturations <95%.
- ☑ Keep warm.
- ☑ Analgesia—Obtain treatment history and locally agreed patient plan. Follow WHO pain ladder. Give paracetamol and NSAIDs if able and then consider:
  - Entonox particularly if no IV access.
  - Morphine 0.1–0.15 mg/kg IV every 20 min until pain is controlled (monitor for respiratory depression), then give 0.05–0.1 mg/kg every 2–4 h.
  - Morphine PCA according to local protocols.
- ☑ Monitor patients every 20 min until pain is controlled and then at least every 2 h.
- ☑ Give antiemetics.

Subsequent management

- ☑ Look for infections, complications, and precipitating factors. Most adults with SCD are functionally asplenic.
- ☑ Most antibiotic treatments are started empirically before culture results are available.

☑ Blood transfusion—indicated when Hb <5 g/dL (or decrease of >2 g/dL) and clinical crisis. Transfuse to Hb >10 g/dL but <12 g/dL. Aim for HbA >70%. Limitation of blood transfusions reduces the risk of long-term complications.

☑ Exchange transfusion is at times indicated for major surgery, but specialist advice must be sought from a consultant haematologist.

Investigations

- FBC—including reticulocyte count and blood film (looking for sickle cells, sideroblasts, and Howell–Jolly bodies). 'Sickledex' test—induces sickling in susceptible red blood cells. Hb electrophoresis—to differentiate between homozygous (sickle cell disease) and heterozygous (sickle cell trait).
- G&S, U&Es, LFT, CXR, ABGs, amylase.
- AXR/CT/MRI if indicated.
- Blood, sputum, urine, stool cultures.

Risk factors

- Patients with sickle cell disease after 6 months of age.
- Sickle cell crisis is extremely rare in those with sickle cell trait.
- Hypoxaemia and acidosis.
- Infection of any cause.
- Cold, hypotension, pain, and dehydration.

Paediatric implications

- ☑ On admission, prescribe oral, or PR medication: paracetamol (20 mg/kg 6-hourly PO/PR), and NSAIDs—diclofenac (1 mg/kg 8–12-hourly PO/PR) or ibuprofen (5–10 mg/kg 4–6-hourly PO).
- ☑ If no improvement or deterioration, give IV morphine 0.05–0.08 mg/kg and repeat at 5 min intervals up to 0.4 mg/kg. Consider prescribing a PCA for those deemed competent.
- ☑ Risk of death from overwhelming Streptococcus pneumoniae sepsis is high. Take cultures and treat all toxic looking children promptly with IV antibiotics.
- ☑ Causes failure to thrive.

Special considerations

- Chronic low haemoglobin levels are normal in those with sickle cell disease. Normal Hb is approx. 6–9 g/dL, therefore a low Hb is not in itself an indication for transfusion or cancellation of elective surgery.
- Patients with sickle cell disease have often had multiple admissions, many insist on pethidine for analgesia. If pethidine is used in high doses, then also prescribe carbamazepine 100 mg tds to reduce the side effects of norpethidine accumulation.
- Many patients have renal impairment therefore use NSAIDs and renally excreted drugs with caution.
- Avoid use of tourniquets, bandages, and so on, as they can promote further occlusion of vessels.
- Caution is needed when considering regional techniques for localized pain. Many patients are started on heparin in view of the vaso-occlusive

nature of this disease, hence regional techniques are relatively contraindicated.
• Sickle cell crisis is rare in those with sickle cell trait only—consider a different cause for their pain.

Anaesthetizing a patient with sickle cell disease

☑ Active management pre-, intra-, and postoperatively of known precipitants—such as dehydration, infection, acidosis, hypothermia, and pain—reduces the likelihood of a sickle crisis developing.

☑ Fasting times should be kept to a minimum.

☑ IV fluids should ideally be established the night before theatre.

☑ Patients should be first on the list.

☑ Liaise with haematology (preferably the patient's physician) with regard to any blood transfusion requirements.

☑ Some patients (those with SCD-SC) may require exchange transfusion to avoid complications associated with hyperviscosity.

☑ Preoxygenate and keep inspired oxygen >40% (correct end-tidal volatile concentration appropriately if you normally use high concentrations of N_2O).

☑ Core temperature measurement—aim for normothermia using warmed IV fluids, forced air warmer, ambient theatre temperature control, and so on.

☑ SCD-related complications have been shown to be more common in those who received regional compared with general anaesthesia.

☑ Use of tourniquets has been described in patients with sickle cell disease, but may increase the risk of crisis. Limbs must be exsanguinated fully as sickling can occur locally in vessels.

☑ Ideally, nurse in a unit experienced at caring for patients with sickle cell disease.

☑ Postoperative oxygen must be prescribed—ideally for 72 h after surgery.

☑ Continue with intravenous fluids until patients are receiving free fluids orally.

☑ Tailor analgesia to the patient's needs—they may require higher than normal doses of analgesics, especially opioids.

☑ Inform outreach/acute pain team.

Further reading

Lucas, S.B., Mason, D.G., Mason, M., Weyman, D. (2008). *A Sickle Crisis: A Report of the National Confidential Enquiry into Patient Outcome and Death*. London, UK: National Confidential Enquiry into Patient Outcome and Death.

National Heart, Lung and Blood Institute (2014). *Evidence-Based Management of Sickle Cell Disease. Expert Panel Report*. Available at: https://www.nhlbi.nih.gov/health-topics/evidence-based-management-sickle-cell-disease

O'Meara, M., Davies, G. (2013). Anaesthesia for patients with sickle cell disease (and other haemoglobinopathies). *Anaesthesia and Intensive Care Medicine*, **14**, 54–6.

Wilson, M., Forsyth, P., Whiteside, J. (2009). Haemoglobinopathy and sickle cell disease. *Continuing Education in Anaesthesia, Critical Care and Pain*, **10**, 24–8.

ⓘ **TURP syndrome**

(➲ See also 'Hyponatraemia', p. 319.)

Definition
Excess absorption of irrigation fluid during transurethral resection of prostate (TURP) causing hyponatraemia.

Presentation
Early
- CVS—bradycardia, hypertension.
- GI—nausea and vomiting, abdominal distension.
- CNS—anxiety/confusion, headache, dizziness, slow waking after GA, restlessness.

Late
- CVS—hypotension, angina, cardiac failure.
- RS—dyspnoea, tachypnoea, cyanosis (pulmonary failure).
- CNS—twitching, visual disturbance (transient blindness due to glycine), seizures, coma.
- GU—renal tubular necrosis, reduced urine output.

Immediate management
☑ ABC—100% oxygen.
☑ Stop intravenous fluids.
☑ Control bleeding, terminate operation, and stop irrigation fluid as soon as possible. Insert urinary catheter.
☑ May require endotracheal intubation and positive pressure ventilation if pulmonary oedema has developed.
☑ Give diuretics (e.g. furosemide 40 mg IV) only if there is acute pulmonary oedema (due to transient hypervolaemia). Furosemide may further decrease Na^+, but it is effective at removing free water. Mannitol (e.g. 100 mL of 20% IV) causes less Na^+ loss than loop diuretics.
☑ Give glycopyrrolate 200–600 µg IV for bradycardia and vasopressors (e.g. metaraminol 0.5–1 mg IV repeated as necessary) for hypotension.
☑ Treat seizures with diazepam 5–10 mg IV. Consider magnesium sulphate 2 g IV if glycine is in the irrigation fluid used.
☑ Check serum Na^+ and Hb regularly.

Subsequent management for severe/late TURP syndrome
☑ Neurological symptoms indicate increasing severity of TURP syndrome. Admit all patients with neurological manifestations to ITU as there is a risk of cerebral oedema and respiratory failure.
☑ Establish invasive monitoring early in severe cases.
☑ Give hypertonic 3% saline 2 mL/kg (or 150 mL) IV over 20 min.

☑ Check the serum Na$^+$ level after 20 min while repeating the second infusion of hypertonic 3% saline 2 mL/kg IV over 20 min.

☑ Repeat twice until a target serum sodium increase of 5 mmol/L is achieved or symptoms improve.

☑ If increase in Na$^+$ of 5 mmol/L is achieved in the first hour, but no change in symptoms, aim to increase Na$^+$ by 1 mmol/L each hour by infusing hypertonic 3% saline. Stop infusion when Na$^+$ increases by 10 mmol/L or reaches Na$^+$ 130 mmol/L.

☑ Monitor electrolytes 2-hourly to avoid overcorrection.

☑ Aim to increase the serum Na$^+$ by 1–2 mmol/L/h for 3–4 h until the neurologic symptoms subside, or until the plasma Na$^+$ >130 mmol/L.

☑ Do not increase Na$^+$ >10 mmol/L in the first 24 h and limit to 8 mmol/L during every 24 h thereafter.

☑ Metabolic acidosis can occur, which may require renal support (i.e. haemofiltration).

Investigations

Serum sodium levels

Risk factors

- Related to speed of absorption of irrigation fluid. Average rate of absorption is 20 mL/min.
- Large prostate (>45 g).
- Prolonged operation time >60 min.
- Hypotonic fluids given IV intraoperatively.
- Volume of irrigation >30 L.
- Inexperienced surgeon.
- Height of irrigation fluid bag >60 cm above the patient.
- Comorbidities (e.g. liver disease, genitourinary stones, UTI).

Exclusions

Congestive cardiac failure

Special considerations

- Elderly population with myocardial impairment may be more symptomatic due to fluid shifts.
- Regional techniques are thought to reduce the incidence of TURP syndrome:
  - conscious level of the patient can be monitored throughout operation and hence early signs can be identified.
  - less absorption of irrigation fluid due to reduced venous pressure in the prostatic bed.
- Clinical signs are absent in those under general anaesthesia—watch for unexplained tachycardia and hypertension. If concerned, check serum sodium.
- Tracer substances—some centres advocate adding ethanol 10% to irrigation fluid and measuring blood level (>0.6 mg/mL indicative of >2 L absorption).

- New techniques have been introduced using bipolar electrosurgery devices and various laser and microwave systems. These devices are compatible with saline. Although hyponatraemia is no longer an issue, there is still a potential problem with fluid overload.

Further reading

Hawary, A., Mukhtar, K., Sinclair, A., Pearce, I. (2009). Transurethral resection of the prostate syndrome: almost gone but not forgotten. *Journal of Endourology*, **23**(12), 2013–20.
O'Donnell, A.M., Foo, I.T.H. (2009) Anaesthesia for transurethral resection of the prostate. *Continuing Education in Anaesthesia, Critical Care and Pain*, **9**(3), 92–6.

☼ Hypothermia

Definition

- Core temperature <35°C
  - mild 32–35°C
  - moderate 28–32°C
  - severe <28°C

Presentation

Varies according to temperature:

- <35°C:
  - apathy
  - confusion and disorientation
  - incoordination
  - shivering
- <32°C:
  - metabolic acidosis and hyperkalaemia
  - hypovolaemia
  - coagulopathy
  - dilated pupils
  - arrhythmias and reduced cardiac output
- <28°C:
  - unconsciousness
  - unresponsive EEG (at 18°C)
  - cardiac dysrhythmias/cardiac arrest, VF, and vasoconstriction
  - ECG—J waves
  - diuresis—but loss of concentrating ability of the kidney
  - apnoea
- <15°C:
  - asystole

Immediate management

☑ ABC—100% oxygen.
☑ Active resuscitation according to ALS guidelines (➲ p. 13).
☑ Drugs and defibrillation may be ineffective below 30°C. Use active and passive warming methods. Withhold adrenaline and other resuscitation drugs until temperature >30°C.
☑ Between 32°C and 35°C, double the time interval between drugs.
☑ Warming may reveal hypovolaemia and patient may require large volumes of fluids.
☑ Aim to correct hypothermia as quickly as it developed. If time frame unknown, then re-warm by 1°C/h.
☑ Modify immediate management according to clinical situation.

Postoperative hypothermia

Ideally—prevention using forced air warming blankets, patient warming mattress, warmed fluids, and HME filters on breathing circuits reduces the chance of post-op. hypothermia. If it does develop:

☑ warm patient using warming blankets.
☑ maintain ambient temperature >21°C.
☑ warm IV fluids and all irrigation fluids.
☑ transfer the patient to recovery, as generally higher ambient temperature than in theatres.
☑ admit to ITU post-op. and warm up slowly prior to waking and weaning.

Emergency surgery patient

☑ ABC—100% O_2 (warmed to 40–42°C and humidified).
☑ Passive re-warming:
  • remove wet clothes and dry patient.
  • turn up ambient temperature.
☑ Active re-warming:
  • radiant heaters.
  • heating blankets and warming mattresses.
  • warmed IV fluids—consider using a rapid infusion system if large transfusions are required.
☑ Humidify inspired gases.
☑ Insert central line and invasive BP monitoring (NB Caution with line insertion, as possible coagulopathy).
☑ Blood gases—interpret uncorrected (for temperature) arterial blood gases as they are easier to understand and can be used for trend analysis during re-warming.
☑ Consider warmed fluid for irrigation of body cavities while in theatre.
☑ Aim to warm to 32–34°C as hyperthermia can be detrimental—hypothermia is thought to be neuroprotective.
☑ Consider the need for postoperative intensive care early.

Cold immersion/submersion

(⊕ See also 'Paediatric drowning', p. 134.)
Immersion—head above water. Patients suffer hypothermia and cardiovascular instability.
Submersion—head below water. Patients develop asphyxiation and hypoxia.
  • Both groups are at risk of traumatic injuries.
  • Manage cardiac arrest and re-warming as above.
  • Vomiting is often seen in submersion victims. If the patient is conscious, place in the recovery position. Unconscious patients require definitive airway control, therefore intubate and ventilate. Decompress the stomach by inserting a large-bore NG tube.
  • Submersion victims suffer a multisystem insult and, as such, require Intensive Care support. Both submersion and immersion patients should be invasively monitored if they arrive unconscious.

Resuscitation in the hypothermic patient

With a continued fall in core temperature, bradycardia, atrial fibrillation, ventricular fibrillation, and finally asystole develop.

☑ ABC—100% oxygen, intubate and ventilate, oesophageal temperature probe. Initiate passive and active re-warming.

☑ Follow ALS protocols, adjusted as follows for hypothermia.

☑ Hypothermia renders the myocardium unresponsive to drugs, defibrillation, and pacemakers; consider withholding drugs until the patient's temperature is above 30°C.

☑ Below 30°C three DC shocks can be tried, but if there is no response then no further shocks should be given until the core temperature is above 30°C.

☑ Between 30°C and 35°C give drugs required, but at twice the time interval and the lowest recommended dose; resume normal drug protocols from ALS as the patient's temperature approaches normothermia.

☑ Chest wall stiffness occurs in hypothermia, which can make chest compressions and ventilation difficult—aim to see the chest move with ventilation, and for 4 cm depression with cardiac massage.

☑ Central access is vital due to peripheral vasoconstriction (poor access, poor flow, and drug accumulation in vessels with sluggish flow).

☑ In specialist centres, cardiopulmonary bypass can be used to actively re-warm patients. If this is not available, standard venovenous haemofiltration can be used, and the replacement fluid warmed. The return line from the filter can also be insulated to prevent passive heat loss. Percutaneous bypass lines reduce haemorrhage. In all cases, beware of coagulopathy.

☑ Active warming causes progressive venous dilation; therefore large volumes of fluids are likely to be required.

☑ Check blood gas and electrolytes/clotting regularly:
  • intra-/extracellular electrolyte shifts can develop rapidly, causing hyperkalaemia. ➲ See p. 313.
  • DIC can also occur, due to failure of the clotting cascade (loss of homeostasis with cold). ➲ See p. 294.
  • hypoglycaemia can develop, requiring glucose-containing fluids. ➲ See p. 297.

☑ Death cannot be confirmed until profound hypothermia is excluded (i.e. the patient has been re-warmed and there is no cardiac output, or attempts at re-warming have failed). Check for a central pulse for at least 1 min with ECG monitoring, and look for signs of life before withdrawing support.

☑ If the patient has other life-threatening injuries, or is completely frozen, active resuscitation should probably not be started.

Subsequent management

☑ Most patients require intensive care as multi-organ failure can develop several days after the hypothermic episode. Watch for neurological sequelae.

☑ Watch limbs, especially digits, for signs of frostbite—amputation may be required.
☑ Treat infections early.
☑ Pancreatitis can develop, but may be masked in the initial stages.
☑ Exclude underlying metabolic disorder (e.g. hypothyroidism, diabetes mellitus).

Investigations

- Core temperature, e.g. oesophageal, rectal, or tympanic (axillary temperature 1°C less than core).
- Thyroid function tests should be considered in patients after successful resuscitation, as undiagnosed hypothyroidism can potentiate hypothermia, especially in older people.

Risk factors

- Extremes of age—elderly and infants can become hypothermic very easily.
- Prolonged exposure/near-drowning.
- Impaired conscious level.
- Trauma victims, including those with head injuries.
- Drug overdose—especially antidepressants.
- Endocrine—hypoglycaemia, hypothyroidism.
- Perioperatively—anaesthesia and surgical exposure promote heat loss from the body.

Exclusions

- Hypothyroid
- Diabetes mellitus

Paediatric implications

Survival from severe prolonged hypothermia in children is much greater than that for adults. A long (>1h) resuscitation time may be required to regain a cardiac output in the hypothermic child.

Special considerations

- Hypothermia occurs all year round and bears no relation to the ambient temperature.
- Hypothermia can be neuroprotective, but hypothermia with comorbidities is a poor indicator of outcome.
- Therapeutic hypothermia (32–36°C) is still considered for 24 h post-admission in out-of-hospital cardiac arrest patients who remain unresponsive after ROSC.

Further reading

Kirkbridge, D.A., Buggy, D.J. (2003). Thermoregulation and perioperative hypothermia. *British Journal of Anaesthesia CEPD Reviews*, **3**, (1), 24–8.
NICE (2016). *Hypothermia: Prevention and Management in Adults Having Surgery. NICE Clinical Guideline CG65*. Available at: https://www.nice.org.uk/guidance/cg65
Nolan, J.P., Soar, J., et al. (2015). European Resuscitation Council and European Society of Intensive Care Medicine guidelines for Post-resuscitation Care 2015: Section 5 of the European Resuscitation Council Guidelines for Resuscitation 2015. *Resuscitation*, **202–222**

! Hyperkalaemia

Definition

- Normal serum potassium 3.5–5.5 mmol/L
- Mild hyperkalaemia 5.5–5.9 mmol/L
- Moderate hyperkalaemia 6.0–6.4 mmol/L
- Severe hyperkalaemia >6.4 mmol/L

Presentation

- Incidental laboratory finding.
- Signs of causative illness: nausea, vomiting, and diarrhoea, dehydration ± renal impairment and acidosis.
- Effects on skeletal muscle:
  - generalized fatigue, weakness, paraesthesia, paralysis
- Effects on cardiac muscle:
  - ECG changes progressing through peaked T waves, prolonged PR interval, widened QRS, loss of P wave, loss of R wave amplitude, sine wave pattern, and asystole.
  - ECG changes are potentiated by low calcium, low sodium, and acidosis.

Immediate management

- ☑ Cardiac monitor. IV access.
- ☑ If hyperkalaemic with ECG changes (peaked T waves, small P waves and wide QRS complexes), give calcium chloride (10 mL 10%) or calcium gluconate (30 mL 10%) over 5 min. Calcium stabilizes the heart by increasing the threshold potential.
- ☑ Give insulin 10 units in 250 mL 10% dextrose over 30–60 min.
- ☑ In addition, give nebulized salbutamol 10–20 mg for severe hyperkalaemia and also consider for moderate hyperkalaemia.
- ☑ Sodium bicarbonate should not be used routinely for the acute treatment of hyperkalaemia.

Subsequent management

- ☑ Re-check K^+ level and blood sugar frequently.
- ☑ Refer all patients with severe hyperkalaemia to the renal/intensive care unit.
- ☑ Ion-exchange resin—calcium resonium 15 g PO (or 30 g PR) 8-hourly.
- ☑ If initial management fails, will need dialysis or haemofiltration.
- ☑ Do not consider elective surgery.
- ☑ For life-threatening surgery, first treat hyperkalaemia. Avoid suxamethonium. An alternative for rapid sequence induction is rocuronium, followed by reversal with sugammadex, which is now widely available.
- ☑ Ascertain and treat cause of hyperkalaemia.

Investigations
U&Es, Ca^{2+}, ABGs, ECG

Risk factors
- Increased intake:
  - ingestion of foods high in K^+ (e.g. bananas), or potassium supplements.
  - rapid blood transfusion.
- Intercompartmental shift:
  - trauma, including crush injuries with rhabdomyolysis, burns.
  - suxamethonium (particularly burns and spinal injuries).
  - malignant hyperthermia.
  - acidosis.
- Decreased excretion:
  - acute or chronic renal failure.
  - adrenocortical insufficiency.
- Medications—potassium-sparing diuretics, renin-angiotensin blocking drugs, NSAIDs, β-blockers, digoxin.

Exclusions
Pseudohyperkalaemia (*in vitro* lysis of cells) occurs most commonly during blood-taking due to tourniquet being too tight, or blood left sitting too long. Also occurs in severe thrombocytosis (platelets >1000 × 10⁹/L) or severe leukocytosis (WBC >70 × 10⁹/L).

Paediatric implications
- Calcium chloride 0.2 mL/kg of 10% solution IV over 5 min, not to exceed 5 mL.
- Calcium gluconate 1 mL/kg of 10% solution IV over 3–5 min, not to exceed 10 mL.
- Glucose (25%) 0.5 g/kg (2 mL/kg) with insulin (0.1 unit/kg) IV over 30 min.

Special considerations
- Do not give Hartmann's.
- Avoid hypothermia and acidosis. Control ventilation to prevent respiratory acidosis.
- Monitor neuromuscular blockade during anaesthesia. Effects may be accentuated.
- If a rapid assessment of K^+ is required, check a venous sample with blood gas analyser on ITU.

Further reading
Elliott, M.J., Ronksley, P.E., Clase, C.M., et al. (2010). Management of patients with acute hyperkalaemia. *Canadian Medical Association Journal*, **182**, 1631–35.

UK Renal Association (2014). *Treatment of Acute Hyperkalaemia in Adults. Clinical Practice Guideline.* Available at: https://www.renal.org/guidelines

① Hypokalaemia

Definition
- Normal serum potassium 3.5–5.5 mmol/L
- Mild hypokalaemia 3.0–3.5 mmol/L
- Moderate hypokalaemia 2.5–3.0 mmol/L
- Severe hypokalaemia <2.5 mmol/L

Presentation
- Incidental laboratory finding.
- Palpitations, muscular weakness, abdominal cramping, nausea, and vomiting, arrhythmias, polyuria, respiratory failure.
- ECG may show small or inverted T waves, prominent U waves (after T wave), prolonged PR interval, and depressed ST segment.

Immediate management
- ☑ ABC including cardiac monitor and IV access.
- ☑ For severe hypokalaemia with cardiac arrhythmias, give KCl at 20 mmol/h via a central line with cardiac monitoring, and in a high dependency setting.
- ☑ If moderate hypokalaemia, use 40 mmol K^+ in 1 L bag and infuse peripherally. Consider oral K^+ supplements, but may not be appropriate in the perioperative setting. Sando K^+ two tablets four times a day = 96 mmol K^+.
- ☑ Withhold loop or thiazide diuretics.

Subsequent management
- ☑ Check K^+ level every 1–2 h initially.
- ☑ Ascertain cause of hypokalaemia.
- ☑ Decision to proceed to surgery depends on urgency of surgery, rate of onset of hypokalaemia, and comorbidity. Chronic hypokalaemia is less significant than that of acute onset.
- ☑ Switch any diuretics to potassium-sparing diuretics (e.g. spironolactone or amiloride).

Investigations
- U&Es, creatinine, Mg^{2+}, Ca^{2+}, PO_4^{3-}, and glucose. ECG. ABGs to check for alkalosis.

Risk factors
- Decreased intake:
  - iatrogenic—No K^+ added to IV fluids
  - malnutrition
- Renal losses:
  - renal tubular acidosis
  - hyperaldosteronism
  - leukaemia
  - magnesium depletion

- GI losses:
  - diarrhoea
  - enemas or laxative use
  - vomiting or nasogastric suctioning
  - intestinal fistula, villous adenoma of rectum
  - pyloric stenosis
- Intercompartment shift:
  - insulin
  - alkalosis
  - hypothermia
- Drug side effects:
  - diuretics (most common)
  - steroids
- β-adrenergic agonists

Exclusions

- Cushing's syndrome
- Conn's syndrome—suspect if hypertensive, hypokalaemic alkalosis in someone not taking diuretics
- Hypomagnesaemia
- Hypocalcaemia

Paediatric implications

- Dose of KCl is 0.5 mmol/kg over 1 h.

Special considerations

- Potassium depletion sufficient to cause a 0.3 mmol/L drop in serum potassium requires a loss of about 100 mmol of K^+ from total body store.
- If bicarbonate is raised, then loss is probably longstanding with low intracellular potassium, and will take days to replace.
- Patients should receive no more than 20 mmol/h potassium, to avoid potential deleterious effects on the cardiac conduction system.
- High concentrations of potassium are damaging to the small peripheral veins, so peripheral infusion of K^+ should always be diluted (max. 40 mmol/L). In theatre/ITU/HDU it is easier to give more concentrated solutions of KCl through a central line, to avoid fluid overload.
- Aim for K^+ of 4.0 mmol/L in a digitalized patient, since hypokalaemia increases the risk of digoxin toxicity. Aim for a K^+ of 4.0–5.0 mmol/L if cardiac arrhythmias are present.
- Always use readymade KCL infusions if possible on safety grounds. If 'strong' KCl ampoules are used, these should be stored carefully to avoid the risk of inadvertent IV injection.
- Resistant hypokalaemia—check magnesium and correct if low.

Further reading

Asmar, A., Mohandas, R., Wingo C.S. (2012). A physiologic-based approach to the treatment of a patient with hypokalaemia. American Journal of Kidney Diseases, **10**, 1053.

Freshwater-Turner, D. (2006). Sodium, Potassium and the Anaesthetist. Available at: https://www.frca. co.uk/article.aspx?articleid=100676

Gennari, F.J. (2002). Disorders of potassium homeostasis. Hypokalaemia and hyperkalaemia. Critical Care Clinics, **18**, 273–88.

① Hypernatraemia

Definition
- Normal serum sodium 135–145 mmol/L
- Mild hypernatraemia 145–150 mmol/L
- Moderate hypernatraemia 151–160 mmol/L
- Severe hypernatraemia >160 mmol/L—high mortality

Presentation
- Depends on the cause—fluid status of patient is important (see next). CNS disturbance likely when >155 mmol/L.
- **Hypovolaemic—low total body sodium, excess water loss**:
  - diarrhoea and vomiting, open wounds (urinary Na^+ <10 mmol/L)
  - osmotic diuresis, e.g. following mannitol (urinary Na^+ >20 mmol/L).
  - ACTH insufficiency.

Clinical features—hypotension, tachycardia, dry mucous membranes.
- Euvolaemic—**normal total body sodium**:
  - insufficient water intake or excessive loss.
  - diabetes insipidus.
  - urine osmolality very high, reflecting intact ADH axis but urinary sodium variable.

Clinical features—normal vital signs, no oedema.
- **Hypervolaemic—increased total body sodium, with excess water**:
  - iatrogenic—sodium bicarbonate or hypertonic saline administration (urinary Na^+ >20 mmol/L).
  - Cushing's syndrome.
  - hyperaldosteronism—serum sodium rarely very high.

Clinical features—peripheral oedema, BP may be variable.

Immediate management

Diagnose underlying cause, assess volume status, estimate volume deficit, select fluid repletion regimen, and subsequently monitor and adjust therapy.

Hypovolaemic hypernatraemia
- ☑ 0.9% saline to correct hypovolaemia.
- ☑ thereafter 0.45% saline or 5% glucose to correct water deficit.

Euvolaemic hypernatraemia
- ☑ Give water to correct deficit—encourage oral intake, 0.45% saline or 5% glucose IV.
- ☑ Monitor serum sodium to avoid water intoxication.
- ☑ Diabetes insipidus—replace urinary losses and give desmopressin 1–4 µg/day IV/SC/IM.

Hypervolaemic hypernatraemia
- ☑ Stop administration of high sodium infusions—use 5% glucose.
- ☑ Consider furosemide (20 mg initially) or dialysis with low sodium dialysate if nothing else works.

Subsequent management

☑ Check serum Na$^+$ every 2–4 h.
☑ Monitor potassium and calcium. Reduce sodium intake.
☑ Investigate most likely cause and treat appropriately.

Investigations

U&Es, urinary sodium levels, serum osmolality, urine osmolality

Risk factors

• Very old and very young—limited water intake.
• Altered conscious level—dehydration.
• Uncontrolled diabetes mellitus.
• Treatment with osmotic diuretics (e.g. mannitol).
• Hypertonic saline infusions.
• Sampling error—'drip arm'.

Exclusions

• Sampling error.
• Acute liver failure—maintain serum Na$^+$ >145 mmol/L to increase osmolality and control ICP.

Paediatric implications

• Dehydration:
    • diarrhoea and vomiting.
    • renal impairment resulting in loss of urinary concentrating ability.
    • severe burns.
• Salt poisoning:
    • accidental excessive intake (e.g. incorrect diet in infants).
    • Munchausen's by proxy—purposeful administration of salt.

Special considerations

• Rapid correction of hypernatraemia can induce cerebral oedema. If chronic, correction should take at least 48 h. Aim to reduce serum sodium level by 0.5 mmol/L per hour and no more than 10 mmol/L in first 24 h.
• Acute hypernatraemia can be corrected over hours rather than days.

In this group the risk of rapid correction causing cerebral oedema is reduced.

Anaesthetic implications

☑ No elective surgery if Na$^+$ >155 mmol/L or hypovolaemic.
☑ For urgent surgery—use CVP monitoring if volume status is uncertain or may change rapidly intraoperatively, and be aware of dangers of rapid normalization of electrolytes.

Further reading

Al-Absi A, Gosmanova EO, Wall BM. (2012) A clinical approach to the treatment of chronic hypernatraemia. *American Journal of Kidney Diseases*, **60**(6), 1032–8.
Bagshaw, S.M., Townsend, D.R., McDermid, R.C. (2009). Disorders of sodium and water balance in hospitalized patients. *Canadian Journal of Anaesthesia*, **56**, 151–67.
Miller, R.D. (2009). Sodium physiology. In: Miller, R.D. (ed). *Miller's Anesthesia*, p. **34**. Philadelphia, PA: Churchill Livingstone.
Reynolds, R.M., Padfield, P.L., Seckl, J.R. (2006) Disorders of sodium balance. *British Medical Journal*, **332**, 702–5.

① Hyponatraemia

(⮡ See also 'TURP syndrome', p. 306.)

Definition

- Normal serum sodium 135–145 mmol/L
- Mild hyponatraemia 130–134 mmol/L
- Moderate hyponatraemia 125–129 mmol/L
- Profound hyponatraemia <125 mmol/L

Presentation

- Important to differentiate between acute (occurred within 48 h) and chronic hyponatraemia (existed for >48 h).
- Depends on fluid status of patient, but commonly nausea and vomiting, headache and weakness, ataxia, psychiatric disturbance, cerebral oedema, and seizures.

Immediate management

Assess:

- ☑ Patient's volume status.
- ☑ Duration and magnitude of hyponatraemia.
- ☑ Degree and severity of symptoms.

Severely symptomatic hypotonic hyponatraemia (usually rapid onset)

- ☑ Admit patient to a high dependency area.
- ☑ Give hypertonic 3% saline 2 mL/kg (or 150 mL) over 20 min.
- ☑ Check the serum Na^+ level after 20 min while repeating the second infusion of hypertonic 3% saline 2 mL/kg over 20 min.
- ☑ Repeat twice until a target serum sodium increase of 5 mmol/L is achieved or symptoms improve.
- ☑ If increase in Na^+ of 5 mmol/L is achieved in the first hour, but no change in symptoms, aim to increase Na^+ by 1 mmol/L each hour by infusing hypertonic 3% saline. Stop infusion when Na^+ increases by 10 mmol/L or reaches Na^+ 130 mmol/L.
- ☑ Alternatively give IV 0.9% saline in combination with a loop diuretic (e.g. furosemide). This is useful in patients with high urine osmolality.
- ☑ Monitor electrolytes 2-hourly to avoid overcorrection.
- ☑ Aim to increase the serum Na^+ by 1–2 mmol/L/h for 3–4 h until the neurologic symptoms subside, or until the plasma Na^+ >130 mmol/L. Do not increase Na^+ >10 mmol/L in the first 24 h and limit to 8 mmol/L during every 24 h thereafter.
- ☑ Start prompt diagnostic assessment and cause-specific treatment.

Acute hyponatraemia with moderately severe symptoms

- ☑ Give a single IV infusion of 2 mL/kg hypertonic 3% saline over 20 min.
- ☑ Aim to correct sodium by 5 mmol/L/day. Do not increase Na^+ >10 mmol/L in the first 24 h and limit to 8 mmol/L during every 24 h thereafter.
- ☑ Ascertain cause and start cause-specific treatment.

Subsequent management
- ☑ Watch for other electrolyte disturbance and treat accordingly.
- ☑ Treat specific cause.

Acute asymptomatic hyponatraemia
- ☑ Stop fluids, medications, and other factors that provoke hyponatraemia.
- ☑ Re-check Na^+ level.
- ☑ Ascertain cause and start cause-specific treatment.
- ☑ If acute decrease in Na^+ >10 mmol/L consider a single IV infusion of 2 mL/kg hypertonic 3% saline over 20 min.

Chronic asymptomatic hyponatraemia
- ☑ Stop fluids, medications, and other factors that provoke hyponatraemia.
- ☑ Treat the cause.
- ☑ Avoid an increase in serum Na^+ of >10 mmol/L during first 24 h and >8 mmol/l for every 24 h thereafter.

Patient with expanded extracellular fluid (hypervolaemic)
- ☑ Fluid-restrict to 1 L/day to prevent further fluid overload.
- ☑ Consider furosemide in the presence of water overload.

Patients with syndrome of inappropriate antidiuretic hormone (SIADH) (euvolaemic)
- ☑ Restrict fluid intake as first-line treatment.
- ☑ Give oral sodium chloride if able with a low-dose loop diuretic (e.g. furosemide).

Patients with reduced circulating volume (hypovolaemic)
- ☑ Restore extracellular volume with IV 0.9% saline at 0.5–1.0 mL/kg/h.

Investigations
U&Es, urinary sodium levels, serum osmolality, urine osmolality.

Causes of hyponatraemia
- Sampling error—'drip arm'.
- Very old and young—excess water administration.
- Diuretics, especially thiazides (e.g. bendroflumethiazide).
- Medical conditions—pancreatitis, cardiac and hepatic failure, renal disease, pneumonia, SIADH.
- Increased ADH secretion due to anaesthesia, pain, and so on.
- Inappropriate fluid administration:
  - excess infusion of hypotonic fluids post-op.
  - glycine absorption during TURP/hysteroscopy.
- Falsely low readings—hyperglycaemia (reduces Na^+ by 1.5 mmol/L per 3.5 mmol/L rise in plasma glucose), paraproteins, and hyperlipidaemia. Define osmolar gap: measure serum osmolality and compare with calculated $[2 (Na^+ + K^+)] + Urea + Glucose$.

Exclusions (pseudohyponatraemia)
Sampling error, hyperglycaemia, hyperlipidaemia.

Special considerations

- **Hypovolaemic—deficiency of total body water and sodium**:
loss of body fluid stimulates secretion of ADH, thus conserving
body water. However, subsequent administration of hypotonic fluid
exacerbates problem.
- Renal (urinary Na$^+$ >20 mmol/L): diuretics, diabetic ketoacidosis,
Addison's disease (raised K$^+$, urea, and creatinine).
- Extrarenal (urinary Na$^+$ <20 mmol/L): gastrointestinal (vomiting and
diarrhoea), third space loss (pancreatitis, burns).
- **Euvolaemic (more common)—normal body sodium with
increase in total body water but little or no oedema**: urinary
sodium is generally >20 mmol/L, serum osmolality <270 mOsmol/kg
and urinary osmolality >100 mOsmol/kg:
  - stress response (e.g. postsurgery, inappropriate ADH secretion,
glucocorticoid deficiency, hypothyroidism, HIV).
- **Hypervolaemic—raised total sodium but total body water
raised further**: generalized oedema is present due to water overload:
  - cardiac and hepatic failure (urinary Na$^+$ <20 mmol/L). Marker of
poor prognosis.
  - renal failure (urinary Na$^+$ >20 mmol/L).
  - measure urinary sodium for an idea as to cause.
- A severely symptomatic patient with acute hyponatraemia is in danger
from brain oedema. In contrast a symptomatic patient with chronic
hyponatraemia is more at risk from rapid correction of hyponatraemia.
Correction of hyponatraemia that is too rapid can induce cerebral
oedema and central demyelination.
- If condition is chronic, correct more slowly.
- Symptomatic patients must be treated immediately (which may be
intraoperatively) and may require Intensive Care support.
- Surgery should not be delayed in those with chronic or asymptomatic
cases of hyponatraemia, but if Na$^+$ <120 mmol/L, proceed cautiously
so as not to exacerbate the situation.
- Emergency cases may require surgery despite low serum Na$^+$.
- Consult with endocrinologists for advice.

Further reading

Reynolds, R.M., Padfield, P.L., Seckl, J.R. (2006). Disorders of sodium balance. *British Medical Journal*,
332, 702–5.

Spasovski, G., Vanholder, R., Allolio, B., et al. (2014). Clinical practice guideline on diagnosis and
treatment of hyponatraemia. Hyponatraemia Guideline Development Group. *Nephrology Dialysis
Transplantation*, **29** Suppl 2, i1.

Tzamaloukas, A.H., Malhotra, D., Rosen B.H., Raj, D.S.C., Murata, G.H., Shapiro, J.I. (2013).
Principles of management of severe hyponatraemia. *Journal of the American Heart Association*.
Available at: http://jaha.ahajournals.org/content/2/1/e005199

① Hypercalcaemia

Definition
- Normal serum calcium 2.2–2.5 mmol/L (ionized 0.9–1.1 mmol/L)
- Mild hypercalcaemia 2.6–3.0 mmol/L
- Moderate hypercalcaemia 3.0–3.4 mmol/L
- Severe hypercalcaemia >3.4 mmol/L

Presentation
- 'Bones, stones, abdominal groans, and psychiatric moans'.
- CVS—dehydration secondary to polyuria, raised BP, bradycardia, dysrhythmias, prolonged PR, and short QT interval.
- GI/GU—nausea and vomiting, abdominal pain, peptic ulceration, constipation, kidney stones and renal failure, pancreatitis.
- CNS—psychiatric disturbance, coma, hyperreflexia, tongue fasciculations.

Immediate management
☑ ABC—100% oxygen.
☑ Rehydrate with IV fluids (0.9% saline).
☑ Once volume is restored, give a loop diuretic (e.g. furosemide 20 mg) which blocks Na^+ and Ca^{2+} reabsorption in the thick ascending limb of the loop of Henle.
☑ Replace ongoing Na^+, K^+, Cl^-, and Mg^{2+} losses.
☑ Ca^{2+} >3.4 mmol/L: give disodium pamidronate 60 mg in 1 L 0.9% saline IV over 4 h. Can take 48 h to work.
☑ If possible, with severe hypercalcaemia (Ca^{2+} >3.4 mmol/L) postpone all elective surgery.
☑ Consider haemodialysis if patient symptomatic.
☑ Malignant disease may warrant surgery in the face of moderate hypercalcaemia (risk/benefit ratio).

Subsequent management
☑ Measure serum PTH levels. If normal or high check 24-h urinary Ca^{2+} level.
☑ Aim to decrease serum calcium by 0.5 mmol/L over 1 to 2 days.
☑ Bisphosphonates, e.g. disodium pamidronate (60 mg in 1 L 0.9% saline IV over 4 h); sodium clodronate (300 mg/day PO for 7–10 days); etidronate sodium (7.5 mg/kg/day PO over 4 h for 3 days).
☑ In renal failure-induced hypercalcaemia—haemodialysis with low-calcium dialysate.
☑ Glucocorticoids are effective in malignancy and granulomatous disease, where gastrointestinal absorption of calcium is inhibited (e.g. prednisolone up to 60 mg/day PO).
☑ Calcitonin increases calcium excretion and inhibits bone resorption—causes moderate and transient decrease therefore little benefit acutely, but give 4 units/kg IM/SC 6–12-hourly.

☑ Phosphate therapy: oral phosphate 3 g/day (causes diarrhoea). IV phosphate must be administered slowly (<9 mmol/12 h). Phosphate increases calcium uptake into bone, reduces calcium absorption from the GI tract, and inhibits bone breakdown. Can be administered to children.

☑ Consult endocrinologist for expert advice.

☑ Ascertain and treat the underlying cause. Investigate if there are clinical features of associated conditions (e.g. cachexia, bone pain with malignancy).

☑ Encourage weight-bearing mobilization as inactivity aggravates hypercalcaemia.

Investigations

- FBC, U&Es, phosphate, albumin, CXR, ECG, PTH levels, amylase.
- Associated low K^+ and Mg^{2+} if on diuretics.

Risk factors

- Primary hyperparathyroidism (most common cause).
- Second most common cause is malignancy—often clinically evident (e.g. squamous-cell lung tumour, metastatic breast cancer, myeloma).
- Renal disease— chronic failure and post-transplantation.
- Drugs—thiazide diuretics, lithium, theophylline toxicity.
- Thyrotoxicosis.
- Phaeochromocytoma.
- Granulomatous disease—sarcoid, TB.
- Hypophosphataemia (<1.4 mmol/L).
- Sampling error—tourniquets used when sample taken.
- Rare—vitamin overdose, excess calcium antacids, milk–alkali syndrome, familial conditions.

Special considerations

- Ionized calcium is physiologically active, therefore measure in preference to total serum calcium. Changes in serum albumin cause changes in total calcium levels, but do not alter the unbound fraction. To calculate the corrected calcium level (mmol/L), deduct 0.1 mmol/L for every 4 g albumin above 40 g/L.
- Hypercalcaemia can cause pancreatitis, therefore check serum amylase regularly. (NB Hypocalcaemia occurs in pancreatitis).
- Anaesthetic agents potentiate the risk of serious arrhythmia in the presence of hypercalcaemia.

Further reading

Joshi, D., Center, J.R., Eisman, J.A. (2009). Investigation of incidental hypercalcaemia. *British Medical Journal*, **339**, b4613.

Khan, M.M., Desborough, J.P. (2003). Calcium homeostasis. *The Royal College of Anaesthetists Bulletin*, **18**, 883–86. Available at: http://cks.nice.org.uk/hypercalcaemia

Maier J.D. Levine S.N. (2015) Hypercalcaemia in the Intensive Care Unit: A review of pathophysiology, diagnosis and modern therapy. *J Intensive Care Med* **30** (5) 235

① Hypocalcaemia

Definition

- Normal serum calcium 2.1–2.6 mmol/L (ionized 0.9–1.1 mmol/L)
- Hypocalcaemia <2.1 mmol/L (ionized calcium <0.9 mmol/L)

Presentation of severe hypocalcaemia

Symptoms usually develop when adjusted calcium levels fall below 1.9 mmol/L, but dependent on the rate of fall.

- CVS—cardiac arrhythmias, short PR, prolonged QT interval, reduced contractility causing reduced cardiac output, hypotension, heart failure.
- CNS—carpopedal spasm, muscle cramps, tetany, convulsions. Chvostek's (facial twitch seen on tapping the facial nerve) and Trousseau's (metacarpophalangeal joints and thumb flexion with hyperextended fingers on occlusion of the brachial artery) signs are pathognomonic of hypocalcaemia.

Subsequent management

- ☑ Biochemical investigations to establish and treat cause.
- ☑ Chronic hypocalcaemia can be treated with oral calcium carbonate and vitamin D supplements.
- ☑ In those with hypoparathyroidism, some vitamin D supplements are inactive, therefore use 1-alfacalcidiol or calcitriol at a starting dose of 0.25–0.5 µg per day PO or IV.

Immediate management

- ☑ ABC—100% oxygen.
- ☑ Calcium intravenous injection:
  - Calcium chloride (10% 5–10 mL) over 10 min ideally through a central line as irritant to veins.
  - Calcium gluconate (10% 10–20 mL)—has to be metabolized by the liver to become active, therefore less effective in the acute setting.
- ☑ If required, start calcium infusion (e.g. 10% calcium chloride at 5–10 mL/h).
- ☑ Support CVS with inotropes if necessary.

Investigations

- FBC, U&Es, phosphate, amylase, vitamin D, serum PTH, magnesium, urine myoglobin, and serum creatine kinase.
- CXR.

Risk factors

- Commonest cause in hospital is disruption of parathyroid gland function after total thyroidectomy.
- Transfusion of blood products, clotting factors—administration of a large quantity of blood products containing citrate can cause an acute reduction in ionized calcium.

- Alkalosis (e.g. hyperventilation—reduces ionized calcium).
- Chronic renal failure—reduced vitamin D activity.
- Calcium channel blocker overdose.
- Post parathyroidectomy—hypo- and pseudohypoparathyroidism.
- Acute pancreatitis.
- Septic shock.
- Rhabdomyolysis.
- Vitamin D deficiency—poor diet, low UV light exposure.
- Hypomagnesaemia—exacerbates low calcium.
- Transient—secondary to drug administration (e.g. protamine, glucagon, or heparin).

Special considerations

- Bolus administration of calcium can cause a transient but dramatic increase in blood pressure and should be administered over 5–10 min, with full monitoring.
- Ideally, calcium should be administered centrally as it can cause vasoconstriction and tissue ischaemia at the injection site. If not possible, administer calcium gluconate (in preference) into a fast-running IVI.
- To calculate the corrected calcium level (mmol/L) add 0.1 mmol/L for every 4 g albumin below 40 g/L.

Further reading

Cooper, M., Gittoes, N. (2008). Clinical review: diagnosis and management of hypocalcaemia. *British Medical Journal*, **336**, 1298–303.

Khan, M.M., Desborough, J.P. (2003). Calcium homeostasis. *The Royal College of Anaesthetists Bulletin*, **18**, 883–6.

Society for Endocrinology (2016). *Emergency Management of Acute Hypocalcaemia in Adult Patients.* Available at: https://www.endocrinology.org/clinical-practice/clinical-guidelines/

① **Hypermagnesaemia**

Definition
- Normal serum Mg^{2+} levels 0.7–1.0 mmol/L (1.8–3.0 mg/dL)
- Hypermagnesaemia—serum level >1.1 mmol/L
- ITU and obstetrics—aim for magnesium level >2.0 mmol/L

Presentation
See Table 10.4.
- CVS—vasodilatation and hypotension (worse with volatile agents and/or narcotics), bradycardia, prolonged PR interval, wide QRS, cardiac arrest.
- RS—bronchodilatation and respiratory depression.
- CNS—sedation, coma, weakness. Reduced acetylcholine at the neuromuscular junction causes potentiation of muscle relaxants. Loss of deep tendon reflexes and facial paraesthesia.
- Metabolic—bone mineralization.
- Coagulopathy—clotting may be impaired.

Immediate management
If Mg^{2+} >4 mmol/L or if patient shows significant clinical features of hypermagnesaemia:
- ☑ Remove source of magnesium.
- ☑ Give 10 mL calcium gluconate 10% slow IV over at least 5 min and repeat if necessary. Use with caution in patients who have renal impairment. Ca^{2+} antagonizes the neuromuscular and CVS effects of magnesium. Effect should be immediate on ECG, but is transient unless serum Mg^{2+} falls.
- ☑ Enhance excretion with IV fluids and forced diuresis (e.g. with furosemide 20 mg initially, repeat according to response).
- ☑ If life-threatening complications +/– renal failure—dialysis with Mg^{2+}-free dialysate.

Subsequent management
- ☑ Biochemical investigations to find possible cause.

Table 10.4 Physiological effects of increasing serum magnesium levels

Physiological range	0.7–1.0 mmol/L
Therapeutic range	1.25–2.5 mmol/L
Knee jerks abolished	3.3–5.5 mmol/L
Respiratory arrest risk	5.0–7.5 mmol/L
Cardiac arrest risk	>15.0 mmol/L

Investigations

- Monitor serum Mg^{2+} levels
- U&Es, creatinine clearance, T_4/TSH, endocrine/hormone screen

Risk factors

- Excessive intake—rare if normal renal function:
  - iatrogenic—excessive administration
  - antacids
  - purgatives—anorexia nervosa.
- Renal failure—especially with dialysis as patients take Mg^{2+} supplements.
- Hypocalcaemia and hyperkalaemia (exacerbate the complications of hypermagnesaemia).
- Adrenocortical insufficiency, hypothyroidism.
- Depression—especially with lithium ingestion.

Special considerations

- 1 g magnesium sulphate = 4 mmol Mg^{2+}.
- Treatment of severe asthma—aim for Mg^{2+} >1 mmol/L.
- Treatment of pregnancy-induced hypertension and eclampsia—aim for serum Mg^{2+} of 2–4 mmol/L.
- Lower dose of muscle relaxants may be required—Mg^{2+} decreases twitch response without train-of-four fade.
- Caution in patients with myasthenia gravis or muscular dystrophy (avoid Mg^{2+} administration in these groups).
- Hypermagnesaemia exaggerates hypotension with GA.
- Phaeochromocytoma—administration of magnesium can improve cardiovascular stability intraoperatively, due to blocking of calcium channels. Effective at serum concentrations exceeding 1.5 mmol/L.

Further reading

Jahnen-Dechent, W., Ketteler, M. (2012). Magnesium basics. Clinical Kidney Journal, 5 Suppl 1, 3–14.
Watson, V.F., Vaughan, R.S. (2001). Magnesium and the anaesthetist. British Journal of Anaesthesia CEPD Reviews, 1(1), 16–20.
Weisinger, J.R., Bellorin-Font, E. (1998). Electrolyte quintet: magnesium and phosphorus. Lancet, 352, 391–6.

① **Hypomagnesaemia**

Definition
- Normal serum Mg^{2+} levels 0.7–1.0 mmol/L (1.8–3.0 mg/dL)
- Hypomagnesaemia <0.6 mmol/L (ionized)

Presentation
- CVS—hypertension with angina due to coronary artery spasm, increased risk of digoxin toxicity, dysrhythmias (VT/VF, torsade de pointes, SVT, AF), ECG changes (increased PR/wide qrs/inverted T waves).
- CNS—abnormal nerve conduction (myoclonus, stridor, cramps), convulsions, coma.
- Psychiatric changes—anxiety, depression, confusion, psychosis, Wernicke's encephalopathy.
- Metabolic—hypokalaemia, hyperinsulinaemia.
- Bone—(chronic signs) osteoporosis and osteomalacia.

Immediate management
- ☑ Acute management (dysrhythmias or acute severe resistant asthma): magnesium sulphate 2 g (8 mmol Mg^{2+}) IV in 5% glucose or saline over 15 min.
- ☑ Torsades de pointes—2 g magnesium sulphate IV over 1–2 min. Continue an infusion 12.5–25 g (50–100 mmol) over 24 h.
- ☑ PIH/eclampsia: magnesium sulphate loading dose 4 g (16 mmol) in 5% glucose or saline over 10–20 min IV. Maintenance infusion 1 g/h (4 mmol/h). Continue for 24 h following last convulsion. If convulsions recur, give 2–4 g (8–16 mmol) IV over 5 min. Aim for plasma concentration of 2–4 mmol/L.

Subsequent management
- ☑ Aim to maintain serum magnesium >0.8 mmol/L.
- ☑ Maintenance dose: 2.5–5 g/day (10–20 mmol/day).

Investigations
Serum Mg^{2+} levels

Risk factors
- Decreased intake:
  - poor diet
  - elderly
  - chronic alcohol abuse
  - excessive administration of IV fluids
  - TPN with inadequate magnesium
- Intensive care patients—multifactorial
- Decreased absorption:
  - pancreatic insufficiency—pancreatitis
  - short bowel syndrome—after small bowel resection

- Excessive renal losses:
  - drugs—loop diuretics, digoxin, gentamicin, ethanol, ciclosporin, amphotericin
  - renal disease—diuretic phase of ATN, interstitial nephritis, excessive diuresis
  - hyperaldosteronism
- Non-renal losses:
  - GI tract—diarrhoea/prolonged NG suctioning/drainage
  - primary hyperparathyvroidism
  - diabetic ketoacidosis with insulin administration
- Massive blood transfusion

Special considerations

- 1 g magnesium sulphate = 4 mmol Mg^{2+}.
- Administration of magnesium can lead to a profound reduction in blood pressure and cardiac output. Care must be exercised in patients who are hypotensive or who have cardiovascular instability.
- Dysrhythmias occurring on ITU, in the presence of likely hypomagnesaemia, should be treated with a loading dose of magnesium as just described.
- Hypomagnesaemia is common after cardiopulmonary bypass and is associated with malignant arrhythmias.
- Pregnancy-induced hypertension and eclampsia—adequate magnesium levels have been shown to reduce intracerebral vascular spasm and decreased resistance in the internal and middle cerebral arteries, thus reducing the incidence of convulsions.
- Low Mg^{2+} increases the risk of stridor/bronchoconstriction at induction of anaesthesia and intubation of the trachea.
- Convulsions—magnesium has been used as a second-line treatment for status epilepticus.
- Asthma—magnesium therapy is used as an adjunct to treat bronchospasm unresponsive to standard treatment. Aim to keep serum Mg^{2+} >1.0 mmol/L.

Further reading

Agus, Z.S. (1999). Hypomagnesemia. *Journal of the American Society of Nephrology*, **10**, 1616–22.
Jahnen-Dechent, W., Ketteler. M. (2012). Magnesium basics. *Clinical Kidney Journal*, **5** Suppl 1, 3–14.
Watson, V.F., Vaughan, R.S. (2001). Magnesium and the anaesthetist. *British Journal of Anaesthesia CEPD Reviews*, **1**(1), 16–20.

Recovery problems

Charles Gibson

⚠ Chest pain

Definition
Discomfort experienced anywhere in the thorax.

Presentation
Patient reports pain, or may appear dyspnoeic, distressed, pale, clammy, and may become hypotensive.

Immediate threats to life
Myocardial infarction (MI), pulmonary embolism, tension pneumothorax, aortic dissection.

Other differential diagnoses
Myocarditis, pericarditis, pneumonia, musculoskeletal pain, referred pain from upper GI system (gastric distension, peptic ulcer disease, laparoscopic banding problem, pancreatitis, biliary disease, ruptured viscus, oesophageal spasm).

Immediate management
- ☑ ABC
- ☑ Establish continuous ECG, NIBP, S_pO_2 monitoring.
- ☑ Call for senior assistance if patient looks unwell.
- ☑ Maintain S_pO_2 >90% with high-flow O_2, non-rebreathing mask, CPAP, or intubation.
- ☑ Examine chest for symmetrical movement, tracheal position, altered percussion resonance, reduced breath sounds.
- ☑ Check 12-lead ECG—new focal ST- and T-wave changes suggests evolving myocardial ischaemia. Tachycardia, new RBBB, and $S_1Q_3T_3$ changes should raise suspicion of PE. Pericarditis and myocarditis and cardiomyopathies often have widespread ST changes across multiple coronary territories.
- ☑ Arrange for an urgent CXR, erect if possible. Pneumothorax and mediastinal widening can easily be missed if the patient is lying supine. A CXR with relatively clear lung fields in a hypoxic patient should raise the suspicion of PE.
- ☑ Take an ABG to look for evidence of hypoxia or lactataemia.
- ☑ Maintain blood pressure and heart rate within the patient's normal range.
- ☑ Analgesics (usually diamorphine 1–5 mg IV, fentanyl 25–100 µg IV).

Subsequent management
- ☑ Disposition and ongoing care will be stratified according to the most likely diagnosis. Most patients will require admission to CCU/HDU/ICU.
- ☑ Consider arterial line and central venous access.
- ☑ **Acute coronary syndromes (ACS)**—➔ see p. 335.

☑ **Pneumothorax**—acutely decompensated patient with clinical diagnosis of tension pneumothorax should receive urgent decompression by placing a 14-gauge IV cannula in the second intercostal space at the mid-clavicular line followed by the insertion of chest drain and underwater seal (➲ see p. 472).

☑ **Pulmonary embolism (PE)**—clinically presents as a shunt (significant hypoxia despite high oxygen flows) in a patient with a relatively clear CXR. Begin treatment with administration of high-flow oxygen and cautious fluid resuscitation (500–1000 mL) +/– noradrenaline. Massive PE (systolic BP <90 mmHg) has a high mortality rate (30%) and usually warrants consideration of mechanical reperfusion strategies (percutaneous or surgical embolectomy) because thrombolysis is usually contraindicated (➲ see 'Pulmonary embolus', p. 41). Submassive PE is defined as a PE with RV dysfunction but no shock. Reperfusion strategies are controversial in these patients and should be considered on a case-by-case basis. Discuss with the surgical team about an IVC filter and early systemic anticoagulation as soon as it is safe to do so (anticoagulation reduces the mortality rate to 3–8% in massive PE). Normotensive PE patients with a normal RV have a low mortality (1%) and should be considered for early systemic anticoagulation ± IVC filter.

☑ **Aortic dissection**—is uncommon and more often seen in elderly or hypertensive patients, but may occur in younger patients with connective tissue disorders (Marfan's syndrome). Severe chest and/or back pain, new neurological deficits, unequal blood pressures in the upper limbs and/or cardiac tamponade. The erect CXR may reveal a widened mediastinum, but definitive diagnosis requires a CT or transoesophageal echocardiography. Control the heart rate and blood pressure with a β-blocker (labetalol or esmolol) aiming for a heart rate <60 bpm and a systolic BP 100–120 mmHg. Add nitroprusside if the BP remains elevated. Control pain with an opiate. Acute dissection of the ascending aorta dissection is a surgical emergency and an urgent opinion from cardiothoracic surgeon should be sought.

☑ **Acute pericardial disease**—examine for friction rub and worsening chest pain on lying flat and improving when sitting forward. The characteristic ECG will show concave ST elevation across multiple chest and limb leads. A normal echocardiogram does not exclude pericarditis. Treatment is of the underlying cause along with colchicine and NSAIDs.

Investigations
• ECG
• CXR
• ABG
• FBC, U&Es, LFTs, amylase
• Consider:
    • troponin levels (may not rise for 6–10 h after MI and can be elevated for reasons other than ACS in approximately one-third of patients, e.g. PE, AHF, CVA, renal failure)
    • CT pulmonary angiogram

- Echocardiography
- Lung ultrasound
- V/Q scan
- Abdominal ultrasound
- Doppler ultrasound of legs (PE)

Risk factors

- Ischaemia/infarction— ➔ see pp. 35, 335.
- Pneumothorax—undiagnosed rib fractures, chest wall or abdominal injury, CVC insertion.
- DVT/PE risk—immobility, obesity, trauma, fractures, pregnancy, pelvic surgery.
- Gallstones, biliary, or peptic ulcer disease.
- Gastric distension—poor nasogastric tube placement.

Paediatric implications

- Chest pain is not usually a feature of cardiac disease.
- Children have difficulty localizing pain. Discuss concerns with parents.
- Usually non-cardiac origin—common causes are musculoskeletal, pulmonary (infection, pneumothorax), or idiopathic (anxiety and hyperventilation in adolescents).

Special considerations

- Thrombolysis is usually contraindicated following surgery because of the bleeding risk.
- If MI is suspected, emergency cardiac catheterization ± coronary angioplasty should be considered prior to ICU/HDU admission.
- PE can be extremely difficult to diagnose. Have a low threshold for further investigation to exclude PE.

Further reading

Erhardt, L., Herlitz, J., Bossaert, L., et al. (2002). Task force on the management of chest pain. *European Heart Journal*, **23**, 1153–76.

☼ Acute coronary syndromes (ACS)

Definition
Acute ischaemic myocardial injury.

Presentation
- Typical MI pain is a central crushing, pressing, or constricting pain or tightness, lasting longer than 20 min, and may radiate to the throat, jaw, arms, or epigastrium.
- Can be 'silent' or atypical (diabetics, elderly, epidural *in situ*, female, perioperative [65%]).
- May present with new arrhythmias, heart failure, or cardiogenic shock.

Immediate management
- ☑ Initiate immediate resuscitation with attention to ABC.
- ☑ Call for senior assistance early.
- ☑ Establish continuous ECG, NIBP, S_pO_2 monitoring.
- ☑ Maintain S_aO_2 >90%.
- ☑ Check temperature, maintain normothermia.
- ☑ Administer 300 mg aspirin chewed/NG, 400 µg sublingual GTN (up to three doses) and titrate morphine to alleviate pain/distress.
- ☑ Stop any NSAIDs or COX-2 inhibitors.
- ☑ Monitor 3-lead ECG and obtain 12-lead ECG—compare with previous records and stratify subsequent management. Patients with STEMI comprise 30% of patients with an ACS and require urgent reperfusion strategies. Thrombolysis is usually contraindicated following surgery, leaving urgent angioplasty as the option. Patients with non-ST-segment-elevation acute coronary syndromes or NSTE-ACS (which includes unstable angina and NSTEMI) should receive adjunctive therapy in accordance with their risk stratification:
- ☑ If there are no signs of heart failure or haemodynamic compromise give β-blockers to keep heart rate <70 bpm but systolic BP >90 mmHg (metoprolol 25 mg PO/NG).
- ☑ Discuss with surgical and cardiological teams about further antiplatelet therapy (ticagrelor 180 mg, prasugrel 60 mg, or clopidogrel 300–600 mg PO/NG) and heparinization (avoid LMWH in unstable patients at risk of bleeding), weighing up the individualized risks of postoperative bleeding with each patient.
- ☑ If hypertensive, maintain adequate systolic BP (100–130 mmHg) using IV metoprolol 5 mg (up to three doses 5 min apart).
- ☑ In hypotensive patients with an inferior STEMI, consider RV or posterior infarction. These patients may respond to cautious fluid boluses providing there are no signs of pulmonary congestion. Otherwise consider cautious use of vasopressors and inotropes (noradrenaline +/– dobutamine) remembering they will increase myocardial oxygen demand and are potentially arrhythmogenic.

☑ Treat arrhythmias (drug therapy, pacing). Be aware of accelerated idioventricular rhythms that can be confused with VT or VF. It is relatively common (~10% STEMIs) within the first 24 h of transmural MI and is usually benign and self-limiting. It is characterized by bizarre widened QRS complexes at a rate of 60–110 bpm.

☑ Manage heart failure with a GTN infusion (1–10 mg/h if blood pressure allows), IV furosemide (20–40 mg) and CPAP (5–10 cmH₂O).

☑ Consider arterial line and central line.

☑ Start/resume a statin as soon as possible (atorvastatin 80 mg).

Subsequent management

☑ Correct electrolyte imbalances, especially potassium (aim >4 mmol/L) and magnesium (aim >1 mmol/L). Maintain good blood glucose control (5–9 mmol/L).

☑ Observe for complications (arrhythmias, heart block, heart failure, shock, acute mitral regurgitation).

☑ Arrange ICU or CCU admission according to hospital procedures.

Investigations

- 12-lead ECG for new ST-segment and T-wave changes or left bundle branch block (LBBB). The ECG is initially normal in 20% of patients with a MI.
- ABG.
- Troponin (starts to rise after 2–3 h after MI).
- FBC, U&Es, LFTs, magnesium, glucose, coagulation profile.

Risk factors

Known history of angina, unstable or poorly controlled hypertension, MI, any vascular disease, chronic renal insufficiency, lipid disorders, diabetes, obesity, hyperhomocysteinemia, advanced age, family history of heart disease, abnormal ECG.

Exclusions

- ST-segment elevation can be seen when early repolarization occurs in normal patients, and is referred to as 'high take off'. It most commonly appears in leads V₂ and V₃ and has a concave upwards appearance.
- Non-ACS causes for ST elevation include coronary vasospasm, acute pericardial disease, LBBB, ventricular paced rhythm, raised ICP, ventricular aneurysm, LVH, Brugada syndrome (an inherited arrhythmia presenting with ST-segment elevation in leads V₁₋₃ and RBBB).
- Cocaine toxicity. Manage symptoms with benzodiazepines.

Paediatric implications

- Causes include illicit drug use, coronary artery anomalies, perinatal asphyxia, myocarditis, Kawasaki syndrome, and obstruction of the coronary arteries following cardiac surgery.
- Infants present with non-specific symptoms, older children complain of prolonged, non-pleuritic chest or abdominal pain.

Special considerations

- Cardiac complications (death, non-fatal MI, heart failure and VT) occur in up to 5% of patients undergoing non-cardiac surgery.
- In-hospital mortality from a perioperative MI is between 12% and 25%.
- Troponin level will often be normal immediately following a period of ischaemic chest pain, therefore subsequent cardiac monitoring and repeat troponin levels may be required. Troponin-T usually peaks at 12 h and persists 4–7 days. Normal range is 1–14 ng/L.

Further reading

Task Force on the management of acute coronary syndromes (ACS) in patients presenting without persistent ST-segment of the European Society of Cardiology (2011). ESC guidelines for the management of acute coronary syndrome in patients presenting without persistent ST-segment elevation. *European Heart Journal*, **32**, 2999–3054.

Task Force on the management of ST-segment elevation acute myocardial infarction of the European Society of Cardiology (2012). Management of acute myocardial infarction in patients presenting with persistent ST-segment elevation. *European Heart Journal*, **33**, 2569–619.

☼ Acute heart failure (AHF)

Definition

AHF is a clinical syndrome representing inadequate systolic or diastolic heart function. If associated with anaerobic cellular metabolism, the terms 'circulatory failure' or 'shock' are often used.

Classification (European Society of Cardiology)

Hypertensive AHF—pulmonary oedema in the setting of relatively preserved systolic left ventricular function and often involving diastolic dysfunction.

Cardiogenic shock—evidence of tissue hypoperfusion after correction of preload. Characterized by systolic BP <90 mmHg and/or urine output <0.5 mL/kg/h with or without organ congestion.

Decompensated AHF—mild signs and symptoms of heart failure that do not meet the definitions for either hypertensive or cardiogenic shock categories.

High output failure—tachycardia, warm peripheries, pulmonary congestion with low to normal BP.

Acute right heart failure—a low output syndrome with raised JVP, increased liver size, and peripheral oedema without pulmonary congestion.

Immediate management

☑ Initiate immediate resuscitation with attention to ABC.

☑ Call for senior assistance early. Many patients will respond quickly to therapy with well-directed management.

☑ Establish patient monitoring with continuous 3-lead ECG, NIBP, and S_aO_2 (and urinary catheter).

☑ Consider early central venous access and arterial line.

☑ Maintain adequate oxygenation (S_aO_2 >90%) with high-flow oxygen, CPAP, or intubation.

☑ If the BP allows, position the patient as upright as possible.

☑ Attempt to normalize the heart rhythm and rate. Acutely decompensated patients with tachyarrhythmias will often need to be electrically cardioverted because most pharmacological agents are negatively inotropic and risk worsening the patient's condition. Amiodarone is probably the safest alternative (300 mg IV loading over 1 h). Digoxin (500 µg IV load) is positively inotropic but results in poor heart rate control in AHF. Bradycardic patients need to be pharmacologically (isoprenaline/dopamine/adrenaline) or electrically paced (external or transvenous).

☑ Aim for systolic BP 100–120 mmHg.

☑ If they are not hypotensive then reduce preload with GTN (50 mg in 50 mL saline, commence at 3 mL/h. Usual range is 1–10 mg/h) plus furosemide 40 mg IV.

☑ CPAP (commence at 10 cmH₂O with 100% O₂) is an effective means of reducing the preload in hypoxic patients.

☑ If hypotensive (systolic BP <100 mmHg) increase afterload cautiously using vasopressors (high-dose dopamine/noradrenaline/vasopressin) ± very cautious fluid boluses (aiming for a maximum of 1.5–2 L in 24 h). Metaraminol is an alternative in the emergency setting until central access can be established.

☑ Optimize cardiac output. Consider inotropic drugs where end-organ perfusion is not adequate—dobutamine (2.5–10 µg/kg/min). Alternative infusions include dopamine and milrinone. Be aware that all these drugs increase myocardial oxygen demand and are potentially arrhythmogenic.

☑ The use of morphine (1 mg IV) should be reserved for those patients with ongoing pain or undue anxiety. It conveys little additional advantage in reducing the preload.

Subsequent management

☑ Search for the underlying cause. Decompensation of pre-existing chronic heart failure, fluid overload, ACS, and acute arrhythmias are the most common causes. Undiagnosed or new valvular lesions (especially aortic stenosis), cardiomyopathies, or tamponade can be easily missed.

☑ Echocardiography (transthoracic, transoesophageal if intubated) is useful to establish segmental or global ventricular dysfunction or valvular pathology and monitor response to treatment.

☑ Correct electrolyte imbalances, especially potassium (aim >4 mmol/L) and magnesium (aim >1 mmol/L).

☑ Maintain good blood glucose control (5–9 mmol/L).

☑ Failure to respond to the above therapies warrants subsequent consultation with cardiology and intensive care. Further monitoring may be warranted with a cardiac output monitor (LiDCO, PiCCO, Vigileo, Swan–Ganz catheter). Additional therapies may include an intra-aortic balloon pump or levosimendan. A bridging mechanical heart device (extracorporeal membrane oxygenation (ECMO) or left ventricular assist device (LVAD)) to recovery or cardiac transplant is rarely required.

Investigations

- FBC, U&Es, LFTs, magnesium, glucose, lactate, troponin
- ABG
- CXR
- 12-lead ECG
- Echocardiography

Risk factors

- Ischaemic heart disease.
- Hypertension (systemic, pulmonary).
- Myocardial, valvular, or pericardial disease or inflammation.
- Obesity, sleep apnoea.
- Acute neurological injuries (head or spinal cord injury, intracranial haemorrhage).
- Thyroid disease.

Differential diagnoses

- Non-cardiogenic pulmonary oedema—sepsis syndrome, allergic reactions, aspiration pneumonitis, multiple trauma, pancreatitis, and others.
- Hypervolaemia.
- Pulmonary embolus, venous air embolism.
- Tension pneumothorax, cardiac tamponade.

Paediatric implications

- Infants with heart failure may have tachypnoea, feeding difficulties, sweating, irritability, and laboured respirations. Hepatomegaly is common.
- Older children often have similar signs and symptoms to adults, although abdominal symptoms may predominate.

Special considerations

- There is no evidence for the use of intra-aortic balloon counterpulsation in patients with cardiogenic shock complicating acute MI for whom an early revascularization is planned.
- Levosimendan (Simdax®) is a calcium-sensitizing agent with inotropic vasodilator properties used for the treatment of heart failure. It has an active metabolite with similar positive inotropic effects to the parent compound exerting pharmacological benefits for approximately 1 week. Its safety and efficacy have not been established. Initiation of levosimendan should only be undertaken after discussion with a cardiologist or intensivist.
- B-natriuretic peptide (BNP) is a peptide hormone released in response to the mechanical stress of heart failure. It plays a homeostatic role as a systemic vasodilator and diuretic. While remaining relatively sensitive and specific for AHF, the diagnosis is normally established by clinical assessment. It may play a clinical role in COPD patients where differentiation between an exacerbation in emphysema and AHF can be difficult. False positives occur in PE, pulmonary hypertension, liver and renal failure.

Further reading

Task Force for the diagnosis and treatment of acute and chronic heart failure of the European Society of Cardiology (2012). ESC guidelines for the diagnosis and treatment of acute and chronic heart failure. *European Heart Journal*, **33**, 1787–847.

① Postoperative hypertension

Definition

BP more than 20% above baseline, systolic BP ≥140 mmHg or diastolic BP ≥90 mmHg.

Presentation

- Primary hypertension is usually asymptomatic.
- Patients with severe acute (systolic BP >180 mmHg or diastolic BP >120 mmHg) hypertension may have headache. Hypertension may precipitate myocardial ischaemia, resulting in chest pain.
- Immediate postoperative hypertension is common. Pain, arousal, and confusion are causative. Moderate hypertension is not usually life-threatening, but when combined with tachycardia is a cardiac stressor. Analgesia and β-blockers are useful.

Immediate management

☑ Initiate immediate resuscitation with attention to ABC.

☑ Call for senior assistance early.

☑ Establish patient monitoring with continuous 3-lead ECG, NIBP, and S_aO_2.

☑ Confirm pressure manually with appropriate-sized cuff, on more than one limb or, if using arterial line, check calibration, tubing, and height of transducer.

☑ Check oxygenation and ventilation to exclude hypoxia and hypercapnia (use PACU capnography machine to sample $ETCO_2$, and consider ABG measurement, especially if MH is suspected).

☑ Treat severe pain with IV opioids.

☑ Exclude bladder/bowel distension (especially if at risk for autonomic dysreflexia).

☑ Drug therapy includes:
- labetalol 50 mg IV then infusion 2 mg/min
- esmolol 0.5 mg/kg IV then infusion 50–200 µg/kg/min
- hydralazine 5 mg IV to maximum 20 mg over 20 min
- GTN infusion (50 mg/50 mL), start 3 mL/h IV and titrate to BP
- sodium nitroprusside (1.5 µg/kg/min up to 8 µg/kg/min)
- magnesium sulphate 2–4 g IV over 10 min, then infusion 1–2 g/h (maintain serum Mg^{++} >1.5 mmol/L)
- phentolamine 1–2 mg IV prn
- clonidine 25–150 µg slow IV

Subsequent management

☑ Referral to physician for investigation and management of persistent hypertension, or to endocrinologist if thyroid disease, primary hyperaldosteronism (Conn's syndrome), or phaeochromocytoma is suspected.

Investigations
Check baseline levels FBC, U&Es, 12-lead ECG, urine for protein/blood.

Differential diagnoses and causes
- **Primary (essential) hypertension**—untreated or preoperative omission of antihypertensive medications.
- **Thyroid storm**—fever, tachycardia, atrial fibrillation, delirium, agitation, or coma, vomiting, diarrhoea, muscle weakness (➲ see p. 288).
- **Phaeochromocytoma**—catecholamine-secreting tumours of the adrenal medulla may present after incomplete surgical removal or *de novo* with severe, paroxysmal, or sustained hypertension (➲ see p. 290).
- **Malignant hyperthermia**— ➲ see p. 280.
- **Pre-eclampsia and eclampsia**— ➲ see pp. 166, 169.
- **Autonomic dysreflexia**—massive sympathetic response to a stimulus below the level of a chronic spinal cord injury (especially above T8). Triggers include bladder or hollow viscus distension or manipulation, temperature changes, surgery without adequate anaesthesia. Phenoxybenzamine is used preoperatively and phentolamine, nifedipine, and clonidine may be used in a hypertensive crisis. β-blocker only if tachycardia (➲ see p. 208).
- **Iatrogenic**—liberal use of adrenaline, cocaine, ephedrine, or other vasopressors during surgery; check intraoperative drug use. Phenylephrine eyedrops may cause hypertension during or before cataract surgery. MAOIs and intraoperative use of indirect sympathomimetics or opioids.
- Pain, agitation, anxiety.
- Full bladder, particularly elderly, confused/agitated males.

Paediatric implications
- Most hypertension in the recovery room is due to pain and is usually associated with tachycardia and agitation.
- Correct cuff size is important—cuff should completely encircle arm to ensure uniform compression. The inflatable bladder should cover at least two-thirds of the upper arm length. The width of the cuff's bladder should be 40% of the mid-circumference of the limb.
- Chronic hypertension in children is usually secondary to renal disease or vascular abnormalities, such as coarctation of the aorta. Adolescents may develop essential hypertension.
- If required, suitable agents for urgent control of BP include labetalol (0.5–3 mg/kg/h), SNP (0.5–8 µg/kg/min).

Special considerations
- Sublingual nifedipine is no longer recommended, as sudden hypotension and cardiac ischaemia may result.

Further reading
Varon, J., Marik, P.E. (2003). Clinical review: the management of hypertensive crises. *Critical Care*, **7**(5), 374–84.

☼ Postoperative hypotension

Definition
BP more than 20% below baseline, systolic BP <90 mmHg or mean BP <60 mmHg.

Presentation
- Typically tachycardia, but dependent upon age and sympathetic/parasympathetic stimulation.
- Signs of reduced cerebral perfusion—altered mental state, nausea, vomiting.
- Weak or absent pulses (brachial, femoral, carotid), reduced urine output.

Immediate management
☑ Initiate immediate resuscitation with attention to ABC.
☑ 100% oxygen.
☑ Call for senior assistance early.
☑ Establish patient monitoring with continuous three-lead ECG, NIBP, and S_aO_2.
☑ Elevate patient's legs.
☑ Consider causes of pulseless electrical activity, since these can all cause severe hypotension (4Hs & 4Ts):
  - hypoxia, hypovolaemia, hypothermia, hyper/hypokalaemia.
  - tension pneumothorax, toxins, thromboembolism, tamponade.
☑ Correct fluid deficit with rapid IV fluid administration— Hartmann's or 0.9% saline. Use O negative blood if there is massive haemorrhage.
☑ Consider vasopressors until suitable circulating volume can be achieved:
  - ephedrine 6 mg IV boluses prn.
  - metaraminol 0.5–1 mg IV prn.
  - phenylephrine 25–100 µg IV prn.
  - pre-arrest or unresponsive—adrenaline 50–100 µg IV prn.
☑ Consider additional IV/CVC access +/– arterial line. Massive blood loss warrants large-bore IV access (PAFC introducer sheath, rapid infusion line) and rapid infusion device.
☑ Inform blood bank of urgent need for blood.
☑ **Anaphylactic/anaphylactoid reaction**—adrenaline IV in increments (50–100 µg) and infusion to maintain BP. ◑ See p. 272.
☑ **Severe blood loss**— ◑ see p. 418.
☑ **Tamponade**—history of chest trauma or cardiothoracic surgery, distended neck veins, 'muffled' heart sounds (unreliable sign). Return to theatre for thoracotomy, pericardiotomy, or, if in extremis, pericardiocentesis.
☑ **Pneumothorax**—deviated trachea, hyperresonance, and reduced breath sounds (on one or both sides), needle thoracentesis (second intercostal space, mid-clavicular line), then follow with chest drain (◑ see p. 485).

Subsequent management

☑ Persistent hypotension requires ICU/HDU admission and consideration of invasive haemodynamic monitoring and inotropic therapy.
☑ Specific therapy according to likely cause.
☑ Coronary angiography for new infarction/ischaemia.

Differential diagnoses and causes

- Most common postoperative cause is a combination of myocardial depression, vasodilatation, and relative volume deficit.
- **Hypovolaemia**—long fasting period, inadequate fluid administration, unrecognized fluid or blood loss, re-warming patient.
- **Inadequate cardiac output**—heart failure, tamponade, arrhythmias, myocardial ischaemia/infarction, PE (venous, air, or amniotic fluid), pneumothorax (chronic lung disease, recent CVC insertion or attempt), fluid overload (TURP syndrome, excessive fluid administration), aortocaval compression (pregnancy, abdominal tumour).
- **Reduced vascular resistance**—anaesthetic drugs, regional blockade (epidural, subdural, high, or total spinal), sepsis (known or suspected infection), toxins, anaphylactic reactions, drug overdose (mechanical pump problem or incorrect programming).
- **Antihypertensive drugs**—particularly ACE inhibitors, angiotensin 2 receptor antagonists.

Exclusions

- Do not delay treatment if there are other signs of low BP. Confirm hypotension by manually checking BP with appropriate-sized cuff, on more than one limb or, if using arterial line, checking calibration, tubing, and height of transducer.
- Check patient's preoperative BP.

Paediatric implications

- Hypotension is a late sign of circulatory failure in children. Earlier signs include tachycardia (up to 220 bpm in infants) and peripheral shutdown. Normal systolic BP can be calculated using the formula: BP = 90 + (age in years × 2). Correct cuff size is important.
- Give 10 mL/kg bolus of crystalloid (lactated ringers or 0.9% saline) and assess response.
- The intraosseous route should be used early if IV access is difficult, and particularly if aged <6 y. The IV/IO adrenaline dose for children in severe shock/cardiac arrest is 10 μg/kg (⊙ see p. 130).

☼ Respiratory failure and hypoxia

Definition

Type 1 (hypoxaemic): P_aO_2 <8 kPa. Normal or decreased P_aCO_2.
Type 2 (hypercapnic): P_aO_2 <8 kPa. P_aCO_2 >6.7 kPa.

Presentation

- Variable, depending on underlying cause. May be:
  - reduced respiratory rate/volume if reduced ventilatory drive or neuromuscular function.
  - tachypnoea and respiratory distress if reduced respiratory function or hypoxia.
- Decreasing S_pO_2, elevated P_aCO_2, reduced frequency, or abnormal pattern in CO_2 waveform.
- Cyanosis (may be seen if S_pO_2 ≤85%, need ≥50 g/L reduced Hb to detect cyanosis).
- Late signs include bradycardia or tachycardia, cardiac arrhythmias or ischaemia, decreased level of consciousness.

Immediate threats to life

- Airway obstruction
- Severe asthma/anaphylaxis
- Tension pneumothorax
- PE
- Neuromuscular blockade

Immediate management

- ☑ Initiate immediate resuscitation with attention to ABC.
- ☑ Call for senior assistance early.
- ☑ Inspect airway and relieve obstruction with suction/Magill forceps—check for dentures, retained pharyngeal ('throat') pack, large clots (nasal, dental surgery).
- ☑ Stabilize airway with oral/nasal airway and jaw manoeuvres.
- ☑ Give 100% oxygen to begin with then titrate to O_2 saturations. If the patient is a CO_2 retainer aim for O_2 saturation of 88–92%.
- ☑ Assess ventilation—observe breathing pattern and frequency. Auscultate lungs (wheeze, absent breath sounds) and percuss chest.
- ☑ Commence bag–valve–mask ventilation with O_2 if spontaneous ventilation inadequate.
- ☑ If bag–mask or spontaneous ventilation inadequate, consider tracheal intubation (or LMA insertion if appropriate).
- ☑ Establish patient monitoring with continuous 3-lead ECG, NIBP, and S_aO_2.
- ☑ Use long suction catheter via tracheal tube to remove secretions.
- ☑ Most patients will respond to IPPV. Those who remain hypoxic, but in whom there are no signs of aspiration or pulmonary oedema, often have lung atelectasis/collapse. Diagnose on CXR. Re-expand by recruitment manoeuvres, suction, and PEEP.

☑ Check intraoperative drug administration (muscle relaxant, opioid, sedative, volatile use). Check for pupil constriction—if opioid overdose, consider ventilation ± naloxone (400 µg in 10 mL saline, administer 100 µg increments). If benzodiazepine overdose, consider flumazenil 0.2–1 mg in IV increments.

☑ Assess neuromuscular function clinically (grip strength, head lift >5 s) and electrically (nerve stimulator: normal train-of-four, sustained tetanus, equal double-burst stimulation). If inadequate neuromuscular function, consider neostigmine (maximum dose 70 µg/kg) with glycopyrronium or atropine, or sugammadex 2mg/kg to reverse rocuronium/vecuronium.

Subsequent management

☑ Persistent or severe hypoxaemia will require admission to ICU/HDU for NIV/invasive ventilation.

☑ If chronic lung disease with CO_2 retention suspected, admit to ICU for ventilation or, if making borderline respiratory effort, admit to HDU for close monitoring of ventilatory function.

☑ Severe bronchospasm— ⊃ see p. 70.

☑ If history of head injury, neurosurgery, or VP shunt *in situ*, perform rapid neurological examination (GCS, pupil inspection), obtain neurosurgical opinion, consider need for CT scan or re-operation.

☑ Upper airway problem— ⊃ see p. 91.

Investigations

- ABG
- CXR
- Peripheral nerve stimulator—post-tetanic count and train-of-four
- Lung ultrasound

Risk factors

- Long-duration or extensive surgery (e.g. thoracoabdominal incision) resulting in atelectasis and lung collapse.
- Underlying severe respiratory disease, especially with abdominal surgery.
- Elderly or cachectic patient.
- Large doses of muscle relaxants (especially in presence of renal or hepatic failure), sedatives, or opioids (remifentanil or other opioids in IV tubing at end of operation).
- Aspiration risk (non-fasted, late pregnancy, obesity, hiatus hernia, trauma, bowel obstruction or impaired gastric emptying, prior gastric surgery).
- Head injury, neurosurgery, VP shunt.
- Obesity (especially morbid obesity: body mass index >35 kg/m²).
- Hypothermia (temperature <35°C).
- Severe pain.
- Recent use of nitrous oxide.

Differential diagnoses

- Residual anaesthetic effects (opioids, neuromuscular, sedatives).
- Heart failure.
- Severe chronic lung disease.
- CNS disorders.
- Phrenic nerve palsy with interscalene block.
- Problems with pulse oximeter—electrical interference, motion, ambient light, metHb (S_pO_2 tend towards 85%), COHb (S_pO_2 falsely high), nail polish, skin pigmentation, methylene blue, indocyanine green, isosulfan blue/patent blue (may also cause artefactual increase in metHb).
- Poor peripheral circulation.
- Chest wall injury.
- Pneumonia.
- Hypotension.
- Congenital heart disease.
- Fatigue.

Paediatric implications

- Respiratory depression or failure can lead to early cardiorespiratory arrest in infants and children, and needs to be managed aggressively and rapidly.
- Infants under 3 months of age are very sensitive to opioids.
- Ex preterm babies can have episodes of apnoea/bradypnoea after anaesthesia.
- Monitor all babies <54 weeks postconceptual age for at least 12 h with apnoea monitor and pulse oximetry.
- Consider the use of caffeine (10 mg/kg IV) if <44 weeks postconceptual age.
- Upper abdominal and chest wall surgery will limit respiratory effort.
- Mild hypoxia in the recovery room is seen in children with a history of recent URTI, who develop V/Q mismatch intraoperatively. Generally resolves within 2 h after child awakens and begins coughing.
- Exclude congenital heart disease and right-to-left shunt.
- Untreated hypoxia can rapidly lead to bradycardia and cardiorespiratory arrest (see p. 125).
- Respiratory reserve limited in neonates and infants due to:
  - reduced FRC.
  - increased oxygen consumption.

Further reading

Canet, J., Gallart, L. (2014). Postoperative respiratory failure: pathogenesis, prediction, and prevention. *Current Opinion in Critical Care*, **20**, 56–62.

ⓘ **Acute confusional state**

Definition

A state of altered consciousness characterized by inattention along with diminished speed, clarity, and coherence of thought.

Presentation

- Disorientation, agitation, abnormal behaviour/movements, fighting with recovery room staff.
- Appear frightened or anxious.
- Picking at bed clothes, dressings, drains, or catheters.

Immediate management

☑ Treat hypoxia and hypotension (➲ see pp. 343, 345).
☑ Reassure and 'orientate' patient to environment. Ensure they have their glasses and hearing aids.
☑ Treat pain (➲ see pp. 364).
☑ Check blood glucose.
☑ Clinical examination/bladder scan for distension and use catheter as needed; check balloon not inflated in urethra.
☑ Measure temperature—actively re-warm as necessary.
☑ Prevent patient from harming themselves or disrupting wounds, removing drains, dressings, catheters. Orderlies or other support staff may be required. Physical restraints remain a last resort.
☑ Rapid neurological examination seeking localizing signs. Perform GCS if regression of conscious state. If stroke or other neurological injury suspected, consult neurologist/neurosurgeon.
☑ Sedation if treatable cause(s) have been corrected and patient at risk of harming himself or others— consider using atypical antipsychotic (olanzapine 2.5–5 mg PO/IM). Incremental haloperidol 0.5–1 mg IV/IM can be used.
☑ If very restless in recovery, a low-dose propofol infusion may allow the patient to wake more slowly and improve.
☑ Physostigmine for anticholinergic syndrome, atropine for cholinergic syndrome (➲ see 'Subsequent management', p. 348).
☑ Avoid benzodiazepines except in cases of drug and alcohol withdrawal or when haloperidol is contraindicated (Parkinson's disease, long QT interval, bradycardia).
☑ Where appropriate, use familiar toys, family members, or known carers as reassurance and support.

Subsequent management

☑ **Anticholinergic syndrome**—consider when confusion is associated with mydriasis, tachycardia, peripheral vasodilatation, dry skin, and facial plethora. Treatment with edrophonium 2 mg IV is diagnostic.

☑ **Cholinergic syndrome**—consider when confusion is associated with muscarinic effects such as bradycardia, miosis, sweating, blurred vision, excessive lacrimation, and/or bronchial secretions, wheezing; or nicotinic effects such as tachycardia, hypertension, muscle weakness. Treat with atropine 0.6–1.2 mg (20 µg/kg in children).

☑ **Serotonin syndrome**—consider when confusion is associated with restlessness, myoclonus, hyperreflexia, tremor, shivering, sweating, fever, and other autonomic nervous system symptoms; following use of serotonin-enhancing drugs (SSRIs, MAOIs, tramadol, pethidine). Treatment is supportive—benzodiazepines may reduce patient discomfort.

☑ **TURP syndrome**—➔ see p. 306.

☑ **Hyponatraemia**—➔ see p. 319.

☑ **Alcohol withdrawal**—IV Pabrinex® (two pairs IV TDS) and reducing dose chlordiazepoxide (initially 10–30 mg PO QDS).

☑ If longer term sedation is needed, consider haloperidol 2–10 mg IV/IM or lorazepam 1–2 mg IV 4–6-hourly.

Investigations

- FBC, glucose, U&Es, LFTs, TFTs.
- Osmolality.
- ABG.
- Temperature.
- Urinalysis.
- CT head if aetiology uncertain.

Differential diagnoses

- Electrolyte disorders: hyponatraemia, hypercalcaemia.
- Hypoglycaemia.
- Sepsis.
- Hypoxaemia.
- Hypothermia.
- Dementia.
- Deafness—locate hearing aid, or person trained in 'signing', or interpreter.
- Full bladder.
- Iatrogenic (ECT, neurosurgery, doxapram, anticholinergic, or acetylcholine esterase inhibitor drugs, benzodiazepines, opioids, ketamine).
- Alcohol withdrawal or drug abuse.
- Postictal.
- Hepatic encephalopathy.
- Hypothyroidism.

Paediatric implications

- Confusion/dysphoria following anaesthesia is common in the paediatric population and generally settles with time.

- Presentation—crying, screaming, agitation, doesn't recognize parents, doesn't make eye contact, won't settle with cuddling, possible evidence of hallucinations in older children. Causes include sevoflurane, ketamine, anxious child preoperatively, pain, hunger, midazolam premedication.
- Consider clonidine 0.5–1 µg/kg IV. If suspect midazolam as cause, consider flumazenil 10 µg/kg IV.

Further reading

Deiner, S., Silverstein J.H. (2009). Postoperative delirium and cognitive dysfunction. *British Journal of Anaesthesia*, **103**, (Suppl 1), i41–6.

! The unrousable patient

Definition
Failure to recover consciousness.

Presentation
- Patient does not recover consciousness after a reasonable period of recovery following general anaesthesia.
- Patient becomes unresponsive following admission to PACU.

Immediate management
- ☑ Initiate immediate resuscitation with attention to ABC.
- ☑ Call for senior assistance early.
- ☑ Establish patient monitoring with continuous 3-lead ECG, NIBP, and S_pO_2.
- ☑ Treat hypoxia and hypotension (→ see pp. 343, 345).
- ☑ Measure temperature—actively re-warm as necessary.
- ☑ Anaesthetic history; check use of opioids (miosis, bradypnoea, apnoea), benzodiazepines (breathing but not awakening), other CNS depressants.
- ☑ Neuromuscular assessment with peripheral nerve stimulator.
- ☑ Reverse suspected drugs (naloxone, flumazenil).
- ☑ Check blood glucose and give 150 mL 10% glucose if hypoglycaemia is suspected.
- ☑ Rapid neurological examination seeking localizing signs. If stroke or other neurological injury suspected, arrange CT/MRI scan, and consult neurologist/neurosurgeon.

Subsequent management
- ☑ Careful check of anaesthetic record; check used ampoules for drug error.
- ☑ According to diagnosis.
- ☑ Admit to HDU or ICU pending investigations.

Investigations
- FBC, U&Es, glucose, TFTs.
- ABG.
- Peripheral nerve stimulator—post-tetanic count and train-of-four.
- CT or MRI scan to exclude stroke or other structural lesion (later, EEG to exclude non-convulsive status epilepticus or metabolic/toxic encephalopathy).
- Osmolality (TURP syndrome, SIADH, diabetes, or alcohol-related complication).

Risk factors
- → See 'Confusion', p. 348.
- Neurosurgery.
- Carotid artery surgery or stenting.

- Long, deep anaesthetics with excess volatile anaesthetics or TIVA.
- Diabetes mellitus (hyperosmolar, hyperglycaemic coma; hypoglycaemia).

Differential diagnoses

- Hypothermia:
  - **iatrogenic hypothermia**—long-duration surgery, use of cool irrigating fluids (TURP, abdominal washouts). Re-warm patient with hot-air warming blanket, warmed IV fluids.
  - **hypothyroid coma**—typically elderly women, with longstanding hypothyroidism, and may be precipitated by infection (pneumonia, UTI), trauma, heart failure, CVA, or drugs (amiodarone). Temperature usually <35.5°C, and there may be hypotension, hypoventilation, hypoglycaemia, hyponatraemia. Admit to ICU for ventilatory and cardiovascular support, temperature and glucose control, slow replacement of thyroid hormones.
- Metabolic/toxic encephalopathy—hypoglycaemia (→ see p. 297), hyponatraemia (→ see p. 319), drug toxicity (e.g. benzodiazepines, opioids, illicit drugs, → see p. 370), sepsis (→ see p. 373).
- Non-convulsive status epilepticus (→ see p. 212).
- Structural intracranial lesion compressing, or involving, brainstem.
- Stroke (ischaemic or haemorrhagic, → see p. 354), subdural haematoma, tumour.
- Pseudocoma—usually a young patient with otherwise normal neurological examination, resists eye-opening, and does not allow arm to fall on face or genitalia.
- Muscle weakness, suxamethonium apnoea or residual curarization (→ see p. 356). Check neuromuscular function with peripheral nerve stimulator.

Paediatric implications

Consider—suxamethonium apnoea, opioid overdose, hyponatraemia, raised ICP, neurological condition (e.g. cerebral palsy).

⊙ Stroke

Definition
Cerebral haemorrhage/infarction resulting in focal cerebral damage.

Presentation
New onset of focal neurological deficit or alteration in mental state.

Immediate management
- ☑ Initiate immediate resuscitation with attention to ABC.
- ☑ Call for senior assistance early.
- ☑ Establish patient monitoring with continuous three-lead ECG, NIBP, and S_pO_2.
- ☑ BP control—arterial line for uncontrolled hypertension or labile BP.
- ☑ Neurological examination.
- ☑ If raised ICP is suspected keep the head in neutral alignment and the head of the bed elevated to 30 degrees.
- ☑ Control ventricular rate in atrial fibrillation.
- ☑ Check glucose and correct rapidly.
- ☑ CT or MRI scan to differentiate type of stroke.
- ☑ Measure temperature and maintain normothermia.

Subsequent management
- ☑ Maintain glucose 5–9 mmol/L.
- ☑ If acute thrombotic stroke <3 h old, consider thrombolysis but it is usually contraindicated following surgery. Liaise with stroke physician. Start aspirin 300 mg/day but don't give it for the first 24 h following thrombolysis.
- ☑ Treat hypertension. In ischaemic strokes the threshold for treatment is lower in patients undergoing thrombolysis (systolic BP >185 mmHg, diastolic BP >110 mmHg) than for those not undergoing reperfusion (systolic BP >220 mmHg, diastolic BP >120 mmHg). Labetalol 10–20 mg IV repeat once) or nicardipine IVI 5–15 mg/h. In haemorrhagic stroke there is a risk of reducing cerebral perfusion if the mean arterial pressure is reduced too much. Treat cautiously and aim for a BP of 160/90 mmHg or MAP 110 mmHg.
- ☑ Admit to Stroke Unit for supportive treatment.
- ☑ Urgent discussion with neurosurgeons if haemorrhagic.
- ☑ Treat atrial fibrillation and other risk factors according to local protocols, and consider anticoagulation in consultation with surgeon and cardiologist.
- ☑ Manage hyperglycaemia with insulin.
- ☑ If the patient is already on a statin then continue treatment. (Current UK guidance advises waiting 48 hrs before starting a statin de novo after stroke—although evidence is emerging suggesting earlier commencement improves outcomes.)

Investigations

- FBC, U&Es, glucose.
- ECG.
- Echocardiography.
- Neurological examination—CT or MRI scan to identify stroke lesion, distinguish infarction from haemorrhage, and help differentiate the aetiological subtype of ischaemic and haemorrhagic stroke (e.g. cardiac embolism, large artery disease, small artery disease). Carotid ultrasound (if carotid territory ischaemic event).

Risk factors

- Cerebrovascular disease (TIAs, migraine).
- Hypertension, smoking, hypercholesterolaemia, diabetes.
- Atrial fibrillation, previous anterior MI.
- Carotid artery surgery or stenting, interventional neuroradiological procedures.
- Cardiopulmonary bypass, induced hypotension.

Differential diagnoses

- Migraine—paroxysmal syndrome characterized by throbbing, pulsatile headache, photophobia, nausea (90%), vomiting (60%), aura (15–25%), and focal neurological signs (<5%). Administer antiemetics and analgesics—aspirin (antiplatelet), NSAIDs, sumatriptan (or analogue), lidocaine infusion—and refer to neurologist.
- Partial epileptic seizures/postictal paresis.
- Hypoglycaemia.
- Subdural haematoma.
- CNS tumour/abscess.
- Multiple sclerosis.
- Systemic infection worsening established neurology.
- Transient global amnesia.
- Parkinson's disease.

Paediatric implications

Predisposing factors include blood dyscrasias, sickle cell disease, migraine, and neoplasia.

Further reading

Royal College of Physicians (2012). *National Clinical Guideline for Stroke*, 4th edition. Available at: https://www.strokeaudit.org/Guideline/Historical-Guideline/National-Clinical-Guidelines-for-Stroke-fourth-edi.aspx

ⓘ **Residual neuromuscular blockade**

Definition
Unexpectedly prolonged neuromuscular blockade following anaesthesia.

Presentation
- Poorly supported or obstructed airway with inadequate breathing/cough, poor hand-grip, head lift <5 s.
- 'Floppy', struggling, jerky, or agitated patient, pseudo-sedation (eyes closed).
- Low S_pO_2.

Immediate management
- ☑ Assess ventilation; if inadequate, commence BLS with bag–mask ventilation and oxygen; apply pulse oximeter.
- ☑ If ventilation adequate, consider jaw support, oral/nasal airway insertion, and assist ventilation as needed with patient on side. Reassure patient, encourage slow inspiratory breaths, and stay with patient until return of full neuromuscular function.
- ☑ Apply nerve stimulator and check train-of-four (TOF) or double-burst stimulation. Absence of fade indicates adequate neuromuscular function. A post-tetanic count can be used when the TOF shows no twitches (reversal is likely when the post-tetanic count is ≥10).
- ☑ Administer further or first dose of reversal agent (max. dose neostigmine 70 µg/kg with glycopyrronium 10 µg/kg) if indicated.
- ☑ If neuromuscular function does not return after reversal, or there are features of Phase II (mixed) blockade, consider IV anaesthesia and tracheal intubation. Transfer to ICU for ventilation.
- ☑ If the patient is conscious but partly paralysed, reassure and consider sedation with small doses of midazolam or propofol.
- ☑ Establish/maintain normothermia and normocarbia.

Subsequent management
- ☑ Pseudocholinesterase genotyping 3 days after suxamethonium, mivacurium, or neostigmine exposure (8 weeks after blood administration) with follow-up by anaesthetist, counselling, and biochemical testing of family members. Organize 'Medic Alert' bracelet or other disease identification system.
- ☑ Referral to neurologist for patients with suspected neuromuscular disease.
- ☑ Explain episode to patient later. Some are terrified and assume this will occur again.

Investigations
- Apply peripheral nerve stimulator and test for residual paralysis.
- Baseline FBC, U&Es, Ca^{2+}, Mg^{2+}, phosphate.

- ABG.
- Core temp (e.g. tympanic).

Risk factors

- Hypothermia.
- Acidosis.
- Hypermagnesaemia.
- Hypokalaemia.
- Known neuromuscular disease (e.g. myasthenia gravis) or symptoms (unexplained weakness) in patient or family.
- Excessive use of neuromuscular blockers or repeated use of suxamethonium (>10 mg/kg).
- Use of aminoglycoside antibiotics (gentamicin, amikacin, tobramycin, neomycin).
- Drugs which act as substrates for/inhibitors of acetylcholinesterase will prolong a suxamethonium neuromuscular block (echothiophate eye drops, metoclopramide, ketamine, oral contraceptive pill, lithium, lidocaine, ester local anaesthetics, cytotoxic agents, edrophonium, neostigmine, and trimetaphan).
- Renal or hepatic impairment (with reduced metabolism/clearance of certain neuromuscular blockers).
- Cholinesterase deficiency (renal failure, hepatic disease, malnutrition, carcinomatosis, pregnancy, cardiopulmonary bypass, cardiac failure, thyrotoxicosis) or reduced activity (abnormal genotypes).
- Lithium therapy.
- Calcium channel antagonists.

Exclusions

- Hypothermia.
- Respiratory depression (⊃ see p. 370).
- Neurological problems, e.g. myasthenia gravis or myasthenic syndromes (Eaton–Lambert syndrome), stroke, laryngeal nerve palsy.
- Metabolic disturbances: hypokalaemia (e.g. hypokalaemic paralysis—rare clinical syndrome of systemic weakness with low K^+), hypermagnesaemia, hypophosphataemia, hypocalcaemia, hyper/hyponatraemia.
- Endocrine: hypothyroidism, Cushing's syndrome.

Special considerations

- Residual neuromuscular block is common (<40%) and can increase the risk of postoperative pulmonary complications.
- Attempted reversal of mivacurium before neuromuscular function starts to return may result in prolonged duration of action and neuromuscular blockade.
- Successful reversal of neuromuscular blockade appears to be dependent upon intracellular pH, therefore correct respiratory acidosis.
- Consider use of sugammadex for reversal of non-depolarizing neuromuscular blockade, especially rocuronium (16 mg/kg for immediate reversal; 4–8 mg/kg for reversal of profound block

(post-tetanic count 1–2), and 2 mg/kg to reverse moderate block, e.g. when T2 is detectable).
• With the exception of rocuronium, do not try to reverse neuromuscular drugs when there are no signs of recovery of the TOF.

Further reading

Murphy, G.S., Brull, S.J. (2010). Residual neuromuscular block: lessons unlearned. Part I: definitions, incidence, and adverse physiologic effects of residual neuromuscular block. *Anesthesia and Analgesia*, **111**(1), 120–8.
Murphy, S.G., Brull, S.J. (2010). Residual neuromuscular block: lessons unlearned. Part II: methods to reduce the risk of residual weakness. *Anesthesia and Analgesia*, **111**(1), 129–40.

ⓘ Oliguria/acute renal failure (ARF)

Definition by RIFLE criteria

- **Risk**— urine output <0.5 mL/kg/h for 6 h, serum creatinine rise ×1.5 or GFR decrease >25%.
- **Injury**— urine output <0.5 mL/kg/h for 12 h, serum creatinine rise ×2 or GFR decrease >50%.
- **Failure**— urine output <0.3 mL/kg/h for 24 h or anuria for 12 h, serum creatinine rise ×3 or GFR decrease >75%.

Presentation

May present as polyuria, oliguria, or anuria. Often classified according to site of lesion: prerenal, renal, or postrenal.

Immediate management

- ☑ Hourly urine output measurement via urinary catheter (exclude blocked catheter by flushing with 50 mL saline via a bladder syringe).
- ☑ Assess volume status and restore normovolaemia:
  - fluid challenge (250–500 mL Hartmann's/0.9% saline over 15 min). Repeat according to response.
- ☑ Maintain BP at normal levels (MAP >70 mmHg) or higher if patient usually hypertensive. Vasopressors may be necessary (➲ see p. 343).
- ☑ Optimize cardiac output.
- ☑ Treat life-threatening complications. These include hyperkalaemia, volume overload, acidosis, and uraemia.

Subsequent management

- ☑ Acute hyperkalaemia (K^+ >6.5 mmol/L)— ➲ see p. 313.
- ☑ TURP syndrome— ➲ see p. 306.
- ☑ Stop or avoid nephrotoxic drugs.
- ☑ Consider using a limited course of furosemide to relieve fluid overload.
- ☑ Refer to nephrologist or intensivist for further management of prerenal or intrinsic ARF.
- ☑ Refer to urologist for postrenal obstruction. Suprapubic catheter or percutaneous nephrostomy may be necessary.

Investigations

- FBC, U&Es, calcium, phosphate, coagulation screen, and consider creatine kinase (rhabdomyolysis).
- ABGs.
- CXR.
- Urinary Na^+ and osmolality. In prerenal ARF the kidney will attempt to retain Na^+ (urinary sodium <20 mmol/L) and concentrate urine (SG >1.015). These patients may benefit from more fluid boluses. In acute tubular necrosis, the kidney will begin to lose this ability (urinary sodium >20 mmol/L and SG <1.015).

Risk factors
- **The 'vulnerable' kidney**—patients with diabetes, hypertension, vasculopathy, and increasing age with a normal creatinine often have a reduced nephron capacity and impaired renovascular response to even modest changes in BP. A total of 75% of the kidneys nephrons need to be impaired before a patient's GFR begins to decline.
- **Pre-existing chronic kidney disease**—glomerulonephritis and/or nephrosclerosis.
- **Prerenal**—hypotension, hypovolaemia/dehydration, cardiac or liver failure.
- **Renal**—nephrotoxins (antibiotics, contrast agents, NSAIDs, ACE inhibitors, ciclosporin, myoglobin), sepsis, obstructive jaundice, ABO blood transfusion reactions.
- **Postrenal**—renal tumours, stones, prostate tumours.
- **Surgery**—aortic, renovascular, prolonged procedures, cardiopulmonary bypass.

Exclusions
- Catheter problems (poorly positioned, obstructed, or kinked urinary catheter). Irrigate catheter to relieve obstruction, dislodge clots or debris.
- If a urinary catheter is not present, or cannot be easily inserted, the presence of a distended bladder should be sought by palpation and/or abdominal ultrasound. Cystoscopy with ureteric stent insertion, suprapubic catheter insertion, or percutaneous nephrostomy may be indicated, according to level and type of obstruction.

Special considerations
- **Optimize volume status** for patients at risk of renal failure.
- **Contrast nephropathy** is a leading cause of in-hospital ARF. Patients with known renal impairment and diabetes are at greatest risk. At present, the most robust evidence suggests a modest fluid load with isotonic sodium bicarbonate (3 mL/kg for at least 1 h before contrast followed by 1 mL/kg until 6 h post procedure) may be beneficial. The role of N-acetylcysteine remains uncertain but can be given in conjunction with sodium bicarbonate (1200 mg bd for the day before and the day of the procedure).
- **Drugs**. Diuretics can be used following appropriate volume replacement. Osmotic (mannitol), loop (furosemide), and thiazide diuretics (and renal dose dopamine) confer no benefit in reducing the incidence of ARF, dialysis, or mortality in oliguric patients. Their role lies in attempting to optimize fluid balance and stratifying patients who respond to diuretics into a more favourable outcome group. Mannitol is most useful in rhabdomyolysis or intracerebral oedema.
- **Abdominal compartment syndrome** occurs in the setting of an intra-abdominal pressure (IAP) >20 mmHg and end-organ dysfunction. A raised IAP may lead to renal and splanchnic hypoperfusion, respiratory embarrassment by inhibiting downward/caudal diaphragmatic movement, reduced venous return to the heart, raised intracranial pressure, and bacterial translocation. This occurs with acute

pancreatitis, large retroperitoneal bleeds, emergency AAA surgery, and abdominal trauma surgery. Urinary manometry is the more reliable method of monitoring IAP. Specific IAP urinary manometry kits exist. Alternatively, connect a manometer to an 18 G needle and insert it into a urinary catheter (which has been clamped distally) with 50 mL of sterile saline in the bladder, to achieve an accurate reading. Zero reference point is pubic symphysis. IAP scale is:

- Normal: 5–7 mmHg
- Grade 1: 12–15 mmHg
- Grade 2: 16–20 mmHg
- Grade 3: 21–25 mmHg
- Grade 4: >25 mmHg

Measure the IAP every 2–4 h. Consider surgical decompression if IAP >25 mmHg and evidence of end-organ dysfunction.

Further reading

Bellomo, R., Ronco, C., Kellum, J.A., et al. (2004). Acute renal failure—definition, outcome measures, animal models, fluid therapy and information technology needs: the Second International Consensus Conference of the Acute Dialysis Quality Initiative (ADQI) Group. *Critical Care*, **8**, R204–12.

⚠ Severe postoperative nausea and vomiting (PONV)

Definition
Persistent nausea ± vomiting despite first-line drug therapy.

Presentation
- Patient reports feeling of nausea.
- Attempted ('dry-retching') or actual vomiting of gastric contents.

Immediate management
- ☑ Check heart rate and blood pressure (nausea often precedes detection of hypotension).
- ☑ Restore intravascular volume and correct electrolyte disturbances.
- ☑ Treat pain and severe anxiety.
- ☑ Drug therapy (treatment cascade will differ according to local protocols):
  - $5HT_3$ antagonists (ondansetron 4 mg IV, granisetron 1 mg IV)
  - phenothiazine (prochlorperazine 12.5 mg IM).
  - metoclopramide 10 mg IV (not with gastric/bowel obstruction).
  - butyrophenone (droperidol 0.625–1.25 mg IV, haloperidol 0.5–2 mg IV).
  - steroids (dexamethasone 4–8 mg IV).
  - antihistamines (cyclizine 25–50 mg slow IV, promethazine 25 mg PO).
  - anticholinergics (hyoscine hydrobromide 0.3–0.6 mg IM/SC/IV).
  - benzodiazepines have been used preoperatively or (rarely) as a low-dose postoperative infusion (midazolam 0.5–1 mg/h) for intractable PONV.
  - small dose of propofol (10–20 mg IV).
- ☑ Consider NG tube if there is gastric outlet obstruction, bowel obstruction, severe retching/vomiting.

Subsequent management
- ☑ Withhold oral fluids and continue IV therapy.
- ☑ Administer antiemetics regularly.
- ☑ Monitor electrolytes, renal and hepatic function.
- ☑ Consider drug side effects.
- ☑ Try alternative opioids for analgesia. Consider regional analgesia/ketamine infusion and NSAIDs if patient intolerant of all opioids used.
- ☑ Consider acupuncture or acupressure (P6 point on wrist—three finger breadths proximal to the wrist, between the flexor tendons for the index and middle fingers).
- ☑ Document severe PONV for future anaesthesia.

Risk factors

- **Patient factors**—baseline risk is 10%. Female sex, history of PONV, or motion sickness, non-smoker, post-op. opioids. Each additional risk factor increases baseline risk to 20%, 40%, 60%, 80% (Apfel score).
- **Anaesthetic factors**—use of certain drugs: opioids, tramadol, N_2O, etomidate, ketamine, neostigmine. Duration of anaesthesia, with each 30 min increasing risk by 60%.
- **Surgical factors**—laparoscopic surgery, laparotomy, breast/plastic/strabismus surgery, gastric dilatation (gastric outlet obstruction, poor bag–mask ventilation).

Exclusions

- Hypotension— ➲ see p. 343.
- Gastric dilatation—difficult bag–mask ventilation, NG tube incorrectly positioned, unrelieved bowel obstruction.
- CNS problem—raised or low ICP, migraine, head injury, neurosurgery, CSF leak. Consider neurosurgical opinion if changed level of consciousness or new CNS signs.
- Consider myocardial ischaemia/infarction. Perform 12-lead ECG.

Paediatric implications—drug therapy

- Ondansetron 0.1 mg/kg IV to maximum of 4 mg.
- Dexamethasone 0.15 mg/kg IV.
- Metoclopramide 0.1 mg/kg IV (cautiously, as prone to extrapyramidal side effects).

Special considerations

PONV (the 'big little problem') is associated with adverse effects (raised intracranial and intraocular pressure), but aggressive perioperative management can reduce morbidity (wound dehiscence, pain), recovery room, and hospital stay.

Further reading

Gan, T.J., Meyer, T.A., Apfel, C.C., et al. (2007). Society for Ambulatory Anesthesia guidelines for the management of postoperative nausea and vomiting. *Anesthesia and Analgesia*, **105**(6), 1615–28.

! Severe postoperative pain

Definition
Severe pain on emergence from anaesthesia or on regression of regional blockade. Pain score ≥7/10 and consistent behavioural score (grimacing).

Presentation
- Patient distress, anger, crying, or reluctance to move.
- Tachycardia, hypertension, sweating, or other sympathetic responses. Agitation, especially in elderly or intellectually impaired.
- Inadequate respiratory effort with arterial desaturation (abdominal/chest wounds).

Immediate management
☑ Start with paracetamol 1 g PO/PR/IV.
☑ Unless contraindicated, give NSAID—ibuprofen 400 mg PO, diclofenac 50–100 mg PO/PR/IV or parecoxib 40 mg IV. (Avoid diclofenac/parecoxib in patients with ischaemic heart disease, renal impairment, peripheral vascular disease, or cerebrovascular disease).
☑ Titrate opioid to analgesia with repeated boluses of: fentanyl 10–30 μg IV, morphine 1–3 mg IV, or tramadol 50 mg slow IV.
☑ Consider clonidine (1–2 μg/kg IV) if associated agitation.
☑ Consider ketamine 10–15 mg IV single bolus for intractable pain, or if patient has implanted/transdermal opioid antagonist. Consider infusion.
☑ Consider pethidine (25–50 mg IV) or hyoscine butylbromide (Buscopan®) if visceral pain (urologic, intestinal, or biliary surgery) or urinary catheter discomfort.
☑ Consider pregabalin (75–100 mg PO) if significant preoperative pain (neuropathic pain component).
☑ Consider temporary use of Entonox® until effect of other analgesics is felt.
☑ Consider regional analgesia (intercostal or nerve block, epidural, paravertebral).
☑ Exclude new or untreated pathology (surgical review if original diagnosis in doubt or possible new pathology, such as compartment syndrome, iatrogenic nerve damage, or ischaemia).

Subsequent management
☑ If there is still significant pain after high-dose morphine, a small dose of midazolam (1 mg) may improve matters—watch respiration and conscious level.
☑ Consider slow IV clonidine 1–2 μg/kg as an adjuvant, observe for sedation, and monitor BP.
☑ Referral to Acute Pain Service to manage postoperative opioid/ketamine infusions or regional block, neuraxial or interpleural infusions, treat complications, and maximize use of multimodal analgesic therapy.

Risk factors

- Preoperative opioid use.
- Poor control of pain prior to surgery.
- Inadequate intraoperative analgesics or exclusive use of remifentanil.
- Implanted opioid antagonist (e.g. naltrexone) or mixed opioid agonist/ antagonist (e.g. buprenorphine, which has a ceiling effect).
- Visceral pain, including bladder spasm (neostigmine) and biliary spasm (morphine).

Exclusions

- Severe anxiety or psychiatric disturbance.
- Acute confusional state.
- Consider full bladder, glucose, or metabolic problem if agitated.
- Opioid-seeking behaviour (advisable to give patient the benefit of doubt, give analgesics, and seek specialist help later).
- Exclude new or untreated pathology.

Special considerations

- **Chronic preoperative opioid use or abuse**—patients may require high opioid dosages that exceed standard protocols. A dedicated pain service can assist with perioperative analgesic therapy.
- **Elderly or intellectually impaired patient**—pain assessment may be difficult and agitation or confusion can be the only indication of pain.
- **Cultural differences**—some cultures show little behavioural evidence of pain. Assessment should include ability to move, breathe deeply, or cough.
- **Severe anxiety**—titrate clonidine 25–50 µg IV every 5 min prn to achieve sedation (maximum 2 µg/kg) or midazolam 1 mg IV every 5 min prn to achieve sedation.

Paediatric implications

Pain scores in preverbal children are difficult. Use observational pain scoring tools (e.g. CHIPPS scale for 0–23 months, FLACC scale for 2–7 y), then self-reporting tools appropriate for age (e.g. Faces pain scale for 4–12 y), and standard visual analogue scales for older children and adolescents.

Further reading

Büttner, W., Finke, W. (2000). Analysis of behavioural and physiological parameters for the assessment of postoperative analgesic demand in newborns, infants and young children: a comprehensive report on seven consecutive studies. *Paediatric Anaesthesia*, **10**, 303–18.

Hicks, C.L., von Baeyer, C.L., Spafford, P.A., van Korlaar, I., Goodenough, B. (2001). The faces pain scale-revised: toward a common metric in pediatric pain measurement. *Pain*, **93**, 173–83.

Merkel, S.I., Voepel-Lewis, T., Shayevitz, J.R., Malviya, S. (1997). The FLACC: a behavioral scale for scoring postoperative pain in young children. *Pediatric Nursing*, **23**, 293–7.

Wu, C.L., Raja, S.N. (2011). Treatment of acute postoperative pain. *Lancet*, **377**, 2215–25.

! Epidural problems

Definition
Any problem related to the epidural technique, catheter, or drugs.

Presentation
Pain, hypotension/bradycardia, headache, nausea/vomiting, itch, shivering, postdural puncture headache, urinary retention.

Immediate management

Hypotension/bradycardia
☑ Associated with total spinal, dural puncture, subarachnoid, or subdural catheter position, high block.
☑ Nausea/vomiting often precedes hypotension (especially parturients).
☑ Stop infusion.
☑ Lay patient flat, elevate legs.
☑ Give ephedrine 3–6 mg IV. Alternatives include metaraminol 0.5–2 mg IV or phenylephrine 100 µg IV (or 5 mg in 50 mL saline at 0–30 mL/h IV).
☑ Give atropine 0.6–1.2 mg IV or glycopyrronium 0.2–0.4 mg IV if bradycardia.
☑ Rapid IV fluid administration (crystalloid 1000 mL).

'Total' spinal
◒ See p. 258 (general) and p. 171 (obstetric).

Local anaesthetic toxicity
◒ See p. 248.

Wound pain
☑ Perform 'ice mapping' to determine extent and quality of block—is the block 'patchy' with missed dermatomes?
☑ Perform catheter aspiration test (absence of CSF or blood, but may be false-negative in 50% of cases).
☑ Consider adjusting catheter position if block too high, too low, or unilateral—withdraw catheter using aseptic technique but leave at least 3 cm in the epidural space. (Do not move the epidural catheter within 12 h of LMWH.)
☑ Administer test dose of local anaesthetic if BP normal (5 ml 0.25% L-bupivacaine), and repeat to achieve analgesia. Consider higher concentration LA ± opioids. If hypotension/bradycardia develop, give opioids only (fentanyl 50–100 µg or diamorphine 2.5 mg).
☑ Consider adding clonidine 1 µg/mL to LA solution to treat patchy block.
☑ Supplement regional analgesia with systemic adjuvant (paracetamol, NSAIDs) or opioid analgesics and remove opioid from epidural solution.

Nausea/vomiting
- ☑ Treat hypotension (➔ see p. 343).
- ☑ Give antiemetics (➔ see p. 362).
- ☑ If symptoms persist, remove opioid from epidural infusion, maintain epidural with local anaesthetic.
- ☑ If epidural infusion has included an opioid, give antiemetics IV according to protocol. Consider naloxone 0.1 mg IV ± naloxone infusion (naloxone 400 µg added to maintenance IV fluids).

Shivering
- ☑ Treat hypothermia with hot-air warming blanket.
- ☑ Warm IV fluids.
- ☑ Pethidine 25 mg IV or tramadol 25 mg IV or clonidine 25–50 µg IV may be useful.

Postdural puncture headache (PDPH)
- ☑ Postural headache relieved by lying and exacerbated by sitting or standing.
- ☑ Risk can be reduced if intrathecal catheter introduced for 24 h at the time of dural puncture. This should be meticulously labelled as 'intrathecal'.
- ☑ Give simple analgesics.
- ☑ Caffeine may be effective.
- ☑ 85% of PDPH resolve by 6 weeks.
- ☑ Definitive treatment is epidural blood patch performed by experienced personnel; but success rate is c.50% (➔ see p. 174).

Subsequent management

- ☑ **Urinary retention**—according to local protocol, the bladder may be catheterized as a single-shot, or an indwelling catheter may be left *in situ* until the epidural catheter technique is discontinued.
- ☑ **Tachyphylaxis**—if sensory block recedes more quickly than expected in patients with an epidural infusion, try an alternative local anaesthetic. Regular testing of sensory level and appropriate increases in infusion rates of the epidural infusion can maintain an effective block. In general, if there are no problems of hypotension or excessive block, an infusion rate of 10 mL/h (lumbar) or 7 mL/h (thoracic) will help to prevent a sudden contraction in block.
- ☑ **Itching**—consider use of naloxone (100 µg IV prn), ondansetron (4–8 mg IV), promethazine (25–50 mg IM), or removing opioid from epidural mixture.

Investigations
MRI if epidural haematoma suspected (➔ see p. 255).

Risk factors
- Previous back surgery
- Obesity
- Kyphoscoliosis

- Inexperienced anaesthetist
- Multiple attempts at insertion
- Poor technique

Exclusions

- **Subarachnoid (spinal) catheter/inadvertent dural puncture**—should be suspected with high block, hypotension, and bradycardia. Treat symptomatically, prepare for airway management if large dose of local anaesthetic has been given or block is ascending. Remove catheter (❯ see p. 258) unless in high-dependency area. If you do leave it in:
  - stop the 'epidural' infusion
  - label the catheter clearly
  - inform the nurse/midwife
  - ensure top-ups are given by anaesthetist only (0.5–1 mL 0.5% bupivacaine as needed).
- **Subdural catheter**—should be suspected when a higher than expected (often patchy) block occurs 15–30 min after injection of local anaesthetic. Remove catheter.
- **Epidural haematoma**—should be suspected if sensorimotor block persists 6 h after surgery—urgent investigation with MRI indicated and proceed with surgical drainage as necessary (❯ see p. 255).

Further reading

Wheatley, R.G., Schug, S.A., Watson, D. (2001). Safety and efficacy of postoperative epidural analgesia. *British Journal of Anaesthesia*, **87**, 47–61.

Emergency department problems

Kath Sutherland, Jim Blackburn, and Neil Rasburn

Major trauma

Definition
Injury to one or more body parts that is potentially life-threatening or life-changing.

Presentation
- Depends on severity of injury.
- Mechanism of injury will give clues to potential injuries.
- Patient may be awake or unconscious.
- A confused patient can make initial assessment, investigation and treatment extremely challenging.
- A similar clinical picture can arise from different injuries, e.g. loss of consciousness (LOC) can result from significant head injury, CVE, or medical coma, major blood loss, or primary cardiac arrest.

Immediate management
- ☑ Ambulance services may move patients direct to a Major Trauma Centre if one can be reached within 1 hour. However trauma units and non-specialist hospitals within regional trauma networks may still receive undifferentiated patients that are too sick to reach the MTC, or where the MTC cannot be reached within 1 hour.
- ☑ Management should be led by a Trauma Team Leader supported by specialists from anaesthesia, emergency medicine and surgical specialties. Effective trauma care requires good teamwork, task management, situational awareness, decision making and good communication.
- ☑ ABC—airway obstruction; chest injuries; catastrophic haemorrhage; circulatory shock.
- ☑ 100% oxygen via a non-rebreathing mask.
- ☑ IV access with two large-bore (14–16 G) cannulae, use humeral intraosseous (IO) if IV difficult.

Airway
- ☑ Cervical spine immobilization with head blocks and tape or manual in-line stabilization (MILS).
- ☑ Establish an airway with jaw thrust if suspected C-spine injury and consider definitive airway if:
  - hypoxic, inadequate respiratory effort, massive blood loss, obstructed airway.
  - agitation
  - confusion/fluctuating LOC requiring head CT—and risk of aspiration.
  - major traumatic injury, GA required on humane grounds ± major surgery imminent.
    - ☑ Balance timing of intubation with ongoing fluid resuscitation using warmed blood products where possible. Ketamine is often the safest choice of induction drug.
    - ☑ Videolaryngoscopy and advanced airway equipment available, with CO_2 monitoring.
    - ☑ Emergency Induction Checklists should be used in all situations except cardiorespiratory arrest.
- ☑ Modified Rapid Sequence Induction. Consider cricoid pressure. Protect cervical spine with MILS.

☑ If major airway trauma, consider surgical airway early with ENT input where possible.

Breathing

☑ Identify major thoracic injuries.
☑ Tension pneumothorax should be diagnosed clinically (◑ see p. 66) and managed early.
☑ If pneumothorax, haemopneumothorax, flail segment, or fractured ribs present consider tracheobronchial injury, pulmonary contusion, diaphragmatic injury, cardiac contusion/tamponade, and mediastinal disruption. Injury to the first rib is an indication of major forces involved in the trauma.

Circulation

☑ Stem major external haemorrhage with direct pressure, haemostatic dressings, tourniquets and limb splintage (inc. pelvic binder) where necessary.
☑ Secure IV access with at least two short, large-bore cannulae (14 G). Consider humeral IO early if peripheral IV access fails. In children consider IO as first line.
☑ Send blood for crossmatch. Activate major haemorrhage call early. Give IV tranexamic acid (1 g) within 1 hour of injury for maximum benefit.
☑ Check pulse rate and volume. Assess peripheral perfusion. Arterial or venous lactate can be a useful guide to volume status. Blood pressure should be low enough in the first 60-90 minutes following injury not to exacerbate bleeding but high enough to maintain major organ perfusion (MAP 50–60 mmHg). Hypotension is a late sign of hypovolaemia, particularly in young and fit patients. Many prescription medications may mask abnormal parameters. Deteriorating conscious level in the absence of primary head injury is suggestive of significant blood loss.
☑ Clinical examination of chest, abdomen, retroperitoneum, pelvis and long bones.
☑ Pelvic injuries can bleed profusely: stabilization with purpose made or improvised binder is critical and may need to precede laparotomy.
☑ Advanced interventions including retrograde endovascular balloon occlusion of the aorta (REBOA) and interventional radiology services are increasingly available for uncontrollable arterial bleeding.
☑ Perform imaging according to resource of institution. The gold standard is a whole body CT scan as soon as possible, if haemodynamically improving or stable. e-FAST scans may direct interventions for active bleeding if indicated and sufficient expertise available.

Disability

☑ Assess with the GCS and observe the pupils.
☑ Assess and document the patient's neurology prior to intubation. The motor component of the score gives the best indication of outcome.
☑ Don't forget to check blood glucose.

Exposure

☑ Examine patient completely and then actively manage patient temperature to avoid hypothermia. Forced air warming blankets and use of fluid warmers are useful.

Fluids

☑ Careful initial fluid resuscitation with blood products. Use 1:1 unit ratio of plasma:red blood cells.

☑ Use a restrictive approach until haemorrhage control is achieved or until 60–90 mins post injury. Titrate fluids to maintain central pulses (carotid and/or femoral). Adequacy of replacement is judged by cardiovascular parameters, urine output, cognitive function, and biochemical improvement (lactate, Base deficit, pH). If Traumatic Brain Injury suspected, use a less restrictive approach to maintain cerebral perfusion.

☑ A rapid infusor should be available and all products should be warmed (➲ see 'Massive transfusion protocol', p. 418).

☑ Once blood product resuscitation commenced use lab results and point of care coagulation testing to guide management at earliest opportunity.

☑ Monitor serum calcium levels closely. Replace calcium using CaCl 10% 10 mmol after approximately every 4 units of pack red blood cells or if ionised calcium falls below 1.1 mmol/L.

☑ Minimal or no response to volume resuscitation suggests concealed bleeding, tamponade, tension pneumothorax, embolism, spinal cord injury, cardiogenic cause, or sepsis.

☑ Consider in context of age, drug therapy, and other comorbidities.

Subsequent management

Secondary survey follows the primary survey and resuscitation, and involves head-to-toe systematic assessment. It may include reassessment of the primary survey and additional imaging/blood tests. Always examine anterior and posterior surfaces of all body areas and axillae, groins and perineum: injuries and wounds are easily missed.

☑ Arterial cannulation will allow close monitoring and give a measure of effectivenss of ongoing resuscitation. Central access would favour the subclavian route, particularly with head or C spine injuries.

☑ Assess the need for 'Damage Control Surgery' rather than concentrating on an absolute diagnosis. This is a measure that can control life threatening injuries in haemodynamically unstable patients not responding to resuscitation.

☑ Rapid CT scan should be performed prior to theatre unless patient very unstable (➲ see 'Investigations', p. 370).

☑ Consider 'occult' chest injuries including pulmonary/cardiac contusion, major vessel transection/rupture, and diaphragmatic/oesophageal rupture.

☑ Consider urethral injury with suspected pelvic injury.

☑ Cervical spine injuries—monitor for loss of motor function, loss of sensation, altered pattern of ventilation, hypotension with bradycardia, loss of signs of peritoneal irritation. Take care not to miss occult blood loss in these patients.

☑ Limb injuries should be assessed for vascular and neurological deficit including compartment syndrome. Avoid regional anaesthesia in the acute phase.

☑ Surgical procedures need to be performed in order of importance.

☑ Consider tetanus status and need for IV antibiotics for any significant open wounds or open fractures

Investigations

- Crossmatch/FBC/U&Es/clotting/LFT/ABG/lactate/Ca
- Whole body, contrast enhanced, multi-detector CT scan of head/neck/chest/abdomen/pelvis and proximal long bones
- CXR (supine)
- Lateral cervical spine X-ray (see Figure 12.1)
- eFAST—Extended Focussed Assessment with Sonography for Trauma. If expertise available can identify chest and abdominal injuries, as well as aiding haemodynamic status. Don't delay CT scan to get this.
- Early C-spine MRI if neurology with no bony injury
- ECG

Risk factors

- Motorcyclists, cyclists, pedestrians, older people, equestrian, agricultural or industrial environments, alcohol or drug usage.

Special considerations

- Severe head injury—see p. 192.

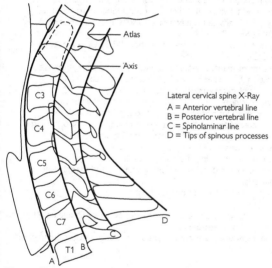

Lateral cervical spine X-Ray
A = Anterior vertebral line
B = Posterior vertebral line
C = Spinolaminar line
D = Tips of spinous processes

Figure 12.1 Lines of alignment on a lateral cervical spine X-ray.

Further reading

NICE guideline [NG39] Major trauma: assessment and initial management. Published February 2016
European Trauma Course – The Team Approach Manual. Ed 4.

☠ Drug overdose

Definition
Deliberate or unintentional consumption of drugs/medication in excess of their therapeutic index.

Presentation
- It may not be obvious what has been taken.
- Presentation can vary from no signs or symptoms to significant cardiovascular disturbance and decreased level of consciousness.
- Polypharmacy is common, the medication consumed may also have been combined with alcohol and illicit drugs.

Immediate management
☑ Always follow ABC, assess neurology, full examination.

☑ Obtain history from the patient, paramedics, witnesses—**'when?', 'what?', 'quantity?'**—past medical history, drug history, psychiatric history.

☑ Initial management is supportive: correct hypoxia, hypotension, dehydration, hypo/hyperthermia, acidosis and control seizures.

☑ Seek specific advice from National Poisons Information Service (TOXBASE).

☑ Monitor temperature, pulse, respiration, BP, ECG, oxygenation, and GCS.

☑ The aims of management are to decrease absorption, increase excretion ± administer specific antidotes (see Table 12.1).

☑ Methods of decreasing absorption include:
- gastric lavage—only if within 1 h of overdose; never with corrosives; intubate if decreased consciousness level.
- activated charcoal—50 g single or repeated dose (also increases elimination). Activated charcoal does not bind heavy metals, ethanol, or acids.

☑ Methods of increasing elimination include:
- charcoal haemoperfusion (for barbiturates and theophylline).
- diuresis.
- urinary alkalinization (for tricyclics).
- dialysis.

☑ All patients who have taken a deliberate overdose should be referred for psychiatric assessment.

☑ In the event of cardiac arrest consider prolonged resuscitation efforts. (seek advice).

Investigations
- Always check blood glucose, paracetamol, and salicylate levels.
- FBC, U&Es, LFT, CK, clotting, bicarbonate, ABGs, ECG, CXR.
- Blood and urine for toxicology screening, specific blood levels.

Table 12.1 Specific antagonists

Overdose drug	Specific antagonist
Opioids	Naloxone
Iron	Desferrioxamine
Lead	Sodium EDTA
Digoxin	FAB (digoxin-specific antibody fragments)
Calcium channel blockers	Calcium
Ethylene glycol	Ethanol
Lithium	Dialysis

Paediatric considerations

- Accidental overdose may have occurred.
- Any safeguarding concerns (neglect or abuse) must be documented and reported.

Special considerations

- In the United Kingdom, drug overdose is responsible for 6300 suicides per annum, and 20% of deaths in young people.
- 140 000 para-suicides occur per annum, most common in young females 14–19 years old. The most common method is poisoning; paracetamol accounts for 50% of cases.

Specific management of toxins

Paracetamol

- Most common drug in overdose, few signs or symptoms early on.
- Toxicity dependent on amount ingested, type of exposure and timing of exposure.
- Hepatic and renal toxin (centrilobular necrosis).
- 150 mg/kg (9 g in a 60 kg adult) can be fatal, more than 75 mg/kg in 24 h needs medical assessment.
- Treatment is with *N*-acetylcysteine (NAC), a glutathione precursor and a source of sulphydryl groups allowing conjugation to non-toxic metabolites. Very high levels (>700 mg/L) associated with coma and high lactate may need haemodialysis (and double doses of NAC).
- NAC dose regimen is 150 mg/kg in 200 mL of 5% glucose over 60 min, then 50 mg/kg over 4 h, then 100 mg/kg in 1 L of 5% glucose over 16 h. Common side effects include flushing, wheeze, hypotension, and anaphylactoid reaction. Hypersensitivity is no longer a contraindication as benefit outweighs risk. Alternative to NAC is methionine PO (<12 h).
- Use nomogram for calculating paracetamol toxic dose (Figure 12.2). Patients with a timed plasma paracetamol level on or above a single treatment line joining points of 100 mg/L at 4 h and 15 mg/L at 15 h after ingestion should receive NAC regardless of risk factors for hepatotoxicity. Note: paracetamol levels can be underestimated if taken when NAC running. If in doubt check with lab.

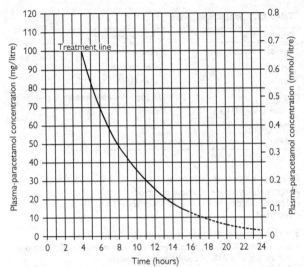

Patients whose plasma-paracetamol concentrations are on or above the **treatment line** should be treated with acetylcysteine by intravenous infusion.

The prognostic accuracy after 15 hours is uncertain, but a plasma-paracetamol concentration on or above the treatment line should be regarded as carrying as serious risk of liver damage.

Graph reproduced courtesy of Medicines and Healthcare products Regulatory Agency

Figure 12.2 Paracetamol poisoning nomogram.

Adapted from Drug Safety Update September 2012, vol 6, issue 2: A1. Open Government Licence v3.0.

- Where there is doubt over the timing or when ingestion has occurred over a period of 1 h or more—NAC should always be given without delay (the nomogram should not be used).
- **Presentation less than 8 h since ingestion**:
    - Activated charcoal if ingestion of >150mg/kg and presentation <1 h.
    - Wait 4 h from last ingestion prior to checking plasma drug levels, and assess risk using normogram (Figure 12.2).
    - Most effective if treatment isstarted <8h post ingestion. Do not delay treatment if 150 mg/kg or 12 g consumed by an adult or if plasma concentration not available in <8h.
    - Check FBC, INR, LFTs, HCO3, U+E, including Creatinine after treatment with NAC.
    - If results are normal, patients usually fit for discharge following psychiatric referral where required and with advice to return if they have symptoms of nausea or abdominal pain.
    - If ALT high start NAC, even if paracetamol concentration is below the treatment line.

- **Presentation 8–24 h since ingestion**:
  - Start NAC.
  - Use nomogram for paracetamol toxic level. Continue NAC if drug level appropriate and admit; if level low, stop NAC unless other bloods abnormal.
- **Presentation >24 h since ingestion**:
  - There is still benefit in starting NAC even after 24 h. Start NAC if jaundiced or hepatic tenderness, high ALT, detectable paracetamol concentration, and/or INR > 1.3.

Aspirin

- Treatment is only likely to be needed after single dose ingestion >125 mg/kg and/or if patients are young or elderly (<10 y or >70 y).
- Early features—hyperventilation, sweating, tinnitus, tremor, nausea/ vomiting, and hyperpyrexia.
- Metabolic features—hypo/hyperglycaemia, hypokalaemia, respiratory alkalosis, metabolic acidosis.
- Other—renal failure, pulmonary oedema, seizures, arrhythmias, coma, and death.
- Specific management:
  - avoid intubation unless respiratory failure—can decompensate rapidly—instigate the following management if possible first.
  - bloods—salicylate level after 2 h >700 mg/L (5.1 mmol/L) is potentially lethal; 300–700 mg/L considered moderate poisoning. Repeat levels 2 hrly if symptomatic, or until levels falling.
  - U&Es, glucose, bicarbonate, ABGs, INR, ECG.
  - consider activated charcoal <1 h after ingestion (>125mg/kg).
  - gastric lavage <1 h after ingestion, only if >500mg/kg and airway can be protected.
  - rehydrate, monitor glucose, correct metabolic acidosis (with 8.4% sodium bicarbonate), and monitor/normalize K^+.
  - monitor urinary pH and alkalinize urine to a pH >7.5 with bicarbonate if plasma salicylate level >500 mg/L and K normal.
  - consider haemodialysis if plasma salicylate level >700 mg/L before rehydration, or if renal failure, severe acidosis, or pulmonary oedema are present.

Tricyclic antidepressants (TCAs)

- Absorbed in GIT, reaches peak levels <6 h after ingestion.
- 10 mg/kg can be fatal.
- Clinical effects:
  - patient may deteriorate rapidly; most major problems occur within the first 6 h.
  - sinus tachycardia, hot dry skin, dry mouth, urinary retention, hypotension, and hypothermia/hyperthermia, rhabdomyolysis.
  - dilated pupils, nystagmus, squint, ataxia, decreased level of consciousness, coma, seizures, increased tone.
  - prolonged PR, QRS, and QT, and ventricular dysrhythmias.
- Management:
  - supportive—check airway, maintain ventilation, correct hypoxia, and hypercarbia. IV crystalloids for hypotension.

- consider activated charcoal if <1 hr after ingestion, and even a second dose at 1-2 hrs if patient intubated or fully awake.

Give sodium bicarbonate in aliquots of (50 mL 8.4%), if QRS >120 msec, hypotension unresponsive to fluids even in the absence of acidosis. Aim for a pH of >7.45 as this limits available free drug. Avoid antidysrhythmic drugs although lidocaine may be useful, and consider inotropic support for refractory hypotension.

Seizures should be treated by correcting hypoxia and acidosis. Check glucose. Give benzodiazepines if seizures frequent or prolonged. Bicarbonate 8.4% 50 mL may also be beneficial in this group.

Active cooling for hyperthermia.

- **Do not** use flumazenil if benzodiazepine also taken—can be fatal.
- continue monitoring ECG, BP, S$_p$O$_2$, respiratory rate, GCS. Check serum creatinine kinase if unconscious.

In cardiac arrest, resuscitation should be continued for >1h, and only stopped after discussion with a senior clinician.

- Consider use of lipid emulsion (i.e. 20% intralipid) if cardiotoxicity unresponsive to other treatments (despite limited evidence).

Selective serotonin-reuptake inhibitors (SSRIs)

- Absorbed in GIT with a peak plasma concentration occurring 3–8 h after ingestion.
- Lipophilic and have long half-lives (4–9 days).
- Clinically:
  - decreased GCS, ataxia, hyperreflexia, hyperthermia.
  - hypotension or hypertension, ventricular tachycardia, and bradycardia.
- Management:
  - supportive care mainstay of treatment activated charcoal and IV fluids for hypotension.
  - ALS protocols for ventricular dysrhythmias. In cardiac arrest, resuscitation should be continued for >1hr.
  - haemodialysis is not indicated.
  - benzodiazepines for CNS manifestations such as agitation or seizures
  - actively cool.
  - check creatinine kinase.

Benzodiazepines

- Often taken in combination with other medications.
- Respiratory and CNS depressant. Arrhythmogenic.
- Management:
  - supportive: maintain adequate ventilation and cardiovascular support.
  - specific: flumazenil is a specific antidote but is not licensed for overdose treatment in the United Kingdom due to risk of cardiac arrhythmias and precipating seziures.

Other specific toxins

See Table 12.1.

initial-medical-management

☣ Massive gastrointestinal bleed

(➲ See also 'Massive haemorrhage', p. 418.)

Definition

Bleeding from any point in the GI tract. Upper GI causes (in order of frequency) are peptic ulcer disease, gastric erosions, oesophageal varices, Mallory–Weiss tears, and oesophagitis. Lower GI causes include diverticulosis, angiodysplasia, cancer/polyps, rectal disease, and irritable bowel disease.

Presentation

- Bleeding: upper GI bleeds present with haematemesis or coffee ground vomit, melaena and occasionally haematochezia (bright red blood per rectum). Lower GI bleeds present with haematochezia, bloody diarrhoea, and less commonly melaena.
- Shock: in early haemorrhage, clinical signs may be subtle or absent. Mildly increased respiratory rate, restlessness and nausea may be the only early signs. The presence of pallor, increased HR, widened pulse pressure, falling BP, cool peripheries or altered conscious level should alert clinicians to significant shock. Clinical diagnosis should be supported by biochemical results. Haemoglobin levels may not fall significantly even in advanced shock.
  Confounders in the assessment of shock include:
  - Age (elderly patients may not exhibit classical signs of shock)
  - Fitness level (athletes)
  - Concurrent medications: beta blockers may mask tachycardia; antihypertensive medications may exacerbate hypotension.
  - Ischaemic heart disease and/or heart failure may lead to significant shock even with only minor shifts in volume status.

Immediate management

- ☑ Appropriate resuscitation followed by endoscopic assessment is the key objective.
- ☑ ABC—100% oxygen. Obtain two large-bore IV access (14 G). Intraosseous access maybe required.
- ☑ Intubate using an appropriate rapid sequence induction of anaesthesia if there is an aspiration risk such as altered mental state or massive haemorrhage. Keep nil by mouth.
- ☑ Commence resuscitation with 500 mL boluses of a balanced crystalloid solution. Give packed red blood cells if Hb <70 g/L. Transfuse to a target Hb of 70-100 g/L. Major haemorrhage protocol may be required.
- ☑ Correct platelets only if active bleeding, haemodynamically unstable and levels <50 x 10⁹/L. Correct clotting if INR >1.5, and fibrinogen <1 g/L.
- ☑ Offer prothrombin complex to patients on warfarin and actively bleeding. Specific antidotes to direct oral anticoagulants (DOACs)

are now available: idarucizumab (Praxabind®) for dabigatran and adexanet alfa (recombinant Xa) for emergency reversal of apixaban and rivaroxiban.

☑ Start an IV PPI if suspicious of peptic ulceration.

☑ If cirrhotic or suspected variceal bleeding, administer terlipressin 2 mg 6-hourly IV to decrease portal blood flow. Give prophylactic antibiotics before endoscopy (follow local guidelines) to reduce risk of re-bleeding and mortality. Sepsis increases portal pressure and endoscopy causes bacteraemia in 50% patients.

Subsequent management

☑ Endoscopy should be undertaken within 24 hours of presentation in all cases. Urgent/immediate endoscopy maybe required if the patient remains unstable and there is risk of ongoing bleeding (80% of ulcers and 60% of varices stop bleeding spontaneously).

☑ May require GA if agitated or there is risk of aspiration. Consider invasive monitoring once airway secure and with concurrent resuscitation.

☑ Ensure adequate blood products available—use local major haemorrhage protocol.

☑ Critical care review should be considered for any patients with instability or requiring emergency anaesthesia or emergency endoscopy for haemorrhage control.

☑ Beware of re-bleeding post endoscopy. Consider repeating endoscopy once the patient has been stabilised.

☑ In uncontrolled bleeding a Sengstaken–Blakemore tube can be placed for tamponade of gastro-oesophageal varices. Sengstaken–Blakemore tubes should only be used in intubated patients and should be placed by experienced staff (risk of oesophageal rupture).

☑ Consider high-dose PPI infusion post endoscopy in patients with peptic ulcer disease (e.g. omeprazole 80 mg slow IV, followed by 8 mg/h for 72 h).

☑ Interventional radiology may be available in high volume centres and could limit or arrest bleeding.

☑ Intra-abdominal surgery is required for 10% of bleeding peptic ulcers.

Investigations

• FBC/U&Es/LFT/clotting (including fibrinogen), thromboelastography, ABGs, ECG, CXR, CT angiography.

Risk factors

• Liver disease, alcohol, infectious (Hepatitides)
• Clotting abnormalities
• Use of anticoagulation medications/NSAIDs
• Comorbidities—liver/heart/renal failure

Exclusions

• Massive haemoptysis, upper airway bleeding

Glasgow-Blatchford score

Should be calculated pre-endoscopy: Score > 1 indicates need for inpatient management. Score of >6 indicates a 50% chance of needing significant intervention, e.g. blood transfusion, endoscopy.
Points in brackets:
- Blood urea (mmol/L): 6.5–7.9 (2), 8–9.9 (3), 10–25 (4), >25 (6)
- Hb (g/L) men: 120–129 (1), 100–119 (3), <100 (6)
- Hb (g/L) women: 100–119 (1), <100 (6)
- Systolic blood pressure (mmHg): 100–109 (2), 90–99 (2), <90 (3)
- Pulse: ≥100/min (1)
- Presentation with melaena (1), presentation with syncope (2)
- Hepatic disease (2), cardiac failure (2)

Special considerations

- Complications of massive blood transfusion.
- Mortality is usually from comorbid conditions (MI, organ failure, aspiration, and sepsis). Rapid correction of haemodynamics results in fewer MIs and fewer deaths.

Further reading

NICE (2012). *Acute Upper Gastrointestinal Bleeding in Over 16s: Management: Clinical Guideline CG141.* Available at: https://www.nice.org.uk/guidance/cg141

Saltzman, J.R. (2019). *Acute Upper Gastrointestinal Bleeding.* Available at: https://www.Uptodate.com

Siau K, Hearnshaw S, Stanley A et al. (2019) UK multisociety consensus care bundle for early clinical management of acute upper gastrointestinal bleeding. Available at: https://www.bsg.org.uk/re-source/bsge-acute-upper-gi-bleed-care-bundle.html

✛ Chemical, biological, radiation and explosive injuries

Definition
Biological, nuclear, radiological, incendiary, chemical, or explosive injury.

Presentation
- Explosive and chemical injuries tend to be immediate, whereas biological and radiation exposure can take some time to reveal any symptoms. Patients may present individually with or without ambulance service assistance (e.g. chemical suicide, domestic explosion, community acquired biohazard) or as part of a major incident response. In this situation patients may be triaged at the scene and decontamination should commence prior to moving patients away from the scene ('hot zone'). Other patients may leave scene without contact with emergency services and self-present to the ED outside of a major incident response.
- If you SUSPECT that a patient has been exposed to a chemical or biological agent or to radiation that could have been released deliberately, IMMEDIATELY alert your local Health Protection Team.
- A single casualty presenting with symptoms should initially be approached with standard precautions and an open mind (alternative diagnoses are more likely). Where 2 casualties present with similar or identical symptoms and over similar time intervals, clinicians should exercise additional precautions (inc. PPE) and inform a senior clinician. Where 3 or more casualties present with similar or same symptoms, over the similar or overlapping time course, initial advice is for staff to withdraw from the area, contain the casualties in a single location, report the occurrence to a senior clinician and involve specialist help (Health Protection Team, Infection Control Team, consider activation of major incident plan).

Immediate management
- ☑ Personal safety is paramount. The risk to responders of secondary contamination through release of chemical or biological agents from clothing, skin, secretions and exhaled gases and must be considered.
- ☑ If specialist personal protective equipment is required this should only be used by those with suitable training and experience.
- ☑ All attempts should be made to determine the identity of the hazardous material. Responders should obtain assistance in identifying chemical(s) from hazchem placards, product information on containers as well as descriptions from incident scene. Further information maybe obtained from observing clinical signs and symptoms of toxidromes. The National Poisons Information Service as well as local specialist advice may be useful.
- ☑ Patients may be able to assist with their own decontamination. Remove and double-bag contaminated clothing and personal belongings. Do not throw these away.

☑ If the victim has ingested a chemical, toxic vomitus may also pose a danger through direct contact or off-gassing of vapour. Consider the level and adequacy of PPE required in this setting - do not approach if not safe to do so.

☑ Victims who were exposed only to gas or vapour and have no gross deposition of the material on their clothing or skin are unlikely to carry significant amounts of chemical beyond the 'hot zone' and are unlikely to pose risksof secondary contamination to hospital personnel. However, victims whose skin or clothing are covered with liquid or solid chemical or those who have chemical vapour condensate on their clothes or skin may contaminate hospital personnel and the emergency department by direct contact or by vapour. In both situations, clothing should be removed early, double bagged and sealed in clinical waste bags and retained.

☑ Flush exposed or irritated skin and hair with plain water for 3–5 min. For oily or otherwise adherent chemicals, use mild soap on the skin and hair. Rinse thoroughly with water. A commercially available neutralising agent - Diphoterine may be effective in removing acidic, alkali or adherent agents including tar and cement and may be available in some specialist settings such as heavy industrial, petrochemical and hazard encountering departments.

☑ Flush exposed or irritated eyes with plain water or saline for at least 5 min. Remove contact lenses if present and easily removable without causing additional trauma to the eye. If a corrosive material is suspected or if pain or injury is evident, continue irrigation while transferring the patient to the critical care area.

☑ In cases of ingestion, do not induce emesis. Administer 125–250 mL of water to dilute stomach contents if the patient is conscious and able to swallow. Immediately transfer the patient to the critical care area.

Chemical agents

Subsequent management
• Depends on the agent used.

Nerve agents (e.g. organophosphates and sarin)
• Sarin is structurally related to organophosphates and inhibits anticholinesterases (AChE).
• Classical presentation of nerve agent poisoning is cholinergic syndrome. Muscarinic features predominate—salivation, bronchoconstriction, bronchorrhoea, bradycardia, diarrhoea, urination, lacrimation, and dilated pupils. Death occurs due to respiratory failure from CNS depression and muscle paralysis.

☑ Treatment follows ABC principles. Airway management is vital and then early administration of antidotes.

☑ Intubate and ventilate if apnoeic or severe respiratory distress (avoid suxamethonium); check ABGs, U & Es, glucose; monitor ECG, treat arrhythmias.

☑ Non-depolarizing muscle relaxants cause prolonged paralysis once AChE is irreversibly inactivated. Reversal with neostigmine is ineffective. Suxamethonium causes prolonged paralysis. Ketamine increases secretions and should be used with caution.

☑ Atropine antagonizes the muscarinic effects, but nicotinic receptors are unaffected and muscle weakness or paralysis will not improve. Administer 0.6–4 mg IV (adult) or 20 micrograms/kg IV (child) every 10–20 minutes until secretions dry up and heart rate 80–90 bpm. Doses of up to 20 mg may be needed to achieve this.

☑ Pralidoxime is a reversible antagonist of AChE. It reverses nicotinic receptor dysfunction and reduces paralysis if given as an infusion. Pretreatment improves survival after nerve agent exposure. Initial dose is 2 g or 30 mg/kg IV (adult) over 4 minutes stat; then 4–6 hourly or infuse IV at 8–10 mg/kg/hour.

☑ Diazepam is indicated to prevent seizures and minimize secondary brain injury. Give 5–10 mg IV (adult) or 1–5 mg IV (child) stat; repeat as required.

Blistering agents (vesicants, e.g. mustard gas)
- Although tissue damage begins immediately, there may be a latent period of between 1 h and 24 h following exposure before symptoms appear. Vapour exposure causes most casualties. More significant exposure leads to shorter latent period. If release occurs anywhere other than a recognised industrial site, assume deliberate release.
- Respiratory symptoms include tracheobronchitis with bronchospasm, epithelial necrosis, ARDS, chemical pneumonitis, pulmonary oedema and haemorrhage. Pseudomembrane formation can cause laryngeal obstruction. Intubation may be required as an emergency intervention.
- Ocular symptoms including pain, lacrimation, and oedema require saline irrigation and petroleum jelly to limit closure.
- Skin becomes oedematous and painful. Fluid loss can be considerable from blisters and full thickness burns. Surgical debridement may be required.
- High-dose exposure can suppress the bone marrow and death can result from secondary infection.
    ☑ No specific antidotes exist to vesicant agents. Treatment is supportive and symptomatic with airway support, bronchodilators, mechanical ventilation as required, judicious analgesia, careful observation and serial laboratory investigation.

Cyanogens (e.g. hydrogen cyanide)
- Hydrogen cyanide is used in industrial manufacture of plastics and nitrites; other cyanide compounds used in printing, dyeing, photography, metal cleaning and manufacturing. They may also be present in smoke from domestic or industrial fires.
- Consider deliberate release if no history of accidental or industrial exposure and/or more than one casualty.
- Cyanogens are rapid metabolic poisons that inhibit mitochondrial cytochrome oxidases leading to inability to utilise oxygen for cellular respiration. They usually result in death within minutes due to

cardiorespiratory arrest. Onset of symptoms is slower following ingestion compared with inhalation or topical absorbtion through skin or eyes.
- Tachypnoea, confusion, dizziness are rapidly followed by convulsions, coma, and cardiac arrest.
- Arterial blood gas analysis shows a metabolic acidosis with a raised lactate level. Mixed venous oxygen saturations are raised due to decreased oxygen uptake.
  - ☑ Early rapid administration of specific antidotes in severe poisoning is essential.
  - ☑ In suspected severe poisoning, dicobalt edetate is the treatment of choice (300 mg followed immediately after with 50 mL glucose 50% infusion, may be repeated).
  - ☑ Hydroxycobalamin should be considered in smoke inhalation victims with signs of significant toxicity (70 mg/kg over 15 min). If contraindicated or not available, give both sodium nitrite (300 mg) which converts haemoglobin to methaemoglobin and binds cyanide, and sodium thiosulphate (12.5 g) which acts as a sulphur donor.

Riot control agents (e.g. CS gas, tear gas)
- Designed to have short acting irritant effects.
- Main effects are very rapid onset eye pain, lacrimation, cough, salivation and bronchospasm.
- High doses can occur if trapped in confined, gas filled space.
- Patients in high dose exposure can develop gradual onset non-cardiac pulmonary oedema with a clinical picture of ARDS results.
  - ☑ There is no specific antidote: treatment is supportive with oxygen, bronchodilators and skin, and ocular decontamination. Remove clothing carefully and double bag as residue can affect staff caring for these patients. In low dose exposure, most patients will recover in minutes to a few hours.

Biological injuries

Immediate management
- ☑ Biological agents could be disseminated via water, food sources or aerosolized/released into atmosphere.
- ☑ Exposure typically results in unusual or unexpected cases, usually with no trauma. Be alert to the case that 'just doesn't fit'. Examples may include abnormal illness severity, number of affected cases, atypical illness for time of year, age, demographic, geographical location, or rapid progression, e.g. young healthy adults presenting in summer with rapidly progressive 'flu', any haemorrhagic fever in the UK without travel history to exposed areas.
- ☑ Other indications of exposure to an infectious agent may include disease within family, friend or work groups and common associations, pets, or surrounding animal contacts.
- ☑ Immediate management should focus on supportive measures, identification of agent and risk management. Take detailed medical

history including: occupation, travel, contact history, hobbies, contact with animals, insect bites, food, what they think might have caused their illness.
☑ Have a low threshold for seeking advice from a senior clinician, consultant microbiologist or infectious disease physician.
☑ Non-infectious agents can be viewed as hazardous (chemical) materials to the extent that decontamination and medical treatment are the mainstay of treatment. However, it is important to note that biological agents may be extremely persistent depending on conditions and mechanism of dispersal. Bio-agents may be 1000 times more potent than chemical agents.

Subsequent management
☑ Supportive management. Treatment depends on causative agent. Follow ID/microbiological advice.
☑ The Health Protection Agency (for UK cases) is a valuable source of advice and support and should be contacted early in suspected biological agent injury.
☑ Consider chemoprophylaxis of contacts.
  • Significant illness and multiorgan failure can result from biological agents.
  • Investigations include FBC, U&Es, LFT, blood/sputum cultures, CXR.

Radiation injuries

Immediate management
☑ Cannot be detected without a radiological survey requiring specialist equipment.
☑ Exposure occurs when any body part is irradiated with any ionizing radiation. Factors to consider are: duration, distance & shielding. If time is halved, exposure is halved. The inverse square law applies to distance. Significant building structures (brick walls, cement, earth etc) will reduce exposure.
☑ Contamination occurs when radioactive material is deposited on a person's skin or clothing, inhaled, ingested or absorbed via a wound.
☑ It is highly unlikely that a contaminated patient would pose a risk to healthcare providers but masks should be worn, outer garments removed when leaving contaminated area, and regular body surveys undertaken. Safety precautions are not required for patients who have been exposed, but <u>not</u> contaminated.
☑ Remove contaminated clothing, double-bag, and store in secure space away from treatment area until specialist disposal can be arranged. Handle foreign objects found on patient with forceps and limit handling and contact time.
☑ Wash any wounds gently with water, followed by soap and water starting from edge and working inwards.

☑ Gastric lavage may be considered in early internal contamination by ingestion.
☑ Radiation experts may recommend administration of specific radionucleotide-specific decorporation agents such as Prussian blue, DTPA or bicarbonate depending on extent of internal contamination.

Subsequent management

☑ Good supportive critical care, with careful fluid and electrolyte balance is vital.
  • Symptoms may be immediate or delayed.
  • Vomiting—time after exposure can estimate radiation dose:
    • <10 min: possible lethal dose
    • 10–30 min: very severe
    • <1 h: severe
    • 1–2 h: moderate
    • >2 h: mild
• Higher radiation doses are associated with bone marrow suppression, gastrointestinal destruction, cutaneous and neurological effects requiring organ support. Those with neurological effects will almost certainly die.
• Cutaneous lesions can be immediate or delayed and can themselves be lethal. Wound healing is delayed.
• The rate of decline of the absolute lymphocyte count is a marker of severity of exposure.

Investigations

• Routine laboratory studies for all exposed patients in a chemical, biological, or radiological incident include FBC, glucose, U&Es, LFTs, ABG, ECG monitoring, CXR, and pulse oximetry.

Paediatric considerations

• Because of their larger surface area:body weight ratio, children are more vulnerable to toxicants absorbed through the skin.

Special considerations

• Explosions may result in blast injury; external injury may not be striking, however shock waves from explosions can lead to significant internal injury. Smaller devices may release shrapnel which cause multiple puncture sites, internal bleeding, and risk of infection from unusual causative organisms. Burns and amputations from explosive devices can be significant distraction from other traumatic injuries: stick to a standardised trauma response recognising that burns care is usually a secondary consideration once traumatic injuries are systematically managed.
• Patients may suffer multiple injuries and appear to require urgent life-saving intervention, but personal safety must be remembered if bioterrorism is suspected.

Further reading

Adalja, A.A. (2019). *Identifying and Managing Casualties of Biological Terrorism*. Available at: https://www.uptodate.com/contents/identifying-and-managing-casualties-of-biological-terrorism/print

Advanced Life Support Group (2005). *Major Incident Medical Management and Support: The Practical Approach in the Hospital*. Oxford, UK: Wiley Blackwell.

Dainiak, N. (2019). *Biology and Clinical Features of Radiation Injury in Adults*. https://www.uptodate.com

Madsen, J. (2019). *Chemical Terrorism: Rapid Recognition and Initial Medical Management*. Available at: https://www.uptodate.com/contents/chemical-terrorism-rapid-recognition-and-initial-medical-managemen

☼ Post-resuscitation care

Definition

Management of patients with return of spontaneous circulation (ROSC) following cardiac arrest.

Presentation

- Patients with ROSC.
- Patients may demonstrate post cardiac arrest syndrome.

This includes any of:
- ☑ myocardial dysfunction, or systemic ischaemia and reperfusion, resulting in shock, bradycardia, or tachydysrhythmias.
- ☑ confusion, agitation, or altered GCS indicating brain injury.
- ☑ persistence of the precipitating pathology, including trauma, sepsis, pulmonary or cardiac disease.

Immediate management

(➔ See also 'Post-resuscitation care', Figure 12.3, p. 391.)

Immediate treatment

- ☑ Give oxygen to achieve S_pO_2 94–98%. Hyperoxia should be avoided.
- ☑ Intubate if significant altered GCS or airway unprotected. Use capnography. Ventilate to low-normal $EtCO_2$ and normal $PaCO_2$ on arterial sample. Hypocarbia and hypercarbia can have adverse effects.
- ☑ Adequate sedation essential for neuroprotection of intubated patients.
- ☑ Obtain reliable IV access. Central venous access will usually be required. Insert arterial line for invasive BP monitoring and sequential arterial blood gas sampling.
- ☑ Aim for SBP >100 mmHg. Restore normovolaemia with boluses of 250–500 mL IV crystalloid (guided by basic monitoring, echo, cardiac output monitoring, lactates).
- ☑ Obtain early echocardiography in the ED if possible. Consider vasopressors/inotropes. Use dobutamine if the ejection fraction is low, and noradrenaline if the ejection fraction is normal.
- ☑ Discuss with cardiology and consider an intra-aortic balloon pump if hypotension persists.
- ☑ Acute Coronary Syndrome (ACS) is the major cause of Out of Hospital Cardiac Arrest (OOHCA). Early angiography and percutaneous coronary intervention (PCI) is beneficial if ST elevation or new LBBB. Discuss with cardiologist also if likelihood of ACS despite normal ECG.
- ☑ Consider GTN and/or furosemide if evidence of pulmonary oedema and MAP >80 mmHg.
- ☑ Once target BP has been achieved the venous saturation should be measured (S_cvO_2). A value of <70% suggests shock. Transfuse packed cells if Hb <100 g/L, consider continuous cardiac output monitoring.

Serial transthoracic echocardiography may be a useful adjunct to assess LV function.

☑ Consider β-blockade (e.g. esmolol) if persistent tachycardia or ACS with normal ejection fraction and central venous saturation ($S_{cv}O_2$) >70%.

☑ Targeted temperature management to maintain a constant core temperature of around 36°C for at least 24 hours; avoid fever at all times.

☑ Diagnose and treat seizures - EEG maybe required. Seizure prophylaxis not usually required.

☑ Maintain normoglycaemia – Keep blood glucose <10 mmol/L: hyperglycaemia is strongly associated with worse outcomes.

Diagnosis

☑ Serial 12-lead ECGs.

☑ Discuss coronary angiography and PCI early with cardiologist: 60% of all cardiac arrests have treatable lesions on angiography irrespective of cause. You may need to transfer while still unstable.

☑ For non-cardiac causes, or when unclear, consider CT brain and/or CTPA. Treat the cause when known.

Subsequent management

Optimizing recovery

☑ Admit to ICU.

☑ Avoid pyrexia for at least 72 h.

☑ Maintain normoxia and normocapnia, and use lung protective ventilation.

☑ Optimize haemodynamics.

☑ Echocardiography and cardiology review.

☑ Maintain normoglycaemia.

☑ Delay prognostication for at least 72 h. No tests, biochemical markers, neurophysiology or imaging can predict neurological outcomes before this point.

☑ Consider organ donation early when withdrawing life-sustaining support.

☑ Consider ICD insertion.

☑ Consider screening for inherited disorders.

☑ Manage risk factors.

☑ Arrange follow-up and rehabilitation.

Investigations

- FBC, clotting, U&Es, LFTs, TFTs, G&S, troponin, lactate
- CXR, serial ECG, echo, coronary angiography
- CTPA, CT head, EEG, core temperature

Risk factors

- Ischaemic heart disease
- Recent myocardial infarction
- Electrolyte disturbance

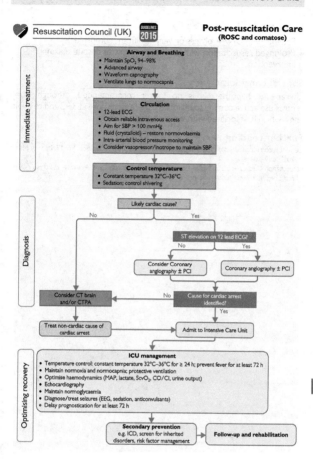

Figure 12.3 Post-resuscitation care.

Reproduced with the kind permission of the Resuscitation Council (UK).

- Hypoxia
- Thromboembolic disease
- Cardiac tamponade
- Hypothermia
- Hypovolaemia
- Tension pneumothorax

Exclusions
- Patients with DNAR orders or very significant comorbidities.
- Prolonged resuscitation with very poor response despite maximal intervention.

Special considerations
Therapeutic hypothermia is no longer recommended, athough many centres use active cooling to maintain core temperature at 36C and to avoid fever which is associated with worse outcomes.

Further reading
Current recommendations on adult resuscitation. Williams S. BJA Education. Vol 17. Issue 3; March 2017, p99–104

Resuscitation Guidelines 2015. Nolan J, Soar J. Post Resuscitation Care: Available at: https://www.resus.org.uk/resuscitation-guidelines/post-resuscitation-care/

⚙ Decreased level of consciousness—requiring anaesthetic input

Definition
Altered mental state, combative, confused, not protecting own airway, reduced Glasgow coma score.

Presentation
- One of the most common referrals for the on-call anaesthetist is to intubate patients for transfer to the CT scanner.

Immediate management
- ☑ History is paramount: search for the cause.
- ☑ Common causes of decreased GCS and request for CT scan include: cerebrovascular event (ischaemia, intracerebral bleed, subarachnoid/extradural bleed); metabolic disorders; post-ictal state (new onset seizures); systemic infections; meningitis; brain tumours; encephalopathy; trauma; following cardiac arrest; poisoning.
- ☑ ABC—100% O_2, obtain 2 points of IV access, send biochemistry blood samples.
- ☑ A definitive airway may be required—RSI.
- ☑ Consider A-a gradient and neuroprotection: ventilate to normal/low normal P_aCO_2.
- ☑ If trauma suspected, minimal handling, protect cervical spine with blocks & tape +/- loosely applied collar according to local protocols.
- ☑ Circulation—hypotension should be corrected and a cardiac cause excluded. Maintain adequate cerebral perfusion pressure (60-90 mmHg), vasopressor infusions are commonly required to achieve this. Consider invasive arterial blood pressure measurement prior to transport.
- ☑ Neurological assessment is vital. Evaluate GCS (with particular attention to motor score as a prognostic factor). Pupil responses should be noted and any focal signs.
- ☑ Serum electrolytes and glucose should be corrected.
- ☑ If the patient is to be intubated and ventilated, initiate contact with the ward/unit where they are to be managed following the CT scan.
- ☑ Intrahospital transfer to CT scanner. Take additional infusions and emergency drugs with you.

Subsequent management
- ☑ If there is evidence of intracerebral or extradural bleed/SAH/tumour, the patient needs urgent referral to neurosurgery and may require further intrahospital or interhospital transfer.
- ☑ 80% of strokes are ischaemic, currently approximately 10% are thrombolysed. New interventions including stroke thombectomy and increased time window for thrombolysis means early referral and

action is vital. Patients requiring anaesthesia for thrombectomy should be managed according to neuroprotective principles and with regard to delivery of anaesthesia outside the operating suite.

☑ HDU/ITU for other appropriate medical causes.

☑ Most ventilated patients should be admitted to ICU for prognostication, family support and consideration of organ donation.

☑ CT normal and/or postictal, consider meningoencephalitis. Give cefotaxime or ceftriaxone 2g IV and load with aciclovir. Consider lumbar punctures (LP) if no evidence of raised intracranial pressure.

Investigations

- FBC/U&Es/LFTs/clotting/glucose, paracetamol/salicylate levels, ABGs, LP, CXR, CT scan.

Risk factors

- Hypertension, ischaemic heart disease, and peripheral vascular disease are risk factors for stroke.
- Decreased conscious level following thrombolysis or antiplatelet treatment may signify the onset of an haemorrhagic conversion or intracranial bleed.
- In general, sedation for CT without intubation should be avoided; general anaesthesia with intubation is often faster, safer and less complicated. Access to patient's airway is much more difficult in transit or in the CT.
- Normal CT head does not exclude raised intracranial pressure—important when considering LP.

Paediatric considerations

- Children with decreased level of consciousness without a history of trauma can pose a diagnostic challenge given the wide variety of causes and the frequent lack of clues as to diagnosis.
- Children can make significant demands on intensive and high dependency resources.

Special considerations

- Malignant cerebral oedema following major cerebral infarcts (particularly middle cerebral artery) may now be considered for decompression by hemicraniectomy, particularly if the patient is <65 years of age.
- These patients may have a reduced GCS 48 h post-event and need urgent referral to neurosurgery.
- If patient has been given muscle relaxants, ongoing seizures may be masked; EEG monitoring may be useful.

⚙ Sepsis

Definition

- Sepsis is characterised by life-threatening organ dysfunction due to a dysregulated host response to infection. It carries a 28.9% mortality.
- Septic shock is a subset of sepsis with increased mortality. Despite adequate fluid resuscitation, there is both persistent hypotension requiring vasopressors to maintain a MAP≥65 mmHg, and a lactate of ≥2.

Presentation

Think of sepsis if there are one or more risk factors (see Table 12.2), a NEWS (National Early Warning Score) of ≥5, and if the patient looks unwell. A robust diagnosis of sepsis can use the SOFA score (Table 12.3). An increase in score of 2 from baseline (or a score of 2 if no previous score known) defines sepsis. SOFA is more complex and Red Flags can be used as a surrogate.

One or more of the following parameters should prompt diagnosis and treatment:

- AVPU (P or U) if changed from normal
- RR ≥25 /min
- Oxygen needed to keep S_pO_2 ≥92% (88% if COPD)
- HR >130 bpm
- Systolic BP ≤90 mmHg (or >40 mmHg drop from normal)
- Not passed urine in last 18hrs (or UO <0.5 mls/kg/hr)
- Non blanching rash (mottled/ashen/cyanotic)
- Recent chemotherapy in last 6 months

Table 12.2 Risk factors for sepsis in table (adapted from NICE guideline NG51)

Risk factors for sepsis

- age <1yr or >75yrs, or very frail patient
- recent trauma or surgery or invasive procedure (within the last 6 weeks)
- impaired immunity due to illness/drugs (long-term steroids, chemotherapy, immunosuppressants)
- indwelling lines, catheters, intravenous drug misusers, any breach of skin integrity

Additional risk factors for women who are/have been pregnant within the past 6 weeks:

- gestational diabetes, diabetes or other comorbidities
- invasive procedure: Caesarean section, forceps delivery, ERPC
- prolonged rupture of membranes
- close contact with someone with group A streptococcal infection
- continued vaginal bleeding or an offensive vaginal discharge

---

Table 12.3 SOFA score (sequential (sepsis-related) organ failure assessment score)

System	Score				
	0	1	2	3	4
Respiration					
P$_a$O$_2$/F$_i$O$_2$ mmHg (kPa)	≥400 (53.3)	<400 (53.3)	<300 (40)	<200 (26.7) with respirator support	<100 (13.3) with respirator support
Coagulation					
Platelets, × 10^3/μL	≥150	<150	<100	<50	<20
Liver					
Bilirubin, mg/dL (μmol/L)	<1.2 (20)	1.2–1.9 (20–32)	2.0–5.9 (33–101)	6.0–11.9 (102–204)	>12.0 (204)
Cardiovascular*	MAP ≥70 mmHg	MAP <70 mmHg	Dopamine <5 or dobutamine (any dose)	Dopamine 5.1–15 or epinephrine ≤0.1 or norepinephrine ≤0.1	Dopamine >15 or epinephrine >0.1 or norepinephrine >0.1

System	Score			
	0	1	2	3	4
Central nervous system					
Glasgow Coma Score	15	13–14	10–12	6–9	<6
Renal					
Creatinine, mg/dL (μmol/L)	<1.2 (110)	1.2–1.9 (110–170)	2.0–3.4 (171–299)	3.5–4.9 (300–440)	>5.0 (440)
Urine output, ml/day				<500	<200

* Catecholamine doses are given as μg/kg/min for at least an hour.

Adapted with permission from Vincent, J. L. et al. (1996). The SOFA (Sepsis-related Organ Failure Assessment) score to describe organ dysfunction/failure. *Intensive Care Medicine*, 22(7):707–10. Copyright © 1996, Springer-Verlag. doi: https://doi.org/10.1007/BF01709751. Updated by Singer JAMA, 2016;315(8):801–10. doi:10.1001/jama.2016.0287.

Immediate management

SEPSIS 6 within 1 h of recognition (as well as ABC) is one of the most effective lifesaving bundles in medicine.

☑ **1.** Administer oxygen. Aim to keep saturations >94% (88–92% if at risk of CO2 retention)

☑ **2.** Take blood culture specimens prior to antibiotics, but do not delay >45 min—at least one peripheral set, plus any other via any vascular device that has been in place for >48 h. Consider urine, CSF, sputum, and pus, cultures.

☑ **3.** Commence antibiotics within 1 h of diagnosis of sepsis or septic shock, empirically as per local guidelines. Each hour delay is associated with significant increase in mortality. Review with results of any positive cultures. Consider antifungal and antiviral agents. Consider allergies prior to administration.

☑ **4.** Resuscitate with IV fluid, up to 30 mL/kg crystalloid bolus if hypotensive or lactate >2 mmol/L.

☑ **5.** Check serial lactates. If lactate >4 mmol/L, recheck after each 10ml/kg challenge and call Critical Care.

☑ **6.** Measure urine output. May require urinary catheter. Commence fluid balance chart and complete hourly. Aim for UO ≥0.5 mls/kg/hr. ARF with sepsis has high mortality.

If poor response (continuing hypotension, high lactate, low urine output):

☑ Correct BP. Start vasopressors if hypotension resistant to initial fluid resuscitation—aim for MAP >65 mmHg (or higher if normally hypertensive). Noradrenaline is normally first line, which will require insertion of a central venous catheter. Metaraminol can be administered peripherally while preparing to obtain central venous access.

☑ Insert an arterial line at the earliest opportunity.

☑ Re-assess volume status and treat accordingly making sure patient is well filled. Assess status and tissue perfusion clinically, by using bedside echo, or assessment of haemodynamic status and cardiac output using equipment such as PiCCO or LiDCO®.

Subsequent management

☑ Transfer to ITU should be arranged for patients who require this level of support. Further management and delivery of care bundles should be carried out in an ITU setting, but aspects can be started in the emergency department.

☑ Consider steroids when hypotension resistant to fluid therapy and noradrenaline.

☑ Blood product administration:

- Give packed RBCs to ensure Hb >70 g/L (>90 g/L if there is concurrent MI, significant IHD, severe hypoxaemia, worsening lactic acidosis or cyanotic heart disease).
- FFP should only be used to correct laboratory clotting abnormalities if there is bleeding or a planned invasive procedure with a risk of bleeding.
- Platelets should be transfused prophylactically if the count is <10 ×10⁹/L, and <20 ×10⁹/L if high risk of bleeding. Higher counts of ≥50 ×10⁹/L should be maintained in active bleeding or if an invasive procedure is planned.

☑ Ventilatory strategies for sepsis-induced ARDS—aim for a plateau airway pressure of ≤30 cmH₂O, use of PEEP, with a target tidal volume of 6 mL/kg. Permissive hypercapnia can be tolerated to facilitate lower tidal volumes, and peak pressures. Manage patient in a semi-recumbent position, and use conservative fluid strategy where hypoperfusion not evident.

☑ Monitor blood glucose, aiming for <8.3 mmol/L. (Avoid hypoglycaemia as this is associated with increased mortality.)

☑ Deep vein thrombosis prophylaxis—use either low-dose unfractionated heparin or low molecular weight heparin unless contraindicated (the latter in high-risk patients). A compression device should be used if heparin is contraindicated, and a combination of both compression device and heparin in high-risk patients.

☑ Stress ulcer prophylaxis depending on local guidelines, but definitely if there are risk factors for bleeding.

Investigations

- FBC, U&Es, CRP, LFTs, clotting, ECG, CXR
- Blood cultures, MSU, LP
- Serial blood gases for lactates, and glucose
- Urine output

Paediatric considerations

➔ See also p. 148

- If decompensated despite 20 mL/kg fluid bolus, involve Critical Care early. Additional boluses to total 60 mL/kg titrating to therapeutic endpoints. Respiratory failure is common after 60 mL/kg resuscitation—consider intubation if not already performed.
- Use dopamine if fluid resuscitation not effective. Noradrenaline and adrenaline should be used for shock refractory to dopamine.
- Consider ECMO if refractory septic shock or sepsis associated respiratory failure.
- Therapeutic endpoints:
  - CRT<2 s
  - normal blood pressure, normal pulses
  - warm peripheries
  - urine output >1 mL/kg/h
  - normal mental status
  - cardiac index 3.3–6 L/min/m²

Further reading

NICE guideline [NG51] Sepsis: recognition, diagnosis and early management.

Daniels R, Nutbeam T. The Sepsis Manual 4th Ed. 2017-18. UK Sepsis Trust.

Singer, M. (2016). The third international consensus definitions for sepsis and septic shock (Sepsis-3). *Journal of the American Medical Association*, **315**(8), 801–10.

Surviving Sepsis Campaign (2015). *Surviving Sepsis Guidelines 2012 and Surviving Sepsis Campaign Revised Bundles* [Revised April 2015]. Available at: https://www.survivingsepsis.org

Equipment problems

Kim J. Gupta

☢ **Leak in anaesthetic breathing circuit**

Definition

Failure of gas delivery from the anaesthetic machine to the patient due to an unintentional leak in the breathing system.

Presentation

- **If the patient is breathing spontaneously**:
  - Reservoir bag empties
  - CO_2 waveform changes
  - F_IO_2 falls, which may cause a fall in S_pO_2
  - Concentration of volatile anaesthetic agent falls, which may cause the patient to wake up.
- **If the patient is on IPPV**:
  - Ventilator bellows empty
  - Reduced or absent chest movements or breath sounds
  - Alarm sounds for low airway pressure, low expired tidal volume/ minute volume, and $ETCO_2$
  - Change in ventilator sounds may be heard
  - Smell of volatile anaesthetic agent may be detectable
  - Audible gas leak may be heard.

Investigations

- Examination of entire breathing circuit and connections, including patient airway device and anaesthetic machine.
- Do not delay immediate management while searching for the leak.

Risk factors

- Inadequate check of breathing system prior to use.
- Moving the patient or the anaesthetic machine.
- Sharing the airway with a surgeon/endoscopist.
- Changing components of the breathing system (e.g. CO_2 absorbers, sampling lines).
- Refilling vaporizers.
- Previously using the fresh gas outlet as an oxygen source without reconnecting the breathing system.
- A machine/workstation returning from a service/repair.

Exclusions

- Fresh gas flow too low, not switched on, or supply failure.
- Endotracheal tube/supraglottic airway misplacement or cuff leak.
- Breathing circuit disconnected from anaesthetic machine.
- Capnograph, oxygen sensor, or other circuit monitoring, disconnected from circuit.
- Split in breathing circuit or reservoir bag (e.g. from tube holder or wheel of anaesthetic machine).
- Leaking or incorrectly seated CO_2 absorber canister, ventilator bellows, or vaporizer (e.g. absent 'O' ring).
- Ventilator/breathing system pressure relief valve set too low or stuck open.

- Ventilator failure or not switched on.
- Placement of nasogastric tube in trachea.
- Tracheobronchial leak.
- Active gas scavenging system ports occluded, causing negative pressure in breathing system.
- APL valve unintentionally open when ventilating with a Bain system.

Immediate management

☑ Scan the breathing circuit for an obvious disconnection.

If a disconnection is not found immediately:
☑ Switch to manual ventilation with 100% oxygen at high flow rates (>10 L/min).
☑ Close APL valve.
☑ Depress oxygen flush (it may then be possible to hear and identify a leak at the point of disconnection).

If reservoir bag fills:
☑ Squeeze bag and check chest expansion and capnograph.
☑ Check that arterial oxygen saturation improves.

If ventilation adequate:
☑ Check for leaks in the breathing system and airway device/ETT seal.

If ventilation unsuccessful:
☑ Abandon breathing system and ventilate with a self-inflating reservoir bag (attached to cylinder oxygen when able).

If ventilation still unsuccessful:
☑ Check the airway device/endotracheal tube for displacement.

If necessary:
☑ Remove the airway device/endotracheal tube and ventilate with a face mask and self-inflating bag.
☑ Maintain anaesthesia intravenously until problem resolved.

Subsequent management

☑ Methodically check entire circuit as detailed.
☑ Once cause of circuit leak is identified and remedied, identify precipitating and background factors to prevent future recurrence.

Paediatric implications

Uncuffed endotracheal tube diameter may be too small.

Special considerations

- In an analysis of 1029 nationally reported incidents of anaesthetic equipment failure in the United Kingdom, 99 (9.6%) were due to a leak in the circuit.
- **If the patient is breathing spontaneously**:
  - the alteration in capnograph trace depends on the site of disconnection. If the sampling port is in a section of circuit

disconnected from exhaled gas, there will be complete loss of the waveform. Otherwise, it will detect a variable amount of rebreathing of carbon dioxide.
- if air is entrained, there may be a fall in inspired/expired oxygen, inhalational agent, or a rise in inspired/expired nitrogen.
- **If patient is positive-pressure ventilated**:
  - bag-in-bottle ventilators—ascending bellows collapse (bag generates 2–4 cmH$_2$O PEEP); descending bellows fall to a fully expanded position and may not reveal disconnection.
  - minute volume dividers—continue to function if disconnection is distal.
  - many ventilators do not have a visible reservoir (e.g. Penlon Nuffield 200).
- **Low-pressure/volume alarms**:
  - breathing system low-pressure alarms are mandatory during IPPV. The alarm trigger limit should be set just below the maximum inspiratory pressure. This alarm is not infallible since resistance distal to the sensor (e.g. partial obstruction at the point of disconnection) may mean that the alarm limit is not reached. Therefore, the optimum location of the alarm sensor is the Y-piece.
  - volumetric devices should usually be located in the expiratory limb.

Further reading

Cassidy, C.J., Smith, A., Arnot-Smith, J. (2011). Critical incident reports concerning anaesthetic equipment: analysis of the UK National Reporting and Learning System (NRLS) data from 2006–2008. *Anaesthesia*, **66**(10), 879–88.

Raphael, D.T., Weller, R.S., Doran, D.J. (1988). A response algorithm for the low-pressure alarm condition. *Anesthesia and Analgesia*, **67**(9), 876–83.

① Ventilator failure

Definition

Unplanned cessation of automatic positive-pressure ventilation.

Presentation

- Bellows stop moving (but may not empty); ventilator cycling stops (may be audible); chest movements stop; absent breath sounds on auscultation.
- Loss of normal breathing system pressure trace; loss of normal capnograph waveform; apnoea, low tidal volume/minute volume alarms sound.
- Switching to manual ventilation restores patient ventilation.

Investigations

- Examination of ventilator hardware, settings, and power supply, as well as breathing circuit, and attached monitoring.
- Do not delay immediate management while searching for the fault.

Risk factors

- Unfamiliarity with ventilator.
- Inadequate machine check.
- Interruption of power supply.
- Power surge and disruption of ventilator programming.
- Recent anaesthetic machine service.
- Brand new equipment.

Exclusions

- Ventilator not switched on.
- Manual/ventilator switch incorrectly set or faulty.
- Improper assembly or failure of ventilator, breathing system, pressure sensors, or pressure relief valves.
- APL valve not closed with Penlon ventilator.
- Ventilator, anaesthetic workstation, or general power failure.
- Ventilator performance or settings insufficient for patient characteristics.
- Inappropriate ventilator settings causing pressure relief valve to open:
  - excessive tidal volume for inspiratory time.
  - excessive inspiratory flow.
  - pressure relief threshold too low.
- Bellows or ventilator mechanism stuck.
- Failure of secondary driving gas to some anaesthetic workstation ventilators.
- Breathing circuit occluded or other cause of high airway pressure (➔ see 'High airway pressure', p. 413).
- Large leaks or inadequate fresh gas flow (➔ see 'Leak in anaesthetic breathing circuit', p. 402).

Immediate management

☑ Check ventilator is switched on.
☑ Check manual/ventilator selector switch is set correctly.
☑ Switch to manual ventilation with a simple breathing system.
☑ Maintain manual minute ventilation and anaesthesia until another suitable checked ventilator is available. Consider allowing return of spontaneous ventilation if appropriate, or call for another ventilator.

If the reservoir bag will not fill or empties quickly:
☑ Check adequacy of fresh gas flow settings.
☑ Check for oxygen pipeline failure (and thus ventilator driving gas failure).
☑ Look for disconnection or large leak in breathing system (➲ see 'Leak in anaesthetic breathing circuit', p. 402).
☑ Look for unintentional extubation, displacement of airway device, and endotracheal tube cuff leak.

If the reservoir bag fills, but there is resistance on squeezing:
☑ Consider the causes and management of high airway pressure (➲ see 'High airway pressure', p. 413).

Subsequent management

☑ Clearly label and remove a faulty ventilator from use until inspected and repaired.
☑ If the ventilator is an integral component of an anaesthetic workstation, take the workstation out of service.
☑ Inform the anaesthetist/manager with responsibility for equipment.
☑ Log the incident with the local incident reporting system.
☑ A qualified/certified person should examine the equipment with the authority of the manufacturer.
☑ Events related to design faults, system faults, and persistently recurring problems should be reported to manufacturers, the National Reporting and Learning System (NRLS), and the Medical and Healthcare Products Regulatory Agency (MHRA).

Special considerations

• In an analysis of 1029 nationally reported incidents of anaesthetic equipment failure in the United Kingdom, sudden failure of the ventilator was the most common (142 reported cases, 13.8%).
• Malfunction of airway pressure or spirometry monitoring alarms may be misinterpreted as ventilator failure.
• Large anaesthetic breathing circuit leaks or breathing circuit obstruction may be misinterpreted as ventilator failure.
• Oxygen pipeline supply-driven ventilators may stop if the supply pressure falls. Some will automatically switch to other piped gases, remaining at sufficient pressure.
• Low-pressure, apnoea, low tidal/minute volume alarms may sound if the ventilator stops at end expiration.

- Continuous positive airway pressure alarm may sound if it fails in inspiration.
- Even though ventilator failure might seem a problem intrinsic to a complex piece of equipment, focusing on fixing a problem with a ventilator can detract from the simple necessity of providing adequate ventilation by hand.

Further reading

Cassidy, C.J., Smith, A., Arnot-Smith, J. (2011). Critical incident reports concerning anaesthetic equipment: analysis of the UK National Reporting and Learning System (NRLS) data from 2006–2008. *Anaesthesia*, **66**(10), 879–88.

! Pipeline oxygen supply failure

Definition
Insufficient pipeline oxygen delivery to the anaesthetic machine.

Presentation
- Oxygen failure alarm sounds and pressure gauge falls.
- Oxygen and linked flowmeters fall, emergency oxygen flush fails, pipeline oxygen-driven ventilators stop.
- Audible escape of gas if pipeline connection leaking.

Investigations
- Examination of main oxygen pipeline supply hose and connections, anaesthetic machine integrity, and power supply.
- Do not delay immediate management while investigating the cause of the oxygen failure.

Risk factors
- Inadequate machine check performed.
- Failure to reconnect pipeline after machine check.
- Unfamiliar pipeline connections.
- Loss of power to an anaesthetic workstation.
- Recent machine or pipeline maintenance, repair, or replacement.
- Exhausted hospital central oxygen source.
- Fault during refilling of central oxygen source.
- Construction work in hospital.

Exclusions
- Obstruction or large gas leak within the anaesthetic machine, e.g. around vaporizers or within the ventilator (◑ see 'Leak in anaesthetic breathing circuit', p. 405).
- Kink or obstruction in supply hose.
- Anaesthetic workstation power failure.
- Oxygen has been shut off at fire safety isolation point.

Paediatric implications
IPPV cannot be delivered via an Ayre's T-piece in the event of a gas failure.

Immediate management
- ☑ Verify pressure failure on the main pipeline pressure gauge.
- ☑ Check for disconnection between the pipeline and wall and reattach it if possible.
- ☑ Turn on the reserve oxygen cylinder **fully**, since the flow from partially opened valves may decrease with cooling as oxygen flows out.
- ☑ Check oxygen analyser confirms return of oxygen flow.
- ☑ Check that the pressure gauge indicates a full or adequately filled cylinder.
- ☑ Use low oxygen flows to preserve available oxygen. If using a circle system, close the APL valve to preserve potentially useful oxygen reserves.
- ☑ Switch to manual ventilation to preserve cylinder oxygen, if ventilator uses oxygen as a driving gas.

Subsequent management

☑ Disconnect the pipeline supply. If the pipeline supply has failed, re-establishment may result in a temporary flow of gas that is contaminated, or the wrong gas may be reconnected at source. As the regulated pipeline pressure is greater than the regulated cylinder pressure, the restored flow will take priority.

☑ Inform the surgeon of the problem and plan to expedite surgery.

☑ Inform other hospital areas where pipeline oxygen is used and the department responsible for the central oxygen supply.

☑ Arrange for an appropriate number of oxygen cylinders to allow completion of surgery.

☑ Find out when the oxygen supply is likely to be reliably restored.

☑ If the cylinder oxygen supply runs out, allow the patient to breathe room air or ventilate using a self-inflating reservoir bag—administer intravenous anaesthesia. Using air alone may render the patient hypoxaemic and should not be used until necessary.

Special considerations

- In an analysis of 1029 nationally reported incidents of anaesthetic equipment failure, 20 (1.9%) were due to a failure of gas supply to the anaesthetic machine.
- If the fresh gas flow to a Mapleson breathing system is interrupted, rebreathing occurs quickly. By contrast, a closed circle system acts as a temporary oxygen reservoir and the absorber prevents CO_2 accumulation. However, be aware that a continuing fresh gas flow containing air from some anaesthetic workstations will pressurize the system and wash out oxygen already present.
- Oxygen supply failure in older anaesthetic machines is heralded by a 'Bosun's' or 'Ritchie' whistle-type alarm. These activate if the supply pressure falls by 50%, sound for at least 7 s, and are silenced by restoring the oxygen supply. Additional fail-safe mechanisms simultaneously stop or adjust the flow of nitrous oxide, preventing the delivery of hypoxic mixtures.
- Modern anaesthetic workstations employ electronic oxygen supply pressure alarms and complex carrier gas management systems in the event of oxygen failure. Some continue to deliver pipeline air even after oxygen pipeline failure.
- Some ventilators are driven by oxygen pipeline supply and stop if it fails. However, some anaesthetic workstations will reroute other available pipeline gases at sufficient pressure to continue driving the mechanical ventilator in this event.

Further reading

Anderson, W.R., Brock-Utne, J.G. (1991). Oxygen pipeline supply failure. A coping strategy. *Journal of Clinical Monitoring*, **7**(1), 39–41.

ⓘ Theatre power failure

Definition
Loss of electrical supply to the operating theatre.

Presentation
- AC power failure alarms sound on devices with charged back-up batteries.
- Devices without charged back-up batteries stop working:
  - anaesthetic workstations (potentially stopping fresh gas flow).
  - monitors.
  - electronically managed ventilators.
  - infusion devices and warming devices.
  - essential surgical instruments (e.g. diathermy), cardiopulmonary bypass machines (may need to be hand-cranked), electrically powered operating tables and beds.
- Lights may go out (in theatres without windows, or at night, darkness may be absolute).
- Theatre air conditioning, heating, laminar flow systems fail.

Investigations
- Investigation of the power failure must not delay immediate management of the problem.

Risk factors
- Lack of back-up batteries or inadequate battery maintenance.
- Injudicious unplugging of theatre equipment—lack of charge.
- Emergency generator tests.
- Hospital construction work.
- Natural disaster.

Exclusions
- Anaesthetic workstation unintentionally unplugged or switched off.
- Workstation electronic failure; failure of electrical leads and fuses.
- Isolated socket power failure.
- Isolated theatre power failure (get help from other theatres).
- Circuit breaker (if fitted) has opened (consider why it has tripped—there may be a potentially dangerous electrical problem).

Immediate management
- ☑ Call for help and light source if necessary (daylight, torches, pen-torches, laryngoscopes, mobile phones). Do not use naked flames.
- ☑ Check mechanical flowmeters or electronic flowmeters (if display remains) and listen and feel for fresh gas flow at the common gas outlet.

If fresh gas flow has stopped:
- ☑ Temporarily continue 'low-flow' spontaneously breathing anaesthesia with a closed circle system if equilibrated.

☑ Switch to a self-inflating reservoir bag with cylinder O_2 and maintain anaesthesia intravenously.

If fresh gas flow is maintained:
☑ Check ventilator is still functioning (if in use).
☑ Begin manual ventilation if necessary.
☑ Maintain clinical monitoring as far as possible:
  • visual—chest rise/fall, cyanosis, pupil size, movement, sweating.
  • tactile—pulses (peripheral or at surgical site), capillary refill time.
  • auditory—stethoscope, sphygmomanometer.
☑ Request easily available battery-powered monitors including:
  • pulse oximeter.
  • defibrillator ECG.
  • transport monitors (for NIBP and CO_2 analyser).

Subsequent management
☑ Obtain information about duration of theatre power failure.
☑ If a hospital-wide power failure, consider nominating a designated crisis manager to disseminate information rather than bombarding a busy engineering department with calls.
☑ If necessary, continue with a pneumatic anaesthetic machine and ventilator if pipeline gas supplies or cylinders allow.
☑ Alternatively, consider establishing spontaneous ventilation if safer.
☑ Be aware of battery life—especially infusion pumps. Make preparations for failure of these. Obtain and prepare volumetric burettes.
☑ Ask surgical team to finish as quickly as possible or abandon operation.
☑ Reallocate personnel and resources to areas where they are needed.
☑ Cancel elective work until a reliable power supply has been restored.
☑ A hospital disaster plan may have to be initiated.

Special considerations
• Power failure ranges from a problem with the anaesthetic workstation to hospital-wide, including back-up generators. Modern machines have integrated battery back-up, but the specific effects of mains power failure depend on the type. Fresh gas flow and volatile delivery may continue but other functions (e.g. monitoring) may cease immediately. Emergency oxygen flush should still work.
• Power fluctuations (lights may flicker) are also capable of causing electronic equipment to switch off or 'hang' in an inoperable state.
• When power is restored, many anaesthetic workstations will be inoperable until an auto-testing process is complete. The start-up process may include leak and compliance tests of the breathing system. These tests should be cancelled if possible. They are time-consuming and require the breathing system to be disconnected from the patient and occluded. If the circuit remains connected to a patient during these tests, there is a risk of barotrauma.
• Pneumatically driven anaesthetic machines and ventilators may continue to function if pipeline supplies are intact or on cylinder oxygen (➲ see 'Pipeline oxygen supply failure', p. 408).

- Operating lights (some have back-up batteries), diathermy, laparoscopic camera and gas delivery equipment, microscopes, lasers, and some drills may stop, as well as theatre air conditioning and heating. Only some hospital areas and power sockets may be supplied with power from an emergency generator.

Further reading

Mitchell, J. (2001). Complete power failure 1. *Anaesthesia*, **56**(3), 274.

Tye, J.C., Chamley, D. (2000). Complete power failure. *Anaesthesia*, **55**, 1133–4.

Welch, R.H., Feldman, J.M. (1989). Anesthesia during total electrical failure, or what would you do if the lights went out? *Journal of Clinical Anesthesia*, **1**(5), 358–62.

☼ High airway pressure

➔ See also 'Difficult controlled ventilation', p. 75 and 'Sudden high airway pressure under one lung ventilation', p. 230.

Definition

An abnormally high positive pressure in the breathing system. A peak inspiratory pressure of more than 30 cmH$_2$O may be considered high.

Presentation

- High measured airway pressure, high airway pressure alarm.
- Audible leaks, abnormal cycling sounds from ventilator, sound of ventilator pressure relief valve.
- Low tidal volume and minute volume alarm, poor chest expansion.
- Diminished cardiac output secondary to raised intrathoracic pressure.

Investigations

- Do not allow investigations to delay immediate management.
- Examination of airway device, breathing circuit, and anaesthetic machine. Examination of patient for signs of light anaesthesia or bronchospasm.
- CXR, ABGs, fibreoptic bronchoscopy.

Risk factors

- Cleaning or re-assembly of the circle system.
- Contamination of breathing system (particularly filter/HME) with condensate, secretions, blood.
- Inadequate breathing system check.
- Re-use of single-use equipment.
- Loose debris on anaesthetic workstation (e.g. cannula caps, needle covers).
- Airway pressure may be appropriate for clinical situation:
  - obesity, severe restrictive lung, or chest wall disease.
  - patient position (e.g. steep Trendelenburg—beware endobronchial migration of endotracheal tube).
  - endotracheal tube resistance (e.g. microlaryngoscopy tube).
  - raised intra-abdominal pressure (e.g. pneumoperitoneum, ileus).

Exclusions

- Surgical team applying retractors or leaning on the patient.
- Airway pressure alarm malfunction or inappropriate setting.
- Ventilator settings inappropriate (excessive tidal volume or inspiratory flow, excessively short I:E ratio or long I:E ratio with gas trapping).
- Mechanical ventilator/manual ventilation selector in the wrong position.
- Ventilator malfunction—expiratory/PEEP valve, pressure-limiting valve.
- Clogged filter/HME—condensate, blood, gastric contents, pulmonary oedema.
- Occult circuit obstruction—kink, foreign body, sputum, clot, secretions, compression (e.g. anaesthetic machine wheel).

- APL valve stuck or unintentionally closed (especially after switching from mechanical ventilation).
- Circle expiratory/inspiratory valve stuck closed.
- Malfunction of scavenging system.
- Oxygen flush depressed inadvertently or stuck open.
- Failure of flow restrictors or machine regulators allowing gas under high pressure to enter breathing system.

Immediate management
☑ Remember: This may be a **clinical** problem, not an equipment fault (➲ see 'Subsequent management', p. 414).
☑ Switch to manual ventilation with 100% oxygen.
☑ Squeeze the reservoir bag and verify difficult ventilation.
☑ Scan the breathing system and the airway device/endotracheal tube for obvious obstructions (e.g. Boyle–Davis gag or foreign body).
☑ Check the filter/HME (heat-moisture exchanger) for any soiling/obstruction—if in doubt remove/replace.
☑ Check for signs of light anaesthesia (laryngospasm/coughing/straining/biting with obstruction of the airway), deepen anaesthesia intravenously.
☑ If ventilation is inadequate, exclude breathing system obstruction by assessing ventilation with an alternative system (e.g. self-inflating reservoir bag) connected directly to the airway device/endotracheal tube.

If ventilation is still difficult, the problem lies in the airway device/endo-tracheal tube or the patient:
☑ Check the airway device/ETT is in the right position and patent—a suction catheter or a gum-elastic bougie should pass easily through the whole length of the airway device.
☑ Manipulate and replace if necessary.

If ventilation is still difficult, the problem lies in the patient:
☑ Proceed to check for specific patient causes of high airway pressure (➲ see 'Subsequent management', p. 414).

Subsequent management
☑ Auscultate for breath sounds and bronchospasm.
☑ Examine chest movement, neck veins, tracheal position.
☑ Lift surgical drapes to look for flushing, urticaria, subcutaneous emphysema.
☑ Consider and rule out:
  - endobronchial intubation.
  - bronchospasm (➲ p. 70) or dynamic hyperinflation (➲ p. 234).
  - anaphylaxis (➲ p. 272).
  - tension pneumothorax (➲ p. 66).
  - lung/lobar collapse.
  - anatomical/pathological obstruction of the trachea or major bronchi.

- opioid-induced chest wall rigidity.
- acute pulmonary oedema, ➔ p. 68.

Special considerations

- Diagnosing the equipment problem can wait if it can be eliminated.
- Capnography and clinical examination may be the only early indicators of inadequate ventilation during pressure-controlled or pressure-limited ventilation. Expired CO_2 may rise or fall, depending on the cause of the high airway pressure.
- During IPPV, expiratory resistance (e.g. an obstructed APL valve, circle expiratory valve, ventilator expiratory valve, or scavenging system) may be diagnosed by raised peak inspiratory pressure, abnormal end-expiratory pressure, or abnormal distension of the reservoir bag during manual (or spontaneous) ventilation.
- Intrathoracic pressure is released by disconnecting the breathing system, unless generated by subtotal obstruction or a 'one-way valve' effect in an airway device.

Further reading

Carter, J.A. (2004). Checking anaesthetic equipment and the Expert Group on Blocked Anaesthetic Tubing (EGBAT). *Anaesthesia*, **59**(2), 105–7.

Keith, R.L., Pierson, D.J. (1996). Complications of mechanical ventilation. A bedside approach. *Clinical Chest Medicine*, **17**(3), 439–51.

Miscellaneous problems

John Isaac, Mark Stoneham, Nerida Williams, and Bruce McCormick

☼ Massive haemorrhage

Definition

Loss of total blood volume in less than 24 h.
Loss of blood >1 mL/kg/min.

Presentation

- Hypovolaemic shock.
- Massive blood loss is usually obvious, but can be concealed intraoperatively or in trauma.

Immediate management

☑ ABC—100% O_2.
☑ Stop bleeding—apply direct pressure, clamp arterial supply, aortic clamp.
☑ Call for help—a team approach is needed.
☑ IV access—14 G × 2, consider using PA catheter sheath (8.5 Fr) in a central vein.
☑ IV fluids—increasing circulating volume is the first priority. Use crystalloid, warmed as soon as practicable.
☑ Re-assess vital signs—pulse, BP, peripheral perfusion.
☑ Activate the Major Haemorrhage Protocol and contact the blood bank, it will speed things up.
☑ Order blood products—designate a named individual to take and label blood samples. Consider likely need for red blood cells, platelets, FFP, cryoprecipitate.
☑ Warn theatres if surgery is likely—prepare fluid warmers, rapid infusion devices, inotropic infusions, transducers.
☑ Anaesthesia—if required, use rapid sequence induction. Reduce doses of induction agents. Consider etomidate (0.1–0.3 mg/kg) or ketamine (1–2 mg/kg). Have intravenous infusions running maximally. Be prepared for hypotension on induction.

Subsequent management

☑ Arterial line, central line, and urinary catheter after definitive treatment started.
☑ Continue to monitor haematocrit, arterial pH, clotting (see resuscitation target values, Table 14.1).
☑ If ACTIVELY bleeding:
  - Administer FFP once the INR >1.5.
  - Administer platelets once the platelet count <80 ×10^9/L.
  - Administer cryoprecipitate if the fibrinogen is <1.5 g/L.
☑ Use near-patient testing whenever available (blood gases, haematocrit, Ca^{2+}, Hemocue®, Coagucheck®, thromboelastography [TEG®], ROTEM®).
☑ Some 'Damage Control Resuscitation' protocols for trauma management advocate early use of red cells and plasma and a formula approach of red cells:FFP:platelets (e.g. 2:1:1).

Table 14.1 Resuscitation target values

Hb	70–80 g/L unless good reason to be higher (severe CVS/respiratory disease)
Platelet count	>80 × 10⁹/L if actively bleeding (or >100 × 10⁹/L if multiple trauma/CNS injury)
Prothrombin time (PT)	<1.5 times control
Partial thromboplastin time (PTT)	<1.5 times control
Fibrinogen	>1.5 g/L

☑ Most cases of massive haemorrhage benefit from IV tranexamic acid (1 g IV over 10 min followed by 1 g IV over 8 h).
☑ Inform ICU early so that they can plan for the admission.

Investigations
• ABGs, haematocrit, clotting screen, cross-match, U&E, TEG/**ROTEM**.

Risk factors
• Surgery (vascular/obstetrics/major cardiothoracic/major GI/major orthopaedic).
• Trauma (especially blunt body-cavity trauma).
• Oesophageal varices in patients with liver disease.
• Ruptured aortic aneurysm.
• Coagulopathy: congenital (e.g. haemophilia), acquired (e.g. advanced liver disease).
• Blind traumatic procedures (e.g. liver biopsy).

Exclusions
• Dehydration
• Sepsis
• Anaphylaxis
• Heart failure

Paediatric considerations
• Get help from experienced colleagues. Paediatricians can come to theatre!
• Intraosseous infusion, external jugular, or femoral vein may help with access.
• Work out blood volume (80 mL/kg). See also paediatric major trauma, ⊃ p. 143.
• Give fluid boluses in aliquots of 10 mL/kg.
• Titrate according to vital signs.
• Keep warm.

Special considerations

- Hypothermia impairs coagulation, so keep warm.
- Hypocalcaemia may occur during very rapid transfusion, causing hypotension. Treat with IV calcium gluconate 10 mL 10%, or calcium chloride 5.0 mL 10% (adult doses).
- During emergency laparotomy, packing abdomen and closing can help control bleeding.
- Remember, platelets can be given via any fresh giving set, but a platelet-giving set has reduced dead space, allowing minimal wastage.
- A 'Cell Saver' should be used whenever possible—avoid in contaminated cases. Needs to be set-up ready and with staff to operate the machine.
- Haematology advice can help—particularly if there is an underlying coagulation disorder.
- The CRASH-2 study found early treatment with tranexamic acid in trauma patients reduces the risk of death from bleeding. Adult dose 1 g IV over 10 min followed by 1 g IV over 8 h.

Further reading

AAGBI (2010). *Safety Guideline: Management of Massive Haemorrhage*. Available at: https://www.esahq.org/~/media/ESA/Files/Downloads/Resources-PatientSafety-PatientSafety-UK%20-%20massive_haemorrhage_2010.ashx

Crash-2 trial collaborators (2010). A randomized placebo-controlled trial. *Lancet*, **376**, 23–32

⑦ Using blood products

Red cell transfusion

- Blood loss of 30–50% can usually be treated with crystalloid solutions (depending on initial Hb concentration). Blood loss of >50% will require red cell transfusion.
- Target red cell transfusion to maintain Hb >70 g/L (CVS disease >90 g/L).
- Use available near-patient testing frequently (blood gases, lactate, haematocrit, Hemocue®).
- Use Group O Rhesus negative blood if anaemia is immediately life-threatening (i.e. Hb <50 g/L with ongoing bleeding). An alternative is uncross-matched group-compatible blood. This can be issued by the blood bank immediately.
- Transfusing SAG-M O-negative blood carries a minimal risk of ABO mismatch as there is so little residual plasma in the bag. Transfusing group-specific blood carries a small risk of the transfused cells being haemolysed due to recipient antibodies. The risk of serious morbidity or mortality from either strategy is very low, and should be weighed against the risk of delaying transfusion until crossmatched red cells become available.

Fresh frozen plasma, platelets, cryoprecipitate

- Coagulation deteriorates after 3–5 L of blood loss. Anticipate changes and measure coagulation regularly. Use near-patient testing if available (Coagucheck®, thromboelastography, ROTEM).
- Transfuse FFP and platelets as guided by tests, this is consistently more appropriate than 'clinical guidance'.
- Prolonged PT and PTT will correct with FFP transfusion.
- Fibrinogen <1.5 g/L with continuing haemorrhage will require cryoprecipitate transfusion.
- There may be considerable delay in obtaining platelets, so you need to plan in advance for their use.
- Platelets are indicated when <80 ×10⁹/L if patient is actively bleeding (100 ×10⁹/L if multiple trauma, CNS disease, or when ineffective due to disease/drugs).
- Transfuse using a standard blood- or platelet-giving set, provided the line has not previously been used for blood transfusion.
- Thawed FFP can be stored safely for 24 h in a blood fridge (4°C).

Other information
See Tables 14.2 and 14.3.

Table 14.2 Cost of various blood products (NHSBT 2019–20)

Component	2019/20 price
Standard red cells	£133.44
Platelets—apheresis	£240.56
Platelets—pooled	£193.14
Fresh Frozen plasma	£31.40
Cryoprecipitate (pooled, UK sourced)	£174.85

ATD, adult therapeutic dose.

Reproduced with permission from NHS Blood and Transplant 2019-20. https://nhsbtdbe.blob. core.windows.net/umbraco-assets-corp/15701/price_list_bc_nhs_2019-20-2.pdf

Table 14.3 Estimated risk of viral infection/million donation tested (NHSBT/Public Health England Epidemiology Unit 2013)

Hepatitis B	1 in 1.27 million
Hepatitis C	1 in 29 million
HIV	1 in 7.04 million

Reproduced from NHSBT/Public Health England Epidemiology Unit 2013. © Crown Copyright 2013. Open Government Licence v3.0.

Further reading

NHSBT Price List 2016–2017. Available at: http://hospital.blood.co.uk/media/28230/component-price-list-2016-2017.pdf

Public Health England (2013). *Safe Supplies: Completing the Picture. Annual Review from the NHS Blood and Transplant/Public Health England Epidemiology Unit, 2012.* London, UK: Public Health England. Available at: http://www.hpa.org.uk/Topics/InfectiousDiseases/ReferenceLibrary/BIBDReferences/

☼ Acute transfusion reactions

Definition

Acute reaction within 24 h of blood/product transfusion.
Acute transfusion reactions vary in severity from minor febrile reactions to life-threatening allergic, haemolytic, or hypotensive events.

- **Febrile non-haemolytic transfusion reactions**—usually clinically mild.
- **Allergic transfusion reactions**—ranging from mild urticaria to life-threatening angio-oedema or anaphylaxis.
- **Acute haemolytic transfusion reactions** (e.g. ABO incompatibility)
- **TACO**—transfusion associated circulatory overload.
- **TRALI**—transfusion-related acute lung injury.
- **Bacterial contamination of blood unit**—range from mild pyrexia to rapidly lethal septic shock, depending on contaminant.

Presentation

- Fever, urticarial rash, dyspnoea, wheeze.
- Anaphylactic shock— ➲ see p. 272.

Immediate management

- ☑ Stop the transfusion—keep the IV line open with crystalloid.
- ☑ Keep the blood/product bag for analysis.
- ☑ Check and record vital signs, including S_pO_2 and temperature.
- ☑ Check for respiratory signs—dyspnoea, tachypnoea, wheeze, cyanosis.
- ☑ If severe, institute ABC—100% O_2.
- ☑ Call for help.
- ☑ Provide further management according to the developing clinical features.
- ☑ Check the identity of patient and blood/product unit and
- ☑ documentation.
- ☑ Check arterial blood gases.
- ☑ Be prepared to manage full-blown anaphylactic shock.
- ☑ Multiorgan failure may ensue—ICU if indicated.

Subsequent management

- ☑ Notify blood bank, they will want the unit returned along with a blood sample from the patient.
- ☑ Consult a haematologist.
- ☑ Inform the Hospital Transfusion Committee.
- ☑ Complete a 'Critical Incident' report.
- ☑ The blood bank will report the case to SABRE and SHOT if appropriate.

Investigations

- S_pO_2, U&Es, LFTs, Haptoglobins, Direct Coombs Test, IgA levels (seek expert Haematology advice).
- Urine for haemoglobinuria.

Exclusions
- Septic shock
- Hypovolaemic shock
- Acute drug reaction/anaphylaxis

Special considerations

Wrong blood transfused
- This is a 'Never Event' and is usually due to cross-match sampling or labelling mistakes, or failure to match the issue form and product with the patient. This occurs with hurried or incomplete checking of blood products with the patient. It is more likely in emergency situations or at night.
- ABO-incompatible transfusion occurs in around 1 in 180 000 red cell units transfused.
- The rapid destruction of the transfused red cells in the circulation (intravascular haemolysis) and the release of inflammatory cytokines leads to profound shock and often acute renal failure and DIC.
- Conscious patients often become unwell very quickly complaining of flushing and or abdominal pain. Anaesthetized patients may present with tachycardia, hypotension, and microvascular bleeding.

Allergic reactions
- If the only feature is a rise in temperature of less than 1.5°C from baseline or an urticarial rash:
  - recheck that the correct blood is being transfused.
  - give paracetamol for fever.
  - give antihistamine for urticaria.
  - recommence the transfusion at a slower rate.
  - observe the patient more frequently than routine practice.

Transfusion-associated circulatory overload (TACO)
- This presents with pulmonary oedema developing within 6 h of transfusion.
- It is a clinical diagnosis, with all the features of circulatory overload including raised JVP, enlarged heart on CXR and echo.
- It is commoner in small and/or elderly patients, especially those with heart and/or renal failure.
- Management is with O_2, fluid restriction, diuretics, and where needed respiratory support.

Transfusion-related acute lung injury (TRALI)
- This presents with pulmonary oedema developing usually within 2 h of transfusion of FFP or platelets.
- TRALI is caused by antibodies in the donor blood reacting with the patient's neutrophils, monocytes, or pulmonary endothelium, leading to non-cardiogenic pulmonary oedema.
- There are no features of circulatory overload and heart size is normal on imaging.
- The patient often has a fever, may have rigors, and may require fluid therapy. Management is supportive with O_2 and when needed respiratory support. Neither diuretics nor steroids are helpful.

- Suspected cases of TRALI should be reported to the National Blood Service and discussed with a transfusion haematologist, as there may be a need to confirm the diagnosis and then investigate the blood donors for specific antigens.

Bacterial contamination of a transfused blood component

- This can cause acute severe septic shock. This occurs rarely, but can lead to mortality. It is commonest with platelet transfusion due to their storage at 21°C. Management is as for septic shock (blood cultures, IV broad-spectrum antibiotics stat) and the suspected component should be sealed and returned to the Blood Service for investigation.

Further reading

Joint United Kingdom (UK) Blood Transfusion and Tissue Transplantation Services Professional Advisory Committee (2014). *Transfusion Handbook*. Available at: http://www.transfusionguidelines.org.uk/transfusion-handbook

☼ Burns

(➔ See also 'Paediatric burns', p. 145.)

Definition
Tissue damage as result of exposure to heat, electrical energy, or caustic agent.

Presentation
- Inhalational burns cause tachypnoea, airway obstruction, and pulmonary oedema.
- Surface burns cause hypovolaemia, pain, and may produce constrictive bands.
- COHb poisoning causes nausea and vomiting, tachycardia, angina, chorea, and convulsions.

Immediate management
The history will help with extent of burn, potential for inhalation injury, and the likelihood of other injuries.
☑ Follow ATLS principles (do not get distracted by the burn and miss other major injuries).

Primary care ABC
☑ Approach with care as a first responder (fire, smoke, electrical shock risk); stop the
☑ Burning process by removing objects that retain heat (e.g. plastic, metal jewellery);
☑ Contamination—not all burns are due to heat. Protect against chemical contamination of the unit and staff.

Secondary care ABC
Airway injury—signs suggestive of inhalational burns include: hoarseness; cough; sooty sputum; singed nasal hair; facial burns; mucosal injury.
☑ If in doubt, intubate early since airway oedema may soon make this impossible.
☑ Anticipate a difficult intubation (➔ see p. 84) but **do not delay**. Suxamethonium is safe initially.
☑ Leave the ETT long and uncut because oedema may displace it later.

Breathing—is the patient breathing spontaneously? Burns caused by electric shock are associated with transient respiratory muscle paralysis.
☑ Give high-flow 100% oxygen as tissue oxygenation may be compromised by carbon monoxide poisoning despite normal S_aO_2 and P_aO_2. High respiratory rate may indicate lower airway damage predisposing to later pulmonary oedema, or it may indicate smoke inhalation with metabolic poisoning.

Circulation:
☑ Check output and rhythm. Electrical burns may cause dysrhythmias by inducing VF or damage to the conducting system. BLS/ALS if necessary.

☑ Establish IV access in an unburnt area if possible. The femoral triangle is often spared.

☑ Fluid resuscitate to normovolaemia. Warmed Hartmann's solution should be started and titrated to cardiovascular response. Burns are not the cause of immediate hypovolaemia.

☑ Check for severe occult injuries sustained during escape from the fire (e.g. by jumping), especially if adequate fluid resuscitation is difficult to achieve.

Subsequent management

☑ Cover exposed burns with 'cling-film'. This limits evaporative loss, conserves heat, and reduces infection risk. Gram-negative sepsis is a major complication.

☑ Give analgesia: full-thickness burns are painless, but there is usually a mixed picture. Titrate morphine IV to response.

☑ Calculate TBSA: burns are classified by total body surface area (TBSA) and depth. There are three simple methods of rapidly estimating burn area:

- Wallace's 'rule of nines'—quick and useful for medium-sized burns, but a tendency to overestimate burn extent by counting erythema (Figure 14.1).
- Lund and Browder charts (◑ see p. 147)—most accurate method if used carefully. Takes into account relative changes in surface area with age.
- Palmar surface = 0.8% of BSA. Useful for very small areas of burn (<15%). This relates to the *patient's* hand, including fingers. Also useful for widespread burns >85% (counting unburnt area).

☑ IV fluid resuscitation is required in adults if the burn involves more than 15% BSA or 10% with smoke inhalation.

- The Parkland formula for fluid management is the most commonly used which calculates 24 h fluid requirement (mL).
- 4 × TBSA of burn (%) × body weight (kg).
- 50% should be given in the first 8 h. Hartmann's is usually the fluid of choice. Subtract any fluid already given (e.g. pre-hospital) and the 24 h period starts at the time of the burn (not the time of presentation).

☑ Insert a urinary catheter to assess adequacy of fluid replacement (urine output >1 mL/kg/h).

☑ Consider escharotomies for patients with circumferential chest wall burns—restrictive respiratory compromise may develop.

☑ Refer to a regional burns centre if complex burn injuries include any of the following:

- Extremes of age—under 5 y or more than 60 y.
- Burn of face or hands or perineum or feet; or any flexure particularly the neck or axilla; or any circumferential dermal or full-thickness burn of the limbs, torso, or neck.
- Inhalation injury Any significant such injury, excluding pure carbon monoxide poisoning.

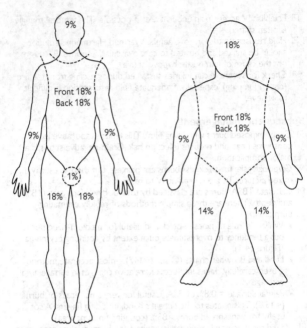

Figure 14.1 Rule of nines burns assessment (➲ see also Lund and Browder charts, p. 147).

Reprinted from *The Lancet*, 257(6653), Wallace, A. B. The Exposure Treatment of Burns, pp. 501–4. Copyright © 1951, with permission from Elsevier Ltd. doi: https://doi.org/10.1016/S0140-6736(51)91975-7.

- Mechanism of injury—chemical injury (>5% TBSA); exposure to ionizing radiation injury; high pressure steam injury; high tension electrical injury; hydrofluoric acid injury (>1% TBSA).
- Suspicion of non-accidental burn injury.
- Size of skin injury with dermal/full-thickness loss <16-year-old with >5% TBSA; 16 y or over >10% TBSA.
- Pre-existing comorbidities (e.g. significant cardiorespiratory disease, diabetes, pregnancy, immunosuppression, hepatic impairment, or cirrhosis).
- Associated injuries—crush injuries, fractures, head injury, penetrating injuries.

Investigations

- Carbon monoxide poisoning (COHb >20%)— standard ABGs will appear normal. S_aO_2 will appear normal because both COHb and oxyhaemoglobin absorb at 940 nm. Bench co-oximetry utilizes an additional wavelength of red light, allowing differentiation.
- Cyanide poisoning (>50 ppm)—causes unexplained metabolic acidosis and high venous oxygen saturation. Common with combustion of plastics. Treat with O_2.
- ECG—for evidence of ischaemia/dysrhythmia/conduction abnormality.
- U&Es—patients may develop hyperkalaemia from release of intracellular K^+.
- Inhalation burns are best documented by later fibreoptic bronchoscopy. CXR is of little help initially as positive findings appear late.

Exclusions

- Inhalational injury should be suspected if there is a history of exposure to smoke, particularly if fire occurred in a confined space, or there is a reduced conscious level.
- Airway injury—careful observation is required following an inhalational injury as severe airway obstruction can develop after a 'free period' of 3–8 h.

Special considerations

- It is easy to confuse full-thickness burns with unburnt skin. Full-thickness burns look dry, waxy/leathery, and are insensitive, but do not bleed on pinprick.
- Following a burn injury, suxamethonium causes acute hyperkalaemia, due to the extrajunctional migration of acetylcholine receptors. It is safe within the first 24 h, but subsequently should not be used for at least 12 months.
- Resistance develops to non-depolarizing relaxants, persisting up to 10 weeks.
- Renal failure may occur secondary to initial hypovolaemia and myoglobinuria.
- While there is no benefit in prophylactic antibiotic or steroid therapy, steroids may be required along with aminophylline if severe bronchospasm develops.
- Enteral feeding has been shown to protect against gut translocation of toxins and micro-organisms, and to reduce the incidence of sepsis.

Further reading

Bishop, S., Maguire, S. (2012). Anaesthesia and intensive care for major burns. Continuing Education in Anaesthesia, Critical Care and Pain, **12** (3), 118–22.

ⓘ Inoculation injury

Definition

An object (e.g. sharp) or substance (e.g. IV fluid) contaminated by blood or other body fluids breaches the integrity of the skin or mucosa (needlestick or subcutaneous exposure), or comes into contact with the eyes, mouth, or broken skin (mucocutaneous exposure).

Presentation

- Usually 'needlestick' injury in the anaesthetic setting.
- Hollow, blood-containing needles present the highest risk to anaesthetists.

Immediate management

☑ Wash the wound liberally with soap and water but without scrubbing.

☑ Exposed mucous membranes, including conjunctivae, should be irrigated copiously with water or saline (remove contact lenses).

☑ If puncture wound, free bleeding should be encouraged gently, but wound should not be sucked.

☑ Hospitals should have an 'inoculation injury' protocol and pack.

☑ Report the exposure **immediately** to occupational health and seek urgent advice on further management and treatment. Local protocols will indicate from whom advice should be sought if the exposure occurs outside normal working hours (usually the emergency department).

☑ If postexposure prophylaxis (PEP) is recommended, it should ideally start within 1 h of the exposure. It may be worth considering up to 72 h after the exposure.

Subsequent management

☑ Further management will involve assessing the potential risk from the patient, seeking consent from the patient to testing for blood-borne viruses (this should not be undertaken by the exposed healthcare worker), and testing the healthcare worker in a similar fashion.

☑ In most circumstances of HBV and HIV exposure, PEP will be offered.

☑ Expert advice should be sought from occupational health/ED.

☑ The exposed person should also be advised to have safe sex for 3 months, not to donate blood until all necessary screening tests are clear, and to see their GP if they develop a fever.

Investigations

- As guided by occupational health.

Risk factors

- The major hazard associated with inoculation injuries is the transmission of blood-borne viruses: HBV, HCV, and HIV.
- A Health Protection Agency (HPA) report regarding healthcare workers, released in 2012, stated that the total number of HCV seroconversions in healthcare workers reported between 1997 and 2011 is 20. The last case of an HIV seroconversion in an occupationally exposed healthcare worker was reported in 1999.

Special considerations

- Always employ 'Universal Precautions':
  - wear gloves
  - handle sharps carefully—do not re-sheath needles
  - dispose of sharps in sharps bin immediately after use. Do not overfill sharps bins
  - discard disposable syringes and needles wherever possible as a single unit
- HBV immunization—all healthcare workers who perform exposure-prone procedures should be immunized against HBV and have their response to the vaccine checked. Advice should be obtained from the occupational health service.
- PEP with HBV immunoglobulin and/or antiretroviral drugs should be recommended to healthcare workers if they have had a significant occupational exposure to blood or another high-risk body fluid from a patient, or other source either known to be HBV/HIV infected, or considered to be at high risk of HBV/HIV infection, but where the result of testing has not or cannot be obtained. PEP should ideally commence within 1 h of the exposure.

Further reading

HPA (2012). *Eye of the Needle: United Kingdom Surveillance of Significant Occupational Exposures to Bloodborne Viruses in Healthcare Workers*. Available at: http://www.hpa.org.uk/Topics/InfectiousDiseases/InfectionsAZ/BloodborneVirusesAndOccupationalExposure

NICE (2012). *Healthcare-Associated Infections: Prevention and Control in Primary and Community Care: Clinical Guideline 139*. Available at: http://www.nice.org.uk/guidance/CG139

⚙ **Bone cement implantation syndrome (BCIS)**

Definition
CVS collapse in response to the insertion of poly methyl methacrylate (PMMA) cement during orthopaedic procedures, most commonly hip arthroplasty procedures.

Presentation
- Hypotension, hypoxaemia, increased PVR causing signs of right heart failure, cardiac arrhythmias, and cardiac arrest.

Classification
Grade 1:
- moderate hypoxia (S_pO_2 <94%)
- or hypotension (systolic BP reduced by >20%)

Grade 2:
- severe hypoxia (S_pO_2 <88%)
- or hypotension (systolic BP reduced by >40%)
- or unexpected loss of consciousness

Grade 3:
- CVS collapse requiring CPR

Data from Donaldson AJ, Thomson HE, Harper NJ and Kenny NW. Bone cement implantation syndrome. *Br J Anaesth* 2009;102:12–22

> **Immediate management**
> ☑ ABC—100% O_2.
> ☑ IV fluids.
> ☑ IV ephedrine (6 mg boluses), α-agonists (e.g. metaraminol IV 0.5 mg boluses) and/or adrenaline (10–50 µg IV boluses).
> ☑ Invasive monitoring (CVP, PA catheter, TOE if available).

Subsequent management
Usually transient reaction which stabilizes. In unfit patients, sudden deterioration may progress rapidly if not managed aggressively.

Investigations
- 12-lead ECG to exclude cardiac event.
- TOE if available

Risk factors
- Clinical experience suggests that the syndrome is rare in healthy patients.
- It is more common in:
  - elderly
  - pre-existing pulmonary hypertension
  - reduced myocardial reserve
  - pathological or intertrochanteric fractures
  - long stem arthroplasty

Exclusions

- Massive pulmonary embolus (↪ see p. 41)—prolonged hypoxaemia.
- Myocardial infarction or cardiac failure (↪ see p. 338)—more prolonged hypotension, pulmonary oedema, little response to fluids and vasopressors, known risk factors.
- Anaphylaxis (↪ see p. 272).

Special considerations

BCIS has been attributed to many things:

- One component of the cement is a liquid monomer which causes vasodilatation and tachycardia when it reaches the circulation.
- Mixing of the cement produces an exothermic reaction, and heat may cause bone marrow and blood cells to release thrombotic and vasoactive substances.
- Embolization of air, fat, bone marrow, and bone debris can occur when the prosthesis is impacted. The embolization of these elements into the right heart can be demonstrated clinically using TOE. It is suggested that these micro-emboli may lead to acute pulmonary hypertension and right ventricular failure. As with most embolic phenomena, TOE reveals many patients with micro-emboli, some of whom develop transient hypoxaemia, but very few of whom develop full-blown BCIS.
- Where possible, consider non-cemented techniques in those at high risk of BCIS.

Further reading

Donaldson, A.J., Thomson, H.E., Harper, N.J., Kenny, N.W. (2009). Bone cement implantation syndrome. British Journal of Anaesthesia, **102**, 12–22.

ⓘ **Extravasation of anaesthetic agents**

Definition
Accidental injection or leakage of iv fluids/drugs from a vein into the surrounding tissue.

Presentation
- Most extravasations have only minor sequelae; however, effects range from mild discomfort and discoloration, through to tissue necrosis with damage to tendons and nerves, compartment syndrome requiring fasciotomy, reconstructive surgery, and even amputation. Serious sequelae are more likely with cytotoxic chemotherapy drugs.
- Most drugs used regularly by anaesthetists do not seem to cause serious sequelae from extravasation.

Immediate management
- ☑ There is no proven definitive treatment for extravasation injury. There is some evidence that early treatment may improve outcome.
- ☑ Stop injecting.
- ☑ Leave the cannula *in situ*.
- ☑ Assess risk of solution injected (➔ see 'Risk factors', p. 435).
- ☑ Elevate the site to reduce swelling where possible (e.g. limb cannula).
- ☑ Hyaluronidase breaks down hyaluronic acid in connective tissue and is used to increase the permeability of tissues to injected fluids (e.g. hypodermoclysis). Subcutaneous infiltration of hyaluronidase (15 units/mL saline) at 5–10 sites along the leading edges of the extravasation has been used successfully. Another approach is to deliver the hyaluronidase into the cannula. Total dose should not exceed 1500 units.
- ☑ Specific local policy should be consulted where a cytotoxic drug has extravasated; active intervention may be indicated (e.g. saline washout under GA or specific antidote administration).

Subsequent management
- ☑ The extravasation injury should be clearly documented in the patient's notes.
- ☑ The patient should be given a full explanation of events and an apology.
- ☑ The site should be observed closely for the first few days.
- ☑ Local blistering suggests partial-thickness injury.
- ☑ Firm induration suggests eventual ulceration.
- ☑ A plastic/reconstructive surgeon should be consulted early.
- ☑ Surgery is usually indicated if full-thickness skin necrosis occurs.

Risk factors

- Site of cannulation—antecubital fossae and dorsi of the hand or foot are the most common sites of extravasation injury. Joints and creases should be avoided as these represent a 'small tissue space', often containing nerves and tendons.
- Patient factors include diabetes, rheumatoid, Raynaud's disease, peripheral vascular disease, lymphoedema, recent surgery to limb, recent radiotherapy to limb.
- Type of drug—the following are all high risk in extravasation injury:
  - high pH (e.g. thiopental, etomidate, phenytoin)
  - vasopressors (e.g. adrenaline, noradrenaline)
  - high osmolality (e.g. mannitol, calcium chloride, potassium chloride, sodium bicarbonate, parenteral nutrition, some antibiotics)
  - cellular toxicity (e.g. chemotherapy)

Exclusions

- IA injection (see p. 436) leads to severe burning pain in the conscious patient. Blanching, hyperaemia, and cyanosis of the distal limb can occur depending upon the drug injected.

Special considerations

- Beware IV cannula inserted prior to arrival in the anaesthetic room. Always test cannulae with a saline flush prior to use, or insert a new one.
- Always use a test dose of 1–2 mL of induction agent and assess the patient and the site of injection.
- Check the cannula if the patient complains of excessive pain at induction. The cannula may well be in an intact vein if using propofol or etomidate, as pain upon injection is common.
- If possible, position the limb so that the cannulation site can be directly inspected throughout the surgical procedure.
- Distrust a positional IV cannula. It may have tissued and fluid may be entering the perivenous space. If the drip does not run freely, assume it has tissued until you can confirm otherwise. Never give drugs via a positional cannula. Insert a new cannula at a different site.
- Topical cooling and topical warming have both been advocated as treatments, although there is little evidence that either is beneficial.

Further reading

Lake, C., Beecroft, C.L. (2010). Extravasation injuries and accidental intra-arterial injection. *Continuing Education in Anaesthesia, Critical Care and Pain*, **10**(4), 109–13.

① **Accidental intra-arterial (IA) injection**

Definition
Accidental injection of an intravenous drug into an artery. Most commonly because of inadvertent administration of drugs via an arterial line.

Presentation
- IA injection leads to severe burning pain in the conscious patient.
- Blanching, hyperaemia, and cyanosis of the distal limb can occur.

Immediate management
☑ Stop injecting immediately.
☑ Leave the cannula in place.
☑ There is no universally accepted treatment protocol. Suggested treatments are aimed at reducing arterial vasospasm (e.g. lidocaine 100 mg and/or papaverine 40 mg in 10–20 mL saline via the cannula).
☑ Consider regional blockade of the upper limb (brachial plexus block or stellate ganglion block) to reduce arterial vasospasm.
☑ Give systemic analgesia.
☑ Consider anticoagulation with IV heparin and subsequently with oral warfarin
☑ Use of intravenous epoprostenol (prostacyclin) has been described.
☑ Seek early guidance from a vascular and/or plastic surgeon.

Subsequent management
☑ Many approaches have been described but none is proven.
☑ No specific treatment recommendations can be given on the available evidence. The few studies available are animal models with small sample sizes.
☑ Formal thrombolysis using urokinase has been described, although an animal model studying IA thiopental injection (using IA urokinase as a therapy) showed a detrimental effect.
☑ **IA thiopental**—causes severe pain and blanching of the distal limb. There is profound constriction of the artery caused by local noradrenaline release. Thiopental may crystallize in arterioles. Thromboses occur and these may embolize to distal parts of the limb (e.g. individual digits).
☑ **IA fentanyl**—has been injected into a conscious patient without causing any symptoms, signs, or sequelae.
☑ **Propofol**—leads to severe distal hyperaemia lasting between a few hours and 12 days. Full recovery is the norm.

Investigations
- Overall diagnosis is clinical, and requires a high index of suspicion.
- Transduce pressure from the cannula and take blood sample for ABGs. If the cannula is kinked, or the patient has an AV fistula, these tests will not be diagnostic.

Risk factors

- Inadvertent IA injection is a rare complication of anaesthesia.
- It can occur due to mistaken injection into an arterial line port, especially if lines are not properly marked or labelled.
- It occurs with cannulae inserted into the antecubital fossa (brachial artery) or into an aberrant radial artery.
- The arterial vascular anatomy of the upper limb is extremely variable, and you cannot assume that arteries occur only as they do in an anatomy text.
- IA injection has been described into cannulae placed in the dorsum of the hand.

Exclusions

- Pain on (IV) injection is common with many anaesthetic induction agents.
- Extravasation from a tissued cannula can cause pain, discoloration, and blanching (⮕ see p. 434).

Special considerations

- Always check for a pulse in the vessel that you intend to cannulate. Ideally this should be performed prior to a tourniquet being applied.
- Ensure that any applied tourniquet is not so tight as to occlude arterial flow in the limb.
- Attaching a drip and allowing it to run prior to induction does not preclude IA placement of the cannula, but may demonstrate backflow of arterial blood (unless you have used a one-way/non-return valve).
- Take great care with all arterial line ports. Label them appropriately, or tape them closed while in theatre.
- Give a test dose of 1–2 mL of induction agent and assess the patient's response before proceeding.

Further reading

Lake, C., Beecroft, C.L. (2010). Extravasation injuries and accidental intra-arterial injection. *Continuing Education in Anaesthesia, Critical Care and Pain*, **10**(4), 109–13.

⑦ What to do in the event of fire

Definition

Fire occurring in a ward area, the theatre suite, or the critical care unit.

The need for fire training

It is important for all staff to understand the need and value of fire training. People, who know what to do if a fire breaks out, can save lives.

There are legal requirements under section 2 of the Health & Safety at Work, Act 1974, and the Regulatory Reform (Fire Safety) Order 2005 which require that all employees receive appropriate instruction and training in what to do in the event of fire.

Presentation

- Most hospitals are now fitted with two-stage fire alarms. When a fire occurs, the alarm will sound continuously in the affected area, but will ring intermittently in adjoining areas.
- Persons in an area where the alarm is sounding intermittently need not evacuate, but should make provisional preparations. Staff should prepare patients and visitors for evacuation should the alarm change to a continuous sound.

Immediate management

- ☑ The person in charge of the department must first determine the exact location of the fire by instructing staff to carry out a rapid visual check of the area.
- ☑ If the fire incident is minor and can be tackled safely by staff, then total evacuation may be unnecessary and the procedures being carried out within the department may continue.
- ☑ If the fire incident is serious, and is within or threatens the department, and cannot be tackled by staff with fire extinguishers, then the safety of staff and patients is paramount. All work should stop and all non-essential persons must be evacuated to an adjoining safe area. While the speedy evacuation of patients is essential, staff must not compromise their own safety to do this.
- ☑ In the event that fire/suffocation is imminent, identify staff and resources that will be required to safely evacuate the patient (e.g. self-inflating bags, oxygen, etc. including an oxygen supply for the staff).
- ☑ Consider the most practical route of evacuation (lifts should not be used, stairs are impassable on ward or ITU beds, but mattresses can be used to move a patient down a stairwell).
- ☑ Establish a route of communication to the outside (telephone, mobile phone, radio, runner).
- ☑ Firemen are trained and equipped to rescue people from burning buildings—doctors are not.
- ☑ It may be that a ventilated patient has a better chance of surviving suffocation if left in the unit than if moved through a smoke-filled exit route.
- ☑ Staff should not risk their lives by staying with a patient who cannot be evacuated.

Special considerations

- Of basic importance to the fire strategy in hospitals is the principle that, should a fire occur, it is rapidly detected, an alarm is given, and the fire brigade is called.
- The immediate and total evacuation of a hospital in the event of fire is usually neither desirable nor necessary.
- In England and Wales, the Regulatory Reform Order (Fire Safety) 2005 (RRO) came into force on 1 October 2006. NHS Trusts have: a duty to ensure the safety of employees; to ensure that the premises are safe; a duty to carry out a fire risk assessment; a responsibility for ensuring that all staff receive basic fire training immediately upon taking up their first appointment and also receive regular updates as part of mandatory training.
- This training should include instruction on fire risk prevention and the action to take in the event of a fire and the emergency evacuation procedures applicable to their actual places of work.
- Fire extinguishers are always red, but have a colour-coded label on the side above the instructions, depending on their contents and intended use. The commonest are:

Red: water

Used for: paper, wood, textiles, furnishings, and other normal combustible materials.

Black: CO_2

Used for: electrical and electronic equipment.

- All staff should seek training in the operation of fire extinguishers available in their workplace.

☼ Bleeding following tonsillectomy

See Table 14.4.

Definition

- Haemorrhage may be early (haemostasis failure) or late (infective).
- Patient may have lost significant amount of blood, but difficult to estimate due to swallowing/vomiting.

Immediate management

☑ ABC—100% O_2. Reassure the patient and relatives.
☑ Ensure senior anaesthetist available.
☑ Check Hb, send sample for cross-match, and start IV resuscitation with large-bore IV access.
☑ May be residual narcosis due to opioids and previous GA. Exclude hypovolaemia as cause.
☑ RSI is usual. Cricoid pressure does not stop blood trickling down pharynx, but does limit the risks from a stomach full of blood.
☑ Alternatively, left side, head down, and gaseous induction—not recommended.
☑ Intubation may well be difficult due to blood and oedema. Have spare suction (in case of blockage with clot) and difficult intubation aids to hand.
☑ Following surgery, use large orogastric tube to wash out stomach (use water at body temperature).
☑ Extubate awake, on left side, head down.
☑ In some patients with adenoidal bleeding a pack may be left *in situ* until the following morning. Keep intubated and ventilated.

Subsequent management

☑ Keep in recovery/HDU for a couple of hours to ensure bleeding has stopped and resuscitation is adequate.

Table 14.4 Outline treatment plan for bleeding following tonsillectomy

Procedure	Re-operation to treat bleeding from adenoid or tonsil
Time	0.5–1 h
Pain	*/**
Position	Supine
Blood loss	May be significant, but difficult to estimate. Cross-match 2 units
Practical techniques	RSI, ETT, IPPV

Paediatric considerations

- Children may compensate for blood loss quite well until anaesthesia is induced, when they may decompensate.
- Be cautious if they have a tachycardia, and ensure sufficient fluid resuscitation before going to theatre.

Special considerations

- The decision to take a patient back to theatre should be made by a senior surgeon.
- Delay should be avoided, but IV resuscitation will usually be required.
- Intubation may well be more difficult than at first operation—do not underestimate risks.

✪ Bleeding following thyroid surgery

See Table 14.5.

Presentation
- Thyroid surgery followed by bleeding into the tissues of the neck.
- More common following large tumour resection (bleeding risk and tracheomalacia).
- The whole neck may be distended and oedematous.

Immediate management

On the ward
☑ Arrange for senior help to be called immediately and urgently.
☑ If stridor and respiratory embarrassment present—remove skin stitch/clips and sutures holding strap muscles together. Manually remove haematoma. This should be performed IMMEDIATELY.
☑ If respiration is not impaired, accompany the patient to theatre and allow surgeon to remove the haematoma under local anaesthesia.

In theatre
☑ After decompression, the patient will need anaesthesia for haemostasis. Intubation may be difficult due to oedema of the upper airway, caused by venous obstruction.
☑ Consider awake fibreoptic intubation (may be difficult due to distortion and swelling) or inhalational induction using oxygen and halothane/sevoflurane. Remember that local anaesthetic for an awake fibreoptic intubation can threaten the airway in patients with stridor.
☑ *In extremis*—either trial of direct laryngoscopy or awake tracheostomy, although the latter may be awkward because of haematoma and/or swelling. Consider LMA for rescue (may also be harder to insert).
☑ If airway obstruction has been severe, keep intubated overnight and give dexamethasone 8 mg IV.

Table 14.5 Outline treatment plan for bleeding following thyroid surgery

Procedure	Return to theatre post thyroid surgery. Haemorrhage may cause airway obstruction
Time	1 h
Pain	*/**
Position	Supine, slight head-up tilt
Blood loss	500–1000 mL
Practical techniques	GA with ETT, may be difficult intubation

Subsequent management

☑ Tracheostomy may be required in a few cases.

Special considerations

- Surgeon should palpate the trachea (partly withdraw the ET tube) to assess degree of tracheomalacia before extubation, although this occurs rarely.
- When decompressing the neck as an emergency procedure, remember that the haematoma may be beneath the muscle layer and simply opening the skin wound may not be sufficient. Even with the haematoma removed, oedema may jeopardize the airway.

☢: Bleeding following carotid endarterectomy

See Table 14.6.

Presentation

Carotid endarterectomy (CEA) earlier in the day. Subsequent distension of the neck that will ultimately compromise the airway. The quoted incidence is 1–4% of CEA patients, most within 4 h after surgery. It increases mortality significantly.

Immediate management

☑ ABC—administer 100% oxygen.

☑ Sit the patient up and reassure them. DO NOT sedate.

☑ Neck wound—if stridor or complete airway obstruction is impending, get a surgeon to open the neck wound **there and then** – even in recovery or on the ward.

☑ Return to theatre.

☑ Call for help—even if you are an experienced vascular anaesthetist, a second pair of experienced hands is vital. Get the difficult airway trolley and make sure all your favourite tools are available.

☑ Consider giving adrenaline nebulizer (5 mg, 5 mL of 1:1000)—this may help to reduce airway oedema, provided it does not delay the patient getting to theatre.

☑ Intubation may be difficult, but with no time for awake fibreoptic intubation—emergency tracheostomy may even be required.

Table 14.6 Outline treatment plan for bleeding following endarterectomy

Procedure	Opening of neck wound, evacuation of haematoma and haemostasis. Airway obstruction can be life-threatening
Time	1–2 h
Pain	*
Position	Supine, head up.
Blood loss	<1000 mL. Check blood is available as patient may only have been grouped and saved prior to CEA.
Practical techniques	If the CEA was performed under regional anaesthesia, the block may still be working sufficiently or can be topped up. Alternatively: ETT, IPPV. NB: intubation may be difficult.

Subsequent management

☑ Once the airway is secure, surgical management is usually straightforward.
☑ Administer dexamethasone (8 mg IV).
☑ Patients intubated due to airway obstruction should be kept intubated overnight on ITU to allow the oedema to settle.
☑ Significant bleeding requiring transfusion is uncommon. However, check the Hb and coagulation.

Further reading

Shakespeare, W.A., Lanier, W.L., Perkins, W.J., Pasternak, J.J. (2010). Airway management in patients who develop neck hematomas after carotid endarterectomy. *Anesthesia and Analgesia*, **110**, 588–93.

☠️ **Emergency aortic aneurysm repair**

See Table 14.7.

Presentation

- Two different clinical presentations:
  - rupture—exsanguinating patient.
  - retroperitoneal leak—hypotensive but stable.
- Ultrasound or CT scan if time available.
- True ruptured AAA has an **in-hospital** mortality of approximately 40%. Survival uncommon >80 y and if CPR has been necessary preoperatively.

Immediate management

- ☑ ABC—100% oxygen.
- ☑ Anaesthetic history—allergies, medications, cardiac history.
- ☑ IV access—two 14 G or PAFC sheath.
- ☑ Activate major haemorrhage protocol: cross-match—8 units packed red cells and warn blood bank about platelets and FFP.
- ☑ Fluids—if hypotensive, warmed fluids and vasopressors to a systolic pressure of 90–100 mmHg.
- ☑ Ephedrine 3–6 mg IV boluses or metaraminol 0.5–1 mg IV boluses.
- ☑ Adrenaline 50–100 µg IV boluses—if resistant hypotension or imminent cardiac arrest.
- ☑ Avoid hypertension, coughing, or straining.
- ☑ Analgesia—IV morphine for pain.
- ☑ Consider tranexamic acid 1 g IV unless very high thromboembolic risk.
- ☑ Inform theatre—phone ahead. Request cell salvage, rapid infusion devices/fluid warmers (Level-1®/Belmont® or equivalent if available), pressure transducers and drugs including vasopressors and inotropic infusion (adrenaline 2 mg in 40 mL = 50 µg/mL).
- ☑ Go directly to theatre.
- ☑ Relatives—speak to (or have someone else speak to) them.

Table 14.7 Outline treatment plan for emergency repair of ruptured abdominal aortic aneurysm

Procedure	Emergency repair of ruptured abdominal aortic aneurysm
Time	3–6 h
Pain	**** (ventilated post-op).
Position	Supine, arms out (crucifix).
Blood loss	1000–10 000 mL (cross-match 8 units packed RBC, order platelets, and FFP). Very suitable for autotransfusion.
Practical technique	ETT, IPPV, arterial, + CVP lines, Level-1®/Belmont® fluid warmer or equivalent.

Perioperative

- ☑ Prepare for induction in theatre.
- ☑ Assign one assistant to manage IV fluids, including organizing supply of fluid/blood.
- ☑ Arterial line pre-induction (upper limbs only). Central venous access rarely needed pre-induction (more commonly after cross-clamp). Urinary catheter.
- ☑ Talk to the patient while he/she is being draped, and preoxygenate.
- ☑ IV infusions running maximally with pressure bags or rapid infuser.
- ☑ When surgeon ready **and blood is available/cell salvage system primed** induce with a suitable hypnotic (e.g. propofol/remifentanil, etomidate/fentanyl, or ketamine with suxamethonium). As soon as intubation is confirmed ($ETCO_2$), surgeons can start. Expect a degree of cardiovascular decompensation on muscle relaxation.
- ☑ Treat further hypotension with rapid infusion of IV fluid and vasopressors/inotropic agents.
- ☑ Clamping the aorta usually allows some measure of haemodynamic stability for the first time. However, collaterals will continue to bleed.
- ☑ IV fluids/blood to maintain Hb 80 g/L. Platelets and FFP as indicated—if in doubt, give them. Use thromboelastography to guide blood replacement therapy. Get a TEG running early and repeat every hour.
- ☑ Unclamping the aorta is hazardous. Fill the patient (CVP >10 mmHg), mildly hyperventilate to P_aCO_2 of 4.2 kPa—but combination of metabolic acidosis, relative hypovolaemia, vasodilatation, and myocardial stunning will usually necessitate inotropic support. Start adrenaline infusion (2 mg/40 mL at 1–10 mL/h). Consider giving calcium gluconate (10 mL 10% IV) and bicarbonate if pH <7.1 (but not simultaneously in the same IV!).
- ☑ Adjunctive therapy for renal protection may include:
  - mannitol (25 g IV)
  - furosemide (20–80 mg IV)

These drugs may increase urine output but there is no evidence that they reduce the incidence of renal failure.

- ☑ Hypothermia is a particular hazard, warm *all* fluids and use warm air blower on upper body (contraindicated on lower body during cross-clamp). Monitor temperature.
- ☑ NG tube (orogastric if severe coagulopathy present).

Subsequent management

- Overnight ventilation in ITU.
- Hypothermia, renal impairment, blood loss, and coagulopathy are common postoperative problems.

Special considerations

- Epidural analgesia rarely appropriate.
- Cardiac output monitoring (e.g. LiDCO Rapid gives useful information during cross-clamping about fluid management).
- However oesophageal Doppler can be misleading during cross-clamp period.

- Be prepared to use group-compatible, non-crossmatched blood if necessary.
- If the bleeding cannot be stopped, the surgeon may pack the abdomen and transfer the patient to ITU. Consider giving recombinant factor 7 (NovoSeven) 2.4 mg which has been shown to be effective in some cases of uncontrolled bleeding. Make every effort to correct other abnormalities first (FFP/cryo/platelets/red cells/temperature).

Emergency endovascular aneurysm repair (EEVAR)

- Many centres are now using endovascular rather than open repair for patients with ruptured AAA.
- A guidewire is passed up the femoral artery which is then dilated up before a balloon is passed up the aorta above the rupture and inflated. This should facilitate haemodynamic stability.
- The stent is then placed appropriately and deployed.
- Anaesthetic techniques vary but it is common to place the balloon under local anaesthesia ± sedation, then once there is haemodynamic stability, if required, induce general anaesthesia.
- A large randomized controlled trial (IMPROVE) of 600 patients was conducted in 2013. Early results indicate the mortality of the two groups was similar, with better outcome from cases done using LA rather than GA.

Further reading

Badger, S., Bedenis, R., Blair, P.H., Ellis, P., Kee, F., Harkin, D.W. (2014). Endovascular treatment for ruptured abdominal aortic aneurysm. *Cochrane Database of Systematic Reviews*, **7**, CD005261.

IMPROVE Trial Investigators (2017). Comparative clinical effectiveness and cost-effectiveness of endovascular strategy v open repair for ruptured abdominal aortic aneurysm: three year results of the IMPROVE randomised trial. *BMJ*, **359**, j4859.

Stoneham, M., Murray, D., Foss, N. (2014). Emergency surgery: the big three-abdominal aortic aneurysm, laparotomy and hip fracture. *Anaesthesia*, **69**, Suppl 1, 70–80.

☼ Emergency laparotomy

Presentation

Patients presenting with non-elective surgical abdominal pathology are a heterogeneous group (see Table 14.8). A minority present with sepsis and a clear diagnosis of perforation, anastomotic leak, or ischaemia. They require rapid diagnostic CT, prompt antibiotics, and emergency surgical source control. A large majority present with bowel obstruction or localized sepsis (e.g. contained perforation) and may undergo a period of conservative management. If and when laparotomy is required it is expedited rather than a true emergency.

Key messages

1. **Rapid accurate diagnosis** with systems to facilitate early CT and early involvement of consultant surgeon.
2. **Administration of broad-spectrum antibiotics within 1 h** of presentation for patients with sepsis or perforated viscus.
3. **Prevention of organ dysfunction** with early goal-directed fluid resuscitation.
4. For emergency cases **time from decision to operate to induction of anaesthesia should be less than 6 h**.
5. **Identification of high-risk cases** using preoperative risk estimation using score such as P-POSSUM.
6. Admission of high risk (>5% mortality) cases to **HDU/ICU** postoperatively.

Key elements of care

In the UK 30-day mortality after non-elective laparotomy is around 15%— far higher than high-risk elective surgery and highly variable between centres (4–44%). Use of care bundles for emergency laparotomy reduces mortality. Bundles should contain the key elements outlined in the Royal College of Surgeons' (UK) recommendations:

Preoperative

- Early identification of sick patients using early warning score (EWS) within 1 h of arrival.
- Early involvement of surgical registrar for sick patients (e.g. EWS >5).
- Rapid accurate diagnosis with systems to facilitate early CT, reported by consultant radiologist and early involvement of consultant surgeon.
- Administration of broad-spectrum antibiotics within 1 h of presentation for patients with sepsis or perorated viscus. In patients with severe sepsis, mortality rises by 7.6% with every hour of antibiotic delay. Choice of antibiotic is guided by local protocols (e.g. amoxicillin 1 g tds/metronidazole 500 mg tds/gentamicin 5 mg/kg od). When presentation has been delayed consider upgrading to Tazocin® (piperacillin/tazobactam 4.5 g tds) +/− antifungal agent such as fluconazole.

Table 14.8 Aetiology and presentation of patients for non-elective laparotomy

Aetiology	Presentation
Emergency laparotomy	Decision to operate to induction of anaesthesia within 2–6 h
Perforated viscus (e.g. caecum, duodenum, diverticular, anastomotic leak).	Septic; risk of organ dysfunction/multiorgan failure. Usually peritonitic. Immediate fluid resuscitation. IV antibiotics within 1 h of presentation and surgical source control within 2 h (max 6 h).
Ischaemic bowel (e.g. discrete SMA/IMA occlusion or part of general hypoperfusion state).	Variable presentation; often difficult to diagnose. CT abdomen may be diagnostic but high false negative rate. Elevated and rising arterial lactate raises suspicion. High mortality.
Abdominal haemorrhage (e.g. spontaneous, or traumatic laceration of liver, spleen, or mesentery).	Conservative management may be appropriate. Interventional radiology has a key role—CT angiogram followed by angiography and coiling.
Failed conservative management (e.g. of contained diverticular abscess, adhesional bowel obstruction, or haemorrhage).	As below, require regular senior surgical review to detect deterioration, sepsis, bowel ischaemia, perforation.
Expedited laparotomy	Decision to operate to induction of anaesthesia within 12–24 h
Bowel obstruction (e.g. adhesional, colonic cancer).	Vomiting, abdominal distension, and pain. CT is essential to differentiate cause. Obstructing cancer will not resolve—surgery when fluid resuscitated and electrolyte abnormalities, anaemia, acute organ dysfunction corrected. High proportion of cases with adhesional obstruction resolve with conservative management. Risk or ischaemia, perforation, aspiration of vomit—must be closely observed with regular senior surgical review and arterial lactate.

- Early aggressive fluid resuscitation to prevent organ dysfunction. Mortality from sepsis increases by 10–15% for each sequential organ failure. Hypoperfusion of organs is detected by end organ damage and high or rising arterial lactate. Aggressive fluid resuscitation should start in the emergency department and continue throughout the perioperative period. Ideally this should be goal-directed, using a cardiac output monitor. Fluid responsiveness is indicated by an appropriate (10–12%) increase in stroke volume after a fluid challenge of 200–300 mL.

- Cardiac output monitor may not be available. Target mean arterial pressure >65 mmHg (higher if normally hypertensive). When patient no longer shows favourable response to fluid, start vasopressor (usually noradrenaline) via central venous catheter. Monitor end organ function, arterial lactate, and pH.
- Transfuse red blood cells if Hb <70 g/L (or <90 g/L if significant ischaemic heart disease)—this will improve oxygen delivery.
- Compromise to be considered between achieving acceptable level of resuscitation and need to allow surgical source control.
- Use scoring system such as P-POSSUM to estimate 30-day mortality. Prior to surgery 'operative findings' are a best guess.
- Plan for high-risk cases (P-POSSUM mortality >5%) to be admitted to HDU/ICU.
- Patients with sepsis and/or perforation should reach theatre within 6 h of decision to operate.

Special considerations—conservative management

- Some patients will undergo a period of conservative management and a proportion will recover without the need for surgery.
- The group that do not resolve are at high risk of rapid and catastrophic deterioration due to sepsis, bowel ischaemia, dehydration, and electrolyte imbalance. Unresolving adhesional bowel obstruction may result in aspiration of faeculent vomit.
- Criteria for close monitoring and regular senior surgical review should be agreed. Any deterioration in condition should be detected quickly and a senior surgeon must decide whether to continue conservative management or proceed to emergency or expedited laparotomy.
- It is important that this group is differentiated from those who are felt to be too high risk for surgery and so take a more palliative pathway of care.

Lung protective ventilation
- Tidal volume 6–8 mL/kg
- PEEP 6 cmH$_2$O and increased as F$_1$O$_2$ increases
- Plateau pressure <32 cmH$_2$O
- F$_1$O$_2$ to achieve adequate oxygenation (P$_a$O$_2$ >9 kPa)
- Slow and gentle lung recruitment manoeuvres to 40 cmH$_2$O for 40 s every 40 min

Perioperative
- Consider arterial line insertion prior to induction. This is essential for real-time BP monitoring and serial lactate measurement (also measurable by VBG). Some cardiac output monitors (e.g. LiDCO rapid and PiCCO Plus) can be connected to a standard arterial line.
- Emergency vasoactive drugs should be prepared prior to induction. Metaraminol (0.5–1 mg IV) if HR >60 bpm, otherwise ephedrine (3–6 mg IV). For those at high risk of cardiovascular collapse adrenaline 1:100 000 can be administered in 0.5–1 mL IV boluses.
- Rapid sequence induction. Ketamine (1–2 mg/kg slowly IV) may be used if marked hypotension or cardiovascular instability.

- Use CO monitoring to guide fluid administration in order to optimize (not maximize) filling. Beware that young fit people will often demonstrate a response to fluid challenge until the point of complete circulatory overload.
- Insert CVC for those with sepsis or haemodynamic stability. Start an infusion of noradrenaline if unresponsive to fluid resuscitation. Mix 5 mg noradrenaline in 50 mL 5% glucose and infuse at 1–30 mL/h to achieve MAP >65 mmHg.
- Lung protective ventilation reduces morbidity, complications, and length of stay, even for patients who will be extubated following surgery.
- If the degree of contamination is gross, the surgeon may elect to leave the abdomen open, for return to theatre in 24–48 h. This is also essential if the abdomen is hard to close and causes abdominal compartment syndrome. This can be detected by monitoring the intravesical pressure via a needle inserted into the sample port of the urinary catheter. Discuss this with the surgeon if the abdominal pressure is >20 mmHg, prior to leaving theatre. Untreated (by leaving the abdomen open) this will cause multiorgan failure.
- Consider postoperative analgesia; rectus sheath catheters, epidural or opioid PCA.

Postoperative management
- Recalculate P-POSSUM score with accurate intraoperative data.
- Admit to ICU/HDU if predicted mortality is >5% or if indicated for other reasons (e.g. respiratory failure or ongoing sedation for open abdomen).

Special considerations
- Highest mortality shown to be for patients who initially go to the ward postoperatively and subsequently deteriorate.

Further reading

Holst, L.B., Haase, N., Wetterslev, J., et al. (2014). Lower versus higher haemoglobin threshold for transfusion in patients with septic shock *New England Journal of Medicine*, **371**, 1381–91.

Huddart, S., Peden, C.J., Swart, M., et al. (2015). Use of a pathway quality improvement bundle to reduce mortality after emergency laparotomy. *British Journal of Surgery*, **102**(1), 57–66.

Pearce, R.M., Moreno, R.P., Bauer, P., et al. (2012). Mortality after surgery in Europe: a 7-day cohort study. *Lancet*, **380**, 1059–65.

Royal College of Surgeons of England and The Department of Health (2011). *The Higher Risk Surgical Patient—Towards Improved Care for a Forgotten Group*. Available at: https://www.rcseng.ac.uk/library-and-publications/rcs-publications/docs/the-higher-risk-general-surgical-patient/

Saunders, D.I., Murray, D., Pichel, A.C., Varley, S., Peden, C.J.; UK Emergency Laparotomy Network (2012). Variations in mortality after emergency laparotomy: the first report of the UK Emergency Laparotomy Network. *British Journal of Anaesthesia*, **109**, 368–75.

Severgnini, P., Selmo, G., Lanza, C., et al. (2013). Protective mechanical ventilation during general anesthesia for open abdominal surgery improves postoperative pulmonary function. *Anesthesiology*, **118**, 1307–21.

Solomkin, J.S., Mazuski, J.E., Bradley, J.S., et al. (2010). Diagnosis and management of complicated intra-abdominal infection in adults and children: guidelines by the Surgical Infection Society and the Infectious Diseases Society of America. *Clinical Infectious Diseases*, **50**, 133–64.

Vincent, J.-L., Sakr, Y., Sprung, C.L., et al. (2006). Sepsis in European intensive care units: results of the SOAP study. *Critical Care Medicine*, **34**, 344–53.

Practical procedures

Louise Cossey and Bruce McCormick

Airway

Breathing

Circulation

Miscellaneous

☠ Cricothyroidotomy

Definition
Airway access via the cricothyroid membrane. Can be needle/cannula cricothyroidotomy, formal cricothyroidotomy, or surgical tracheostomy.

Indications
- Last resort in failed intubation in order to achieve oxygenation.
- Bronchial toilet in patients with poor clearance of sputum (e.g. Mini-Trach®).
- Administration of supplemental oxygen.
- Administration of nebulized drugs.

Contraindications
Relative
- Unclear or distorted anatomy.
- Surgical cricothyroidotomy not recommended in children <12 y.

Anatomy
- Cricothyroid membrane lies between thyroid cartilage superiorly and cricoid cartilage inferiorly.
- Palpate anterior part of neck in the midline. Most prominent cartilaginous point is thyroid cartilage. With index finger, palpate downwards until you feel a hollow between the thyroid cartilage and cricoid cartilage—the cricothyroid membrane (Figure 15.1).

Scalpel cricothyroidotomy
Description
- Insertion of a cuffed ET tube through the cricothyroid membrane.
- For management of unanticipated difficult tracheal intubation, ➔ see p. 84.

Technique
- After cleaning the neck, follow the Difficult Airway Society guidelines in Figure 15.2.

Complications
- Aspiration
- Creation of false passage

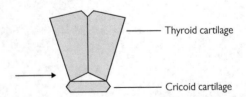

Figure 15.1 Cricothyroid membrane (arrow).

Failed intubation, failed oxygenation in the paralysed, anaesthetised patient

CALL FOR HELP

Continue 100% O$_2$
Declare CICO

Plan D: Emergency front of neck access

Continue to give oxygen via upper airway
Ensure neuromuscular blockade
position patient to extend neck

Scalpel cricothyroidotomy

Equipment: 1. Scalpel (number 10 blade)
2. Bougie
3. Tube (cuffed 6.0mm ID)

Laryngeal handshake to identify cricothyroid membrane

Palpable cricothyroid membrane
Transverse stab incision through cricothyroid membrane
Turn blade through 90°(sharp edge caudally)
Slide coude tip of bougie along blade into trachea
Railroad lubricated 6.0mm cuffed tracheal tube into trachea
Ventilate, inflate cuff and confirm position with capnography
Secure tube

Impalpable cricothyroid membrane
Make an 8–10cm vertical skin incision, caudad to cephalad
Use blunt dissection with fingers of both hands to separate tissues
Identify and stabilise the larynx
Proceed with technique for palpable cricothyroid membrane as above

---

Post-operative care and follow up
• Postpone surgery unless immediately life threatening
• Urgent surgical review of cricothyroidotomy site
• Document and follow up as in main flow chart

This flowchart forms part of the DAS Guidelines for unanticipated difficult intubation in adults 2015 and should be used in conjunction with the text.

Figure 15.2 Emergency front of neck access.

- Tracheal transection
- Haemorrhage
- Oesophageal/tracheal laceration
- Mediastinal emphysema
- Vocal cord damage
- Subglottic stenosis (late)

Needle/cannula cricothyroidotomy

Description

- Insertion of a wide-bore cannula through the cricothyroid membrane.
- Allows oxygenation via a 14 G cannula for up to 30 min.
- Usually achieved via Sanders injector or, where not available, using the system described next.
- Ventilation is not adequate and hypercapnia will occur.
- ENT/Maxillofacial surgeon should be called urgently to carry out emergency tracheostomy.
- Cannula can be upgraded to a wider bore airway using formal cricothyroidotomy kit.
- Be prepared! Familiarize yourself with the equipment available in each department of your hospital for:
  - gaining access to the trachea
  - connecting a cannula to an oxygen supply
  - ventilating the patient.

Equipment checklist

- Antiseptic solution.
- Scalpel blade (not essential).
- 14 G cannula attached to 10 mL syringe containing 3–4 mL sterile saline.
- System for connecting cannula to oxygen delivery device—usually a Sanders injector or Manujet® (a Sanders injector with a pressure gauge and adjustable driving pressure, Figure 15.3).
- Where an injector is not available, the following alternative can be used:
  - remove the drip chamber of an IV giving set and attach the end to the common gas outlet of an anaesthetic machine using the connector from a size 3.0 mm endotracheal tube. Attach the Luer lock end to a three-way tap and then the cricothyroidotomy cannula (Figure 15.4).

Technique

- Patient supine. Clean and extend neck.
- Ensure muscle relaxation. Continue to give oxygen via upper airway.
- Fix skin with traction. Identify the cricothyroid membrane and stabilize trachea with thumb and forefinger.
- Insert cannula/syringe directing needle 45° caudally, aspirating as cannula advances. Aspiration of air shows tracheal entry.
- Remove syringe and withdraw stylet, advancing cannula downwards.
- Hold cannula securely to patient's neck *yourself* and avoid kinking.
- Attach oxygen delivery system as previously described. Oxygenation achieved by directing oxygen flow through cannula for 1 s and then allowing gas to escape for 3 s. Expiration of gas should occur through the patient's airway—it may be useful to ensure this is possible by inserting an oropharyngeal airway or LMA.
- In emergencies, if cricothyroid membrane cannot be felt (e.g. obesity), insert needle in midline below thyroid cartilage. Insertion between tracheal rings is acceptable.

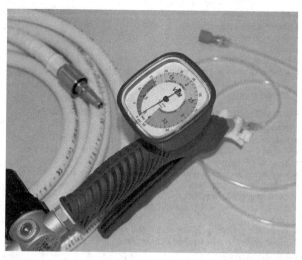

Figure 15.3 Manujet (VBM, Germany).

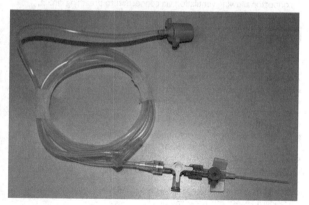

Figure 15.4 Alternative oxygen delivery system.

- Resistance to needle insertion is usually due to cricoid cartilage or tracheal ring if too far caudal. Withdraw needle 5 mm, and redirect 3 mm caudally.

Complications
- Kinking:
  - Failure of expiration (may occur if airway not patent)
- Inadequate ventilation:
  - Bleeding from skin (use pressure—rarely life-threatening)

- Airway soiling (blood)
- Oesophageal laceration
- Pneumothorax
- Haematoma
- Posterior tracheal wall perforation:
  - Subcutaneous and mediastinal emphysema (beware use of Sanders injector with cannula misplaced outside trachea)
- Thyroid damage

Formal/Seldinger cricothyroidotomy (e.g. Mini-Trach®)

Description

- Inserted using commercially available kits—usually 4.0 mm ID tube.
- Allows ventilation using Sanders injector or attachment to anaesthetic breathing circuit via 15 mm connector.
- In an emergency, can be used as first line by anaesthetists familiar with technique and equipment.
- Used to upgrade needle/cannula cricothyroidotomy.
- May be used electively to aid bronchial toilet (e.g. Mini-Trach II®, Portex).
- Principal disadvantage is lack of cuff seal (may need to manually occlude upper airway to achieve adequate ventilation of lungs).

Equipment checklist

- Seldinger technique—most sets have cannula with 15 mm standard connector allowing ventilation via connection to breathing circuit, e.g. Cook Melker catheter. In the elective situation, Mini-Trach® kit is usually used.
- QuikTrach® kit—a sharp, curved, conical needle tip allows insertion through the skin without a scalpel incision and immediate connection to breathing circuit.

Technique

- Patient supine. Clean and extend neck.
- Ensure muscle relaxation if used for airway rescue. Continue to give oxygen via upper airway.
- Scalpel incision to skin.
- Passage of Seldinger wire into trachea allows insertion of a wider gauge cannula (4.0 mm ID) mounted on a dilator.
- Shoulder of tube may cause it to catch on the cricothyroid membrane. Try twisting to and fro while inserting, or cut through membrane alongside wire using scalpel.
- Standard 15 mm connector allows oxygenation and ventilation using standard anaesthetic breathing circuit.
- Use local anaesthetic when inserting Mini-Trach® electively.

Paediatric implications

- Needle or cannula cricothyroidotomy is preferred to surgical cricothyroidotomy in children under 12 years of age.
- Use a 20 or 18 G cannula for an infant, a 16 G cannula for small children, and 14 G cannula for children over 12 y.

ⓘ Intubating laryngeal mask airway (ILMA)

Definition
Variant of LMA that is wide and short enough to allow passage of a specialized ETT into the trachea (Figure 15.5). Success rate for intubation is 88% in routine cases.

Indications

Elective use
- Anticipated difficult intubation where ventilation is not a problem.

Emergency use
- Failed intubation— ➲ see p. 84.

Contraindications

Absolute
- Limited mouth opening, severe trismus.

Relative
- Does not guarantee ventilation will be possible—does not replace fibreoptic intubation.
- Cervical spine injury.
- Prior radiotherapy or abnormal neck anatomy (use fibreoptic guidance).

Equipment checklist
- Appropriately sized ILMA (see Table 15.1).
- Specialized, silicone reinforced ETT. Diameter of all sizes of ILMA allows passage of sizes 6.0, 6.5, 7.0, 7.5, or 8.0 mm.
- Stabilizing rod—aids removal of ILMA over ETT after placement (alternative is bougie with several layers of tape applied to one end).

Preparation
- Patient anaesthetised.
- Apply lubricant to posterior surface of ILMA and completely deflate cuff.
- Check chosen lubricated ETT fits smoothly into ILMA, removing it before use.

Technique
- Head in neutral position.
- Holding device by handle, insert ILMA.
- Inflate ILMA cuff to recommended volume. Ventilate patient via breathing circuit.
- Adjust position to achieve best capnography trace (a long horizontal plateau on expiration).

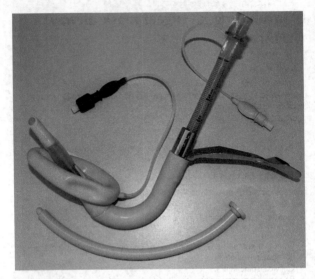

Figure 15.5 Intubating laryngeal mask airway.

Table 15.1 LMA-Fast Trach™ sizes

LMA-Fast Trach™ size	Patient weight
3	30–50 kg children
4	50–70 kg adult
5	70–100 kg adult

- Alternatively, confirm position using bronchoscope or transilluminate neck using lightwand.
- If correctly positioned, patient can be intubated blindly by passing lubricated ETT through ILMA. If necessary, rotate ETT 90° anticlockwise to negotiate right arytenoid cartilage. Attach 15 mm connector to ETT, confirm correct positioning in standard way and oxygenate patient. The LMA can either be left in position for the duration of the case or removed.
- Remove ILMA using tube stabilizer with 15 mm connector unattached.

Failed intubation using ILMA

- If it is not possible to intubate the patient after two attempts, check ILMA position and glottic orientation with bronchoscope, or try larger ILMA. Some anaesthetists prefer to mount the ETT on a bronchoscope routinely.
- Avoid prolonged intubation attempts, which will cause bleeding and swelling. Emergency cricothyroidotomy (● see p. 454) should not be delayed if oxygenation is inadequate.

Complications

- Sore throat
- Hoarse voice
- Epiglottic oedema
- Oesophageal intubation (5%)
- Oesophageal rupture

Paediatric implications

- The smallest available ILMA is a size 3, which may be used for children of >30 kg.
- Intubation of children smaller than this may be achieved through a standard LMA, although correct LMA positioning is more difficult with the smaller LMA sizes (Table 15.2).

Intubation through a classic LMA

- The fenestrations of the laryngeal aperture of the LMA may need to be removed to allow passage of the ETT.
- Position laryngeal mask in the normal fashion and use as a guide for blind intubation by passing an appropriately sized ETT through laryngeal mask.
- Recommended maximum tube sizes are shown in Table 15.3.
- In about 70% of cases the ETT will be guided directly into the trachea (but only 50% with cricoid pressure applied).
- The ETT can be stabilized in position as the LMA is removed, using the plunger from a 5 mL syringe.
- Bronchoscopy may both enhance placement and confirm correct positioning. Mount the ETT on the bronchoscope, which is then used as a bougie for insertion of the tube. The bronchoscope and then the laryngeal mask are removed.

Table 15.2 Paediatric LMA sizes

Size 2.5	20–30 kg
Size 2	10–20 kg
Size 1.5	5–10 kg
Size 1	<5 kg

Table 15.3 Maximum ETT size vs. LMA size

Laryngeal mask size	ETT size (ID, mm)
1	3.5
1.5	4.0
2	4.5
2.5	4.5
3	5.0
4	6.0 cuffed
5	7.5 cuffed

• An alternative is to insert an airway exchange catheter (Cook®) through the LMA. After removal of the LMA, oxygenation is possible while an ETT is railroaded over the catheter. A gum elastic bougie can be used, but without the facility for oxygenation during the exchange.

Further reading

Kihara, S., Watanabe, S., Brimacombe, J., Taguchi, N., Yaguchi, Y., Yamasaki, Y. (2000). Segmental cervical spine movement with the intubating laryngeal mask during manual in-line stabilization in patients with cervical pathology undergoing cervical spine surgery. *Anesthesia and Analgesia*, **91**, 195–200.

① Awake fibreoptic intubation

Definition

Fibreoptic endotracheal intubation in an awake patient.

Indications

- Known or suspected difficult intubation.
- Known or suspected cervical spine injury (fracture or ligamentous injury).
- Morbid obesity.
- Poor mouth opening (rheumatoid arthritis, TMJ trauma).
- Full stomach, but difficult intubation anticipated or suxamethonium contraindicated (burns, spinal injury).

Contraindications

Absolute

- Uncooperative patient.
- Severe stridor secondary to perilaryngeal obstruction.
- Known mid- or low-tracheal stenosis.
- Allergy to local anaesthetics.
- Fibreoptic intubation is not indicated in the 'can't intubate . . . can't ventilate' situation.

Relative

- Airway soiling (bloody airway).
- Children.

Preparation

- Full clinical assessment of airway.
- Explanation and consent—cooperation essential. During passage of the ETT through the vocal cords over the bronchoscope, the patient will feel they cannot breathe and should be warned of this.
- Assess nasal passages for patency (on history and unilateral occlusion).
- Calculate maximum dose of local anaesthetic – 9 mg/kg of lignocaine
  - Antisialogogue to reduce secretions and optimize effect of local anaesthetic. Either 400 µg IM 1 hour before or 200 µg IV in the anaesthetic room, and xylometazoline 0.1% nasal spray.
- IV access.
- Oxygen via nasal catheter.

Technique

See Table 15.4.

Multiple variations exist—➐ see under 'Special considerations', p. 465.

- Use mild sedation—midazolam (1–2 mg) and fentanyl (50–100 µg) or remifentanil infusion (<0.2 µg/kg/min). Verbal contact must be maintained at all times.
- Determine more patent nostril, and spray with cocaine solution (1 mL 5%).

Table 15.4 Checklist

Decongestant	Xylometazoline—0.1% or phenylephrine 1% nasal spray—administer in advance if possible
Local anaesthetic drugs	Cocaine 5–10%
	Cocaine and lidocaine gel 2%
	Lidocaine spray 10%
	Four syringes of 1.5 mL lidocaine 2%
Sedative drugs	Midazolam, fentanyl/remifentanil
	Induction agents and neuromuscular blockers
Equipment	6.0/6.5 mm nasal ETT
	6/7 mm nasopharyngeal airways (cut along length)
	Forrester spray/atomizer
	Safety pin
	Warm water in container
	Nasal oxygen catheter
Equipment checks	Check bronchoscope light functions properly, clean tip, and focus
	Check oxygen can be delivered down suction port, and lidocaine injected freely

- Dilate nasal passage with warmed 6 mm then 7 mm nasopharyngeal airway lubricated with cocaine or lidocaine gel (cut 7 mm along long axis and insert safety pin to aid grip during manipulation of scope).
- Spray oropharynx with lidocaine 10% and use Forrester spray/atomizer to topically anaesthetise pharynx using lidocaine 2% (2–4 mL) as far back as possible.
- Instil oxygen (2 L/min) through bronchoscope to oxygenate patient, clear secretions from the tip, and aid atomization of injected local anaesthetic.
- Pass **lubricated** bronchoscope through the nasopharyngeal airway and, having visualized the vocal cords, instil 1.5 mL lidocaine 2% directly onto the cords. Pass through the cords and repeat for tracheal inlet. The trachea can be identified by circular rings of cartilage.
- Load warmed, lubricated ETT onto bronchoscope and re-insert through nasal airway into trachea.
- Remove the 'split' 7 mm nasopharyngeal airway and advance the ETT over the scope, maintaining the view of the trachea as you advance—be careful not to advance too far or irritation of the carina will cause coughing.
- 90° turn of ETT anticlockwise allows leading edge of bevel to pass between cords (i.e. bevel facing posteriorly).

- Remove bronchoscope, carefully visualizing correct tube placement, and confirm with capnography and bag movement. Do not inflate cuff yet as this may cause panic (increased resistance to respiration).
- Induce anaesthesia, inflate cuff, and fix tube securely.

Complications

Poor compliance/coughing, bleeding in airway (from nasal dilatation), excess secretions, laryngospasm, vomiting, and aspiration.

Special considerations

- Where it is not possible to instil oxygen through the bronchoscope, administer oxygen 2–4 L/min via nasal cannula or sponge.
- **Cricothyroid puncture**—this technique may be used, but tends to cause vigorous coughing. Identify the cricothyroid membrane (between thyroid cartilage and cricoid ring) and raise a small subcutaneous wheal with 2% lidocaine. Vertically insert a 20/22 G cannula attached to a 5 mL syringe containing 2.5 mL lidocaine until air can be freely aspirated. This confirms placement within the trachea. The cannula sheath may not pass easily through the membrane, in which case a 23/25 G needle can be used instead. Inject 2–3 mL 2% lidocaine.
- **Choice of ETT**—the Portex preformed nasal 'Blue Line' ETT is extremely pliable when warmed. A 6.5 mm tube fits most people, although occasionally a 6 mm may be needed. Shorten proximally by 3 cm to prevent the tube impinging on the nasopharyngeal airway before removal. An alternative would be a 6 or 6.5 mm armoured tube. Standard ETT's will tend to cause nasal bleeding.
- **Difficulty in visualizing larynx**—ask the patient to protrude their tongue, swallow, or phonate (may improve view).
- 'Red out' indicates too far (oesophagus) or not midline (piriform fossa). Pull back to soft palate and ensure fibrescope is midline. Dimming room lights may allow transcutaneous visualization of the tip.
- **'Tube first' technique**—use 6/7 mm nasopharyngeal airways to dilate nasal passage, then insert ETT 10 cm to back of nasal cavity. Pass bronchoscope through ETT and position with good view of laryngeal inlet. If required, spray further 2% lidocaine onto cords at this stage. Advance bronchoscope into trachea (view tracheal rings). Use bronchoscope as bougie, advancing tube over bronchoscope and into trachea (tip of the bronchoscope in neutral position).
- **Considerations for oral route**—use fibrescopic oropharyngeal airway (e.g. Berman airway®, Vital Signs, or Ovassapian intubating airway, Hudson; Figure 15.6) which protects fibrescope, holds tongue forward, and keeps scope in midline. NB: Use airway of correct size to ensure tip is just above the laryngeal inlet. Technically much more difficult.
- Contraindications to nasal insertion include coagulopathy, basal skull fracture, CSF leak, and severe nasal disease.
- Positioning depends on preference, either:
  - patient sitting at least 45° upright with operator facing them
  - patient supine with operator in normal intubating position

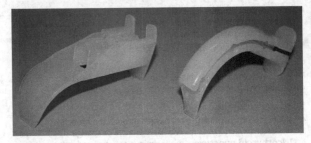

Figure 15.6 Berman airway and Ovassapian intubating airway.

⑦ Lightwand intubation aids

Definition
Stylet with an end-light to guide intubation by transillumination of the soft tissues of the neck.

Indications
Anticipated or unexpected difficult airway, especially poor mouth opening or neck movement.

Relative contraindications
- Environments with excess ambient light.
- Any facial hair or neck pathology that hinders transillumination.

Complications
As for any attempted oral or nasal intubation.

Equipment
- Lightwands are mouldable fibreoptic stylets with external (Imagica™) or internal (Trachlight™, Laerdal) light sources. They may also be combined with fibreoptic technology and attached to a laryngoscope handle, e.g. Levitan FPS, Clarus medical (Figure 15.7).

Preparation
- Load ETT on to the lubricated stylet with the end of the stylet remaining just inside the tube.
- Mould the tube into the 'hockey stick' position by bending it to 90° 3–6 cm from the end.
- Keep ambient light to a minimum.

Technique
- Administer induction of anaesthesia.
- Slightly extend the patient's head unless the cervical spine is at risk.

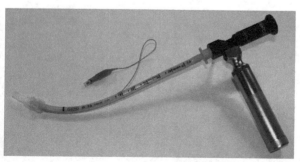

Figure 15.7 Lightwand.

- Ensure the lightwand is turned on and hold in a pencil grip.
- Open the mouth and provide jaw thrust to elevate the epiglottis with non-dominant hand.
- Introduce the stylet into the oropharynx from the side but rotate into the midline as it passes posterior to the tongue.
- A circle of light in the midline at the level of the hyoid indicates that the tip is lying in the vallecula.
- The light will remain continuously bright as the stylet and tube are advanced successfully into the trachea.
- The stylet is removed and placement confirmed in the usual manner.

Troubleshooting

- Red glow seen off midline—tip in piriform fossa and stylet should be withdrawn and repositioned.
- Briefly losing light and then recovering a dissipated glow indicates oesophageal intubation.

① Retrograde intubation

Definition

Intubation of trachea achieved by passing a guidewire through crico-thyroid membrane and out of the mouth. This acts as a guide for the ETT.

Indications

- Management of predicted difficult intubation.
- Emergency airway access where laryngoscopy is difficult but mask ventilation is possible.

Contraindications

Relative

- Coagulopathy.
- Obscure cricoid or cricothyroid anatomy.
- Infection of cricothyroid membrane.
- Goitre.

Equipment checklist

- Antiseptic solution and fenestrated drape.
- Gauze swabs.
- Scalpel blade.
- Retrograde intubation kit:
  - commercially available kits avoid difficulties with equipment (e.g. Cook Retrograde Intubation Set®).
  - 16 G epidural (Tuohy) needle or 16 G cannula, 10 mL syringe containing 3–4 mL sterile saline, guidewire.
- Appropriately sized lubricated ETT (min. ID 4 mm for Cook set).

Preparation

- In predicted difficult intubation, airway is anaesthetised as described for awake fibreoptic intubation (➲ see p. 463).
- Patient supine, neck extended.

Technique

See Figure 15.8.

- Clean and drape area.
- Aseptic technique.
- Advance needle or cannula, with 10 mL syringe attached, through cricothyroid membrane in midline.
- Aim slightly cephalad (compared to caudad for cricothyroidotomy).
- Entry into trachea indicated by aspiration of air into syringe.
- Remove syringe and stylet if using cannula.
- Insert J-end of guidewire aiming cephalad, until tip can be retrieved from mouth, using a tongue depressor and Magill forceps. Rolling the wire between your fingers makes it stand away from the mucosa in the oropharynx, aiding retrieval.

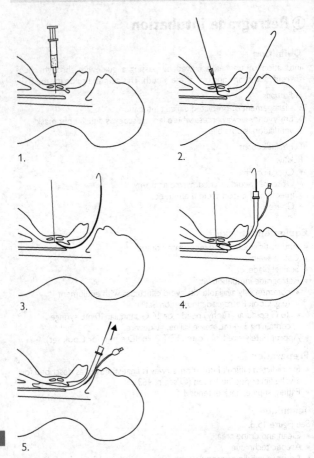

Figure 15.8 Technique of retrograde intubation.

- In specialized sets, black mark on wire should be visible at access site, to ensure sufficient length of wire is available in mouth to manipulate the ETT.
- Remove cannula. (A bronchoscope can be placed onto wire at this point, via the suction port, to assess wire placement.)
- Cook set allows anterograde passage of an 11 Fr catheter, which aids subsequent passage of ETT. Internal diameter of ETT must be at least 4 mm to use this device.

Table 15.5 Appropriate dilator sizes for retrograde intubation

ETT size (ID/mm)	Ureteric/nephrostomy dilator size [French gauge (OD/mm)]
3.5–4	10F (3.3)
4.5	12F (4.0)
5	14F (4.7)
>5	16F (5.3)

- The ETT can be mounted on a ureteric or percutaneous nephrostomy dilator (Boston Scientific, MA, USA) to aid passage through the vocal cords. The nephrostomy dilators are shorter (35 cm) and more easily used with a relatively short guide wire. Appropriate sizes are shown in Table 15.5.
- Pass ETT over wire with 90° turn anticlockwise—allows leading edge of bevel to pass between cords (i.e. bevel facing posterior). When tenting is noted at the cricothyroid access site, rotate the tube 180°.
- Maintain control of wire throughout placement.
- Remove guide wire through ETT to avoid soiling neck puncture site.
- Inflate cuff and confirm placement in the usual manner.

Complications

- As for needle/cannula cricothyroidotomy (see p. 456).
- Bleeding in airway, difficulties passing the ETT past the vocal cords, epiglottis, or glottic structures.

Paediatric implications

Compliance difficult in younger children. May be possible in children over 12 y.

! Chest drain insertion

Definition
Insertion of catheter into pleural cavity.

Indications
- Pneumothorax.
- Traumatic haemothorax or haemopneumothorax.
- Pleural effusion.
- Empyema.
- Postoperative drainage (e.g. thoracotomy, oesophagectomy, cardiac surgery).

Contraindications
Absolute (without further investigation)
- Unclear clinical and radiological diagnosis (e.g. bullous lung disease or pneumothorax).
- Lung adherent to chest wall.

Relative
- Tension pneumothorax should initially be treated by needle thoracocentesis.
- Coagulopathy, thrombocytopenia, anticoagulation.
- Drainage of postpneumonectomy space is relatively contraindicated.

Note
The National Patient Safety Agency (UK) advises that:
- Chest drains are only inserted by staff with relevant competencies and adequate supervision.
- Ultrasound guidance is strongly advised when inserting a drain for fluid.

Anatomy
- Awake patient 45° head up. Anaesthetised patient may be supine.
- Place ipsilateral arm behind head to expose axillary area.
- Triangle between anterior border of latissimus dorsi, lateral border of pectoralis major, and horizontal line at level of nipple indicates safest area, with minimal risk of damage to underlying structures.
- Insertion site:
  - mid-axillary line, fifth intercostal space.
  - 'triangle of safety' lies between the lateral border of pectoralis major, the anterior border of latissimus dorsi and above the nipple line (see Figure 15.9).
  - pneumothoraces may be treated by catheter inserted apically (mid-clavicular line, second intercostal space). This is also the site for emergency needle thoracocentesis.

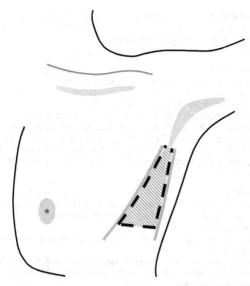

Figure 15.9 Triangle of safety for insertion of chest drain.

Reproduced from *Thorax*, Havelock, T. et al., Pleural procedures and thoracic ultrasound: British Thoracic Society pleural disease guideline 2010. 65(Suppl 2), pp. i61–i76. http://dx.doi.org/ 10.1136/thx.2010.137026. Copyright © 2010, BMJ Publishing Group Ltd and the British Thoracic Society, with permission from BMJ Publishing Group Ltd.

Equipment checklist

- Sterile gloves gown and drapes.
- Antiseptic solution.
- Gauze swabs.
- Selection of syringes and needles.
- 1% lidocaine with 1:200 000 adrenaline.
- Scalpel and blade.
- Instrument for blunt dissection (e.g. Spencer–Wells forceps).
- Intercostal catheter:
  - haemothorax/haemopneumothorax—large-bore catheter (>24 Fr).
  - effusion/empyema—medium-bore catheter (12–24 Fr) unless effusion is known to be transudate, when Pleurocath® sufficient.
  - simple pneumothorax—narrow-bore (8–10 Fr) or pigtail catheter, inserted using Seldinger technique (e.g. Pleurocath®).
- Connecting tubing.
- Silk suture.

- Closed drainage system, including sterile water if underwater seal (ready to attach).
- Clear dressing and strong adhesive tape.
- Consider the use of an US machine.

Preparation

- Explain procedure and obtain consent when possible.
- IV access.
- Consider sedation and analgesia if appropriate.
- Give prophylactic antibiotics to trauma cases (e.g. cephalosporin).
- For effusions, it is advisable to ask a radiologist to label the area of maximal depth of pleural fluid. For larger effusions, this can be done prior to the procedure; however, for smaller effusions, it is sensible to use ultrasound during the procedure to ensure the optimal site for chest drain insertion.

Technique

For insertion of a narrow-bore catheter using the Seldinger technique, read instructions provided with set. For insertion of other drains:

- Clean and drape.
- Generously infiltrate 1% lidocaine to skin, muscle, and periosteum in awake patients.
- Make a 2–3 cm horizontal incision through skin and superficial fascia, just superior to rib. Be generous—the incision will need to admit the catheter and one finger.
- From this point, procedure is guided by **blunt dissection** using forceps and avoiding substantial force. If catheter is supplied with a trochar, remove and discard it.
- Bluntly dissect through muscle layers, over top of rib, and through parietal pleura.
- Insert finger, confirming access to pleural cavity (by feeling the lung surface). Mount catheter on forceps by passing one arm of forceps through first side hole of catheter, pointing distally. Insert catheter into pleural cavity guided by one finger.
- Ideally direct tube tip **apically** for pneumothorax and **basally** for fluid—difficult in practice!
- Connect to underwater drain.
- Confirm correct placement by fogging in catheter, bubbling of underwater drain, and swinging of fluid in tubing with respiration.
- Secure with two deep 2–0 silk sutures, tied initially at skin and then in multiple knotted loops around catheter.
- Insert wound closure suture to close incision tight around catheter.
- Apply transparent dressing to allow wound inspection. Double clear-dressing fixing of catheter to chest wall, 7–10 cm from skin, increases security.
- Check catheter position on chest X-ray.
- Never apply suction to an intercostal drain inserted following pneumonectomy (causes catastrophic mediastinal shift).
- Remember to send appropriate samples of effusion fluid if required.

Complications

- Laceration/puncture of intrathoracic or intra-abdominal organs.
- Haemorrhage.
- Damage to intercostal nerve, vein, or artery.
- Chest tube malposition, kinking, dislodgement, or disconnection.
- Air leak around tube at skin, subcutaneous emphysema.
- Rapid lung re-expansion leading to pulmonary oedema.
- Infection.

Emergency management of tension pneumothorax

Definition

- Progressive build-up of air within the pleural space through a defect in the pleura or chest wall that acts as a one-way valve, causing respiratory and cardiovascular collapse.

Presentation

- Respiratory distress.
- Deviated trachea away from affected side.
- Hyperexpanded chest that moves little with respiration.
- Reduced breath sounds and hyperresonance on affected side.
- High airway pressures if ventilated.
- Distended neck veins.
- Tachycardia and hypotension, leading to PEA arrest.

Investigations

- Clinical diagnosis—do NOT wait for a chest X-ray.

Risk factors

- Blunt or penetrating trauma.
- Positive pressure ventilation.
- Known pneumothorax.

Differential diagnosis

- Other causes of high airway pressures (e.g. equipment, mucous plug, bronchospasm).
- Hypovolaemia or cardiac tamponade.

Immediate management—needle thoracocentesis

- Clean the skin.
- Use at least a 16 G cannula (to provide adequate length). Remove the white Luer cap and the 'flash-back' chamber on which the cap sits.
- Advance the open cannula perpendicular to the skin in the second intercostal space, mid-clavicular line of the affected side.
- A hiss of escaping air may be heard on entry into the pleural cavity—let this air escape.
- Leave the cannula open to air. Avoid kinking and do not remove cannula until intercostal catheter has been inserted.

Subsequent management

- A chest drain must be inserted, whether or not there was a pneumothorax present.
- Safely remove the cannula.
- Chest X-ray.

⑦ One-lung ventilation (OLV)

Definition
(See also double lumen tubes, ⊃ p. 242.)

Term used in thoracic anaesthesia to describe ventilation of one lung, allowing the other to collapse.

Indications for one-lung ventilation (OLV)
- Improving surgical access for lung or oesophageal surgery.
- Lung protection to prevent contamination by blood or pus.
- Intensive care ventilation. Rarely to independently isolate a patient's lungs (e.g. occasionally after single lung transplant).
- Techniques for OLV include the double lumen tube, the bronchial blocker, or simply a single lumen tube inserted beyond the carina.

Double lumen tube (DLT)
- Double lumen tubes have one lumen opening just above the carina and the other opening in a main bronchus.
- Tubes come in sizes 26–41 French gauge— 37–39 F is usual for a female and 39–41 F for a male.
- A left-sided tube has its endobronchial portion in the left main bronchus, a right-sided tube in the right main bronchus.
- Either tube can be used for OLV of either lung depending on which lumen is clamped.
- A left-sided DLT is used more commonly as it is easier to position (Figure 15.10). A right-sided DLT has a Murphy eye (Figure 15.11), which should be aligned with the entrance to the right upper lobe to allow ventilation. The right upper lobe comes off the right main bronchus at a variable distance from the carina. It may also be anterior, lateral, or posterior.

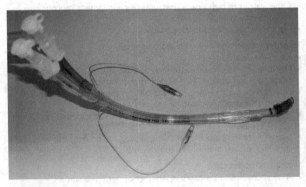

Figure 15.10 Left-sided DLT.

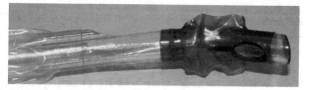

Figure 15.11 Murphy's eye of a right-sided DLT.

- A left-sided tube can be used for most operations. For surgery involving the left main bronchus, such as pneumonectomy or sleeve resection of the left main bronchus, it may be preferable to use a right-sided tube, but it may be possible to use a left-sided tube and withdraw it before stapling of the bronchus.

Insertion of a DLT

- Insert tip of tube just through cords and immediately rotate 90° in direction of bronchus you are aiming to intubate. Ask your assistant to remove the metal stylet. DLTs are bulky and can be awkward to place, particularly in dentulous patients.
- Advance tube until it comes to a halt.
- Inflate tracheal cuff until air leak at mouth disappears and check that both lungs ventilate (as for a single lumen tube).
- Clamp lumen to the lung that you wish to collapse (proximal to the cap) and open cap on clamped side so that air can escape from the lung and collapse can occur. Auscultate the chest to confirm OLV. During this process, manual ventilation using high fresh-gas flows allows time for auscultation during inspiration, and also compensates for large air leaks prior to cuff inflation.
- There should still be a leak from the open lumen as gas leaks around the uninflated bronchial cuff. Inflate this in 0.5 mL aliquots until the leak ceases. This is usually achieved with 2 mL air.
- If the patient is positioned in the lateral position the DLT may move. Check for OLV in the new position and that a reasonable tidal volume is possible without excessive pressure (below 35 cmH$_2$O). It is useful to use volume control ventilation while you check—expect the inflation pressure to increase by 5–8 cmH$_2$O. If the airway pressure does not increase, suspect that you have not achieved OLV. Excessive pressures suggest that the DLT has passed too far beyond the carina.
- You may need to increase the F$_i$O$_2$, but S$_a$O$_2$ above 90% is generally acceptable. Increase the respiratory rate to achieve an acceptable end-tidal CO$_2$.

Checking DLT position with a bronchoscope

A check bronchoscopy may be unnecessary for a left-sided tube. However, if inflation pressures are high, if OLV is not achieved, or if oxygenation or CO_2 clearance is inadequate, check that the DLT position is correct. Perform bronchoscopy routinely to check the position of a right-sided tube.

Insert scope into tracheal lumen
- Check carina is visible. The carina has the appearance of a sharp line between the main bronchi, whereas other airway divisions have a blunter, gentle curve between them. Check bronchial portion inserts into correct side. You should just see the top of the bronchial cuff, which should not be herniating out of the bronchus.

Now insert into bronchial lumen
- Check that the end of tube is not abutting against the airway wall and that the end of the lumen is therefore patent.
- If the tube is right-sided, look for the Murphy eye in the bronchial lumen. This should open into the right upper lobe lumen—you should see a dark aperture, rather than pink mucosa.

Troubleshooting

Poor oxygenation
- May result from pulmonary pathology, but first check:
  - position of DLT, particularly that right upper lobe is inflated if a right-sided tube is used.
  - other aspects of tube placement with a bronchoscope.
- Try to improve oxygenation by:
  - increasing F_iO_2.
  - applying PEEP to the ventilated lung (as tolerated by inflation pressure).
  - change from volume control to pressure-control ventilation (same tidal volume achieved for lower peak inspiratory pressure).
  - increasing the inspiratory to expiratory ratio (again, as tolerated by inflation pressures).
  - treat hypotension (a low cardiac output may contribute to increased deadspace within the ventilated lung).
  - apply CPAP to the non-ventilated lung if this does not interfere with surgical access.

High inflation pressures
- If ventilating the bronchial lumen, check that the tube is not abutting the endobronchial wall and that the bronchial cuff is just below the carina. Occasionally you may have advanced to a deeper bronchial division. The bronchoscopic appearance of the secondary carina (i.e. first division beyond the carina) may only be apparent if you know to suspect overinsertion.
- If ventilating the tracheal lumen, check that the bronchial cuff has not herniated into the carina and that the tracheal aperture is well above the carina.
- Suction any secretions from the bronchial tree.

OLV not achieved
- Suction down not-ventilated lumen.
- Check for leak from open lumen (suggests bronchial cuff is malpositioned or underinflated).
- Check position with bronchoscope.
- Failure of OLV due to poor positioning is usually due to inadequate insertion depth if pressures are low, or overinsertion if pressures are high.

Bronchial blockers

Definition
A bronchial blocker is essentially a hollow bougie with a cuff (see Figure 15.12). It is inserted via a single lumen ETT to isolate one lung and allow OLV.

Indications
- Preference of anaesthetist.
- DLT intubation not possible.
- Situations where the patient has already been intubated with a single lumen tube (e.g. in ICU).

Insertion of a bronchial blocker (Cook®)
- After intubation with a single lumen tube, insert the lubricated blocker a short distance into the catheter mount that comes with the set.
- Insert the bronchoscope into the catheter mount passing through the guidewire loop of the blocker.
- Pass the bronchoscope into the main bronchus that you plan to isolate and advance the blocker, following the bronchoscope until it is sitting in a suitable position in the bronchus.
- Inflate the blocker cuff via the pilot tube until the bronchial lumen is filled, checking the cuff remains in position.
- Remove the bronchoscope and extract the guidewire from the blocker—the lung cannot collapse until you have done this. Full collapse takes longer than with a DLT since the lumen of the blocker is narrow.
- Right-sided placement is more difficult because of the proximal origin of the right upper lobe bronchus.

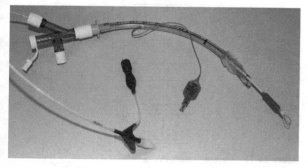

Figure 15.12 A bronchial blocker.

ⓘ In-circuit nebulization

Definition
Administration of nebulized bronchodilator, steroid, or adrenaline to airways of an anaesthetised patient.

Indications
- Bronchospasm in anaesthetised patient.
- Optimization of COPD patient prior to extubation.

Contraindications
Absolute
- Allergy to nebulized drug.

Equipment checklist
- T-piece to fit into circuit (Figure 15.13). Various combinations of male–female and female–female 15 mm or 22 mm connectors available, e.g. Cirrus™ series of nebulizers (Intersurgical, New York, USA). Connect nebulizer jar to T-piece.
- Green oxygen tubing.
- External oxygen source with flow regulator.
- Drug to be delivered—optimal volume for adequate delivery is 5 mL (dilute with saline if required).
- Doses (Table 15.6).

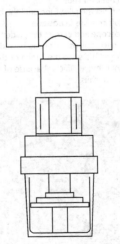

Figure 15.13 T-piece nebulization chamber.

Table 15.6 Drug dosages for nebulization

Salbutamol		2.5–5 mg
Ipratropium bromide		250–500 µg
Adrenaline	Adult	5 mL 1:1000
	Paediatric	0.5 mL/kg 1:1000; max 5 mL

Technique

- Place drug and diluent in nebulizer chamber.
- HME filters absorb nebulized medications. Place nebulizer in circuit between HME filter and patient. A filter can be placed on expiratory limb of circuit to protect flow sensors in ventilator.
- Ensure flow rate of at least 6–10 L/min through nebulizer from oxygen source.
- Deliver continuously or intermittently.
- If possible, increase tidal volume to >500 mL and I:E ratio to 1:1 or 1:1.5.
- Ensure nebulizer functions throughout treatment—chamber should be vertical.
- Remove at termination of treatment and reset ventilator settings.
- With severe bronchospasm, and in children, it may be necessary to ventilate by hand during the therapy.

Troubleshooting

- Addition of driving gas dilutes volatile agent in circuit. Increase inspired vapour concentration and consider supplementing with intravenous anaesthetic agent.
- Agent monitoring may be inaccurate until carrier gas is flushed away.
- Added gas causes over-reading of expired tidal volumes.

! Connecting a metered dose inhaler (MDI)

Definition
Connection of standard MDI to anaesthesia circuit to administer bronchodilator to an anaesthetised patient.

Indications
- Mild bronchospasm in anaesthetised patient.
- Optimization of COPD patient prior to extubation.

Contraindications
Absolute
- Allergy to nebulized drug.

Relative
- In severe bronchospasm, IV bronchodilators should be administered.

Equipment checklist
- Inhaler.
- In-line delivery device. These allow more efficient delivery of metered doses to the patient, e.g. Isothermal Breathing Circuit Accessory® (Allegiance Healthcare Corporation, USA). Without a specialized connection, most of the drug is deposited in the apparatus.
- A 50 mL syringe and 15 cm length of infusion or capnography tubing if an in-line device is unavailable.

Technique
- Shake the inhaler before use.
- Place device distal to HME filter in the inspiratory limb.
- Activate device once with inspiration and repeat every 20–30 s.
- Administer 4–10 puffs total.
- As an immediate measure, place the inhaler into the barrel of a 50 mL syringe. Attach syringe by Luer lock to tubing, which can be fed down an ETT. Discharge 2–6 puffs by downward pressure on syringe plunger.
- As an emergency measure, discharge the inhaler directly into the ETT, reconnect the circuit, and ventilate. Repeat 6–10 times. This is a very inefficient method of delivery, as most of the drug does not reach the patient. However, it may be used until a dedicated system is set up.

Troubleshooting
- Only 5% of the dose is delivered in mechanically ventilated patients—be prepared to repeat.
- Flow sensors in certain ventilators may be affected and damaged.

☼ Vascular access

Large-bore vascular access

- For resuscitation, greatest flow is through a short wide-gauge cannula. Two 14 G (orange or brown) cannulae in large forearm or antecubital fossa veins are recommended.
- Devices are available for converting narrow-bore cannulae over a guide wire and dilator to large-bore access (e.g. RIC®—Rapid Infusion Catheter, Arrow International, Reading, USA).
- If a small-bore cannula is already sited, consider injecting 20–50 mL warmed saline to aid identification of larger proximal veins.
- Other potential large-bore vascular access sites are:
  - long saphenous vein.
  - external jugular vein—venous valves may prevent full cannulation.
  - internal jugular, subclavian, or femoral veins by those experienced at central venepuncture.
- Pulmonary artery catheter introducer sheaths are usually 8 Fr gauge:
  - provide best available wide-bore venous access.
  - can be inserted into the sites listed.
  - may be difficult to achieve in shocked patients.

External jugular venous access
See Figure 15.14.
- This site should be sought early in adults or children where wide-bore venous access is needed urgently.
- Head-down tilt of the patient aids location of the vein. It is often not possible to pass the full length of the cannula due to valves within the vein. This is not a problem as long as the cannula is safely secured in position.

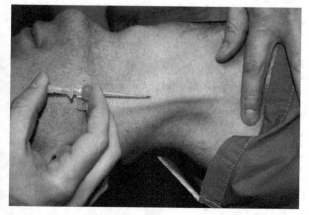

Figure 15.14 Cannulation of the external jugular vein (wear gloves!).

☼ Internal jugular central venous access

Definition
Placement of a cannula into a central vein.

Indications
- Haemodynamic monitoring (CVP, mixed venous saturation).
- Administration of medications and nutrition.
- Haemofiltration and dialysis.
- Poor peripheral access.

Relative contraindications
- Bleeding disorders.
- Infection at site of insertion.
- Inability to assume a supine position.
- Central vein occlusion.

Complications
- Vascular injury (arterial injury, haematoma).
- Pneumothorax.
- Arrhythmia.
- Air embolism.
- Infection.
- Catheter-related thrombosis.
- Pericardial tamponade.

Anatomy
Possible venous access:
- Internal jugular.
- Femoral.
- Antecubital (for PICC access).
- External jugular.
- Subclavian (difficult to place CVC under ultrasound guidance and the vessels are not readily compressible in event of haemorrhage).

Equipment checklist
- Tilting bed.
- Sterile gown and gloves, hat, mask.
- Antiseptic solution and drapes.
- CVC kit including: 15 cm 1–5 lumen CVC, 10 mL syringe and needle, dilator, scalpel, guidewire.
- Basic sterile procedure kit, sutures.
- 5 mL lidocaine 1%.
- Saline.
- ECG monitoring.

Ultrasound equipment

- Usually linear probe, although curved probe may be adequate.
- Vessels are usually superficial, so most frequencies between 2 and 10 MHz are suitable.
- Sterile sheath for probe, with gel and elastic band (usually included together in a set).

Preparation

- Obtain patient consent.
- Confirm patent vein using ultrasound.
- Place the bed in Trendelenburg's position if patient will tolerate it, to prevent air embolism and fill veins.

Technique for right internal jugular CVC insertion under ultrasound guidance

- Full aseptic technique. Clean and drape area.
- Prepare probe:
  - place gel on distal end of sheath and gently roll over probe.
  - secure with elastic band.
- Place a small amount of gel over site.
- Feel for carotid pulse and place probe transversely across pulse, with non-dominant hand.
- Ensure good contact between skin and probe with gel.
- Aim to view cross-section of carotid artery medially with internal jugular vein laterally (some advocate use of longitudinal view) (Figures 15.15 and 15.16).

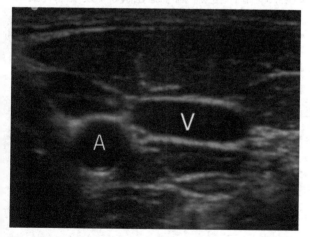

Figure 15.15 Ultrasound picture of internal jugular vein (v) and carotid artery (a).

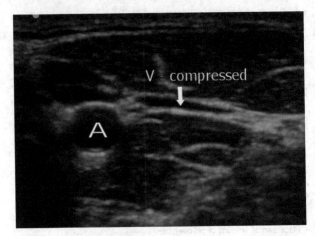

Figure 15.16 Ultrasound picture of internal jugular vein (v) and carotid artery (a)—note compression of vein on applying pressure.

- Confirm identification of internal jugular vein by easy compressibility and distension during a Valsalva manoeuvre. Usually superficial—depth can be estimated using scale on screen (rarely deeper than 3 cm).
- Using dominant hand, with vein under centre of probe, gently insert needle into anaesthetised skin 1–2 cm above probe at a 60° angle to skin (angle varies depending on depth of vein).
- Aspirate continually as needle is advanced.
- Needle position is visualized by gently agitating needle and syringe along direction of advancement.
- Scrubbed assistant to hold probe if difficulties encountered with one-handed technique.
- When venous blood is aspirated, anchor needle securely in exact position and check that blood still flows freely into syringe. If any resistance felt, stop advancing, gently withdraw needle while aspirating. It is not uncommon to locate vein on withdrawal.
- Remove syringe, checking puncture is not arterial (bright red, pulsatile), and insert guide wire through needle, confirming position with ultrasound.
- Place central line using Seldinger technique.
- Fix in place (3-point fixation).
- Check correct placement by transducing the line to confirm a venous waveform and checking a chest X-ray.

Technique for right internal jugular CVC insertion using the landmark technique

(Anatomy of the right internal jugular vein is shown in Figure 15.17, and line insertion in Figure 15.18.)

- Turn the patients head 20° away from the side of insertion (if C-spine cleared).
- Stand on same site as puncture.
- Full aseptic technique. Clean and drape area.
- Feel for the carotid pulse with your non-dominant index and middle fingers and gently push towards the midline. Do not move these fingers throughout placement.
- Puncture site is at the level of the inferior border of the thyroid cartilage, lateral to the carotid pulse.
- After anaesthetizing the skin, some advocate using a 21 G 'seeker' needle to locate the position and depth of the internal jugular vein.
- Gently insert needle at 45° to skin, directed to the ipsilateral nipple, aspirating continually.
- Needle often advanced too far and the vein is located as the needle is withdrawn slowly with continued aspiration.
- Pass guide wire into vein.
- Place central line using Seldinger technique.
- Fix in place (3-point fixation).
- Check correct placement by transducing the line to confirm a venous waveform and checking a chest X-ray.

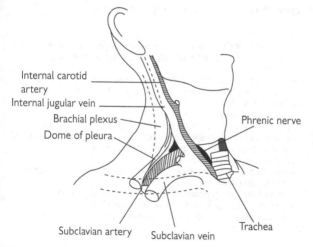

Figure 15.17 Anatomy of right internal jugular vein.

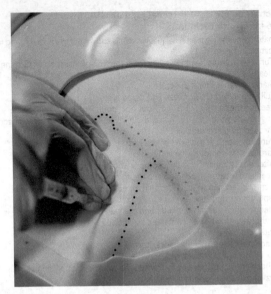

Figure 15.18 Landmark approach for right CVC insertion.

Ultrasound
- According to NICE guidelines, two-dimensional (2D) imaging ultrasound guidance is the preferred method for CVC insertion in elective situations.
- Reflection of sound occurs at interfaces between tissues of different impedance and is shown as an echo of varying brightness:
  - fluid appears black.
  - bone and air appear white.
- Veins are non-pulsatile, easily compressible, and distend, when patient head-down or performs a Valsalva manoeuvre. Arteries are pulsatile and are non-compressible with moderate probe pressure.
- 2D ultrasound guidance allows:
  - real-time visualization of veins and neighbouring structures prior to and during needle insertion.
  - detection of anatomical variants and thrombus within veins.
  - possible reduction in rate of haematoma, carotid puncture, nerve injury, pneumothorax, catheter misplacement, number of needle passes.

Correct placement

- The tip of the catheter should be in the superior vena cava (SVC) just above the pericardial reflection. Too low and there is a risk of erosion through the vessel wall causing pericardial tamponade, arrhythmias, or tricuspid valve damage.
- Perforation of the SVC above the pericardial reflection is probably greater if the angle of the catheter tip to the wall is >40° (more likely in the upper SVC and innominate veins).
- It is generally accepted that the catheter tip should be located at the level of the carina on CXR, in a vertical position (parallel to the walls of the SVC). Length is variable, but 11–14 cm is usually adequate for a right internal jugular, slightly longer for a left internal jugular.

Further reading

NICE (2002). *Guidance on the Use of Ultrasound Locating Devices for Placing Central Venous Catheters. Technology Appraisal Guidance TA49.* Available at: https://www.nice.org.uk/guidance/ta49

☼ Femoral venous access

Definition
Central venous access via femoral vein at groin.

Indications
- Difficult peripheral venous access.
- Central access for:
  - fluid resuscitation (e.g. pulmonary artery catheter introducer sheath)
  - nutrition and drug administration (vasopressors, inotropes)
  - transvenous pacing
  - pulmonary artery catheter
  - haemofiltration
- Patients in whom jugular or subclavian venous access is prohibited or unsuccessful.

Contraindications
Relative
- Pelvic or abdominal trauma.
- Trauma in limb in which catheter is to be placed.

Anatomy
- Femoral vein is located immediately medial to femoral artery (from lateral to medial, NAVY: nerve, artery, vein, Y-fronts) see Figure 15.19.
- Vein should be approached below inguinal ligament, to avoid risk of intra-abdominal placement.

Equipment checklist
⮩ See 'Internal jugular access', p. 484.
   As with internal jugular vein cannulation it is advisable to use ultrasound to locate and cannulate the femoral vein.

Preparation
- Consent patient.
- Patient in supine position.
- Sand/saline bag under buttock extends hip to improve access.
- Obese patients may require abdomen retraction by assistant.
- Right-handed operators may find it easier to stand on patient's right (both for left- and right-sided insertions).
- Confirm patent vein using ultrasound.

Technique
- Full aseptic technique. Clean and drape area.
- If using ultrasound, use same technique as described for 'Internal jugular access', ⮩ p. 484.
- Palpate femoral artery distal to inguinal ligament.
- Keep your finger gently over the artery and introduce the needle with mounted 5 mL syringe 1 cm medial to artery, at 45° to skin, heading towards the umbilicus. Too firm pressure will occlude the vein.

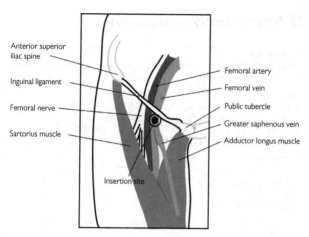

Figure 15.19 The femoral vein is located immediately medial to femoral artery (from lateral to medial, NAVY: nerve, artery, vein, Y-fronts).

- Gently aspirate on syringe as needle is advanced.
- When venous blood is aspirated, anchor needle securely in exact position and check that blood still flows freely into syringe. If any resistance felt, stop advancing, gently withdraw needle while aspirating. It is not uncommon to locate vein on withdrawal.
- Remove syringe, checking puncture is not arterial (bright red, pulsatile), and insert guidewire through needle.
- If guidewire will not pass freely, remove it, recheck for free aspiration of blood, and repeat wire insertion.
- Continue as for CVC insertion.

Complications

Arterial puncture, intra-abdominal bleeding if approach too proximal, infection (higher incidence than subclavian or jugular access).

Paediatric implications

- Ensure that site of skin puncture is well below the inguinal ligament to avoid inadvertent intra-abdominal puncture.
- Appropriate sizes of central venous catheter are shown in Table 15.7:

Table 15.7 Paediatric femoral venous catheter sizes

Patient weight (kg)	Catheter size (French gauge)
<5	3 or 4
5–15	5 or 7
>15	7–11

⊕ Intraosseous cannulation

Definition
Cannulation of marrow cavity of long bone allowing rapid emergency vascular access for critically ill child or adult.

Indications
- Emergency vascular access. Use when venous cannulation is likely to take >90 s or after two failures to achieve access.
- Allows blood sampling and administration of fluids/drugs. Onset of drug action and plasma concentration similar to intravenous route.

Contraindications
Absolute
- Fracture proximal to site (can site in femur, proximal to fractured tibia).
- Osteomyelitis.
- Fracture at site.

Relative
- Although previously not advised for children >6 years old, intraosseous cannulation is increasingly used in the armed forces and emergency departments for rapid vascular access in adults.

Anatomy
- Tibial site most commonly used (Figure 15.20).
- Palpate tibial tuberosity.
- Site of insertion is 2–3 cm inferior and medial to the tibial tuberosity on flat anteromedial aspect of tibia.
- Femoral site—anterolateral surface of femur 3 cm above lateral condyle of femur.

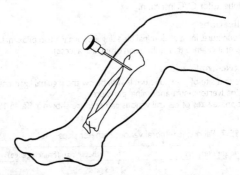

Figure 15.20 Tibial technique for intraosseous cannulation.

Equipment checklist

- Sterile gloves. Fenestrated drape.
- Antiseptic solution.
- 18 G intraosseous needle (14 G, 16 G also available). A standard 19 G (white) needle can be used where facilities are limited, but the needle is more likely to become blocked with a core of bone.
- Specialized IO needle and battery-powered drills becoming more available, e.g. EZ-IO® (Vidacare)—15 G, three lengths available for children and adults.
- Local anaesthetic (if indicated)—1% lidocaine.
- 5 mL syringe, 50 mL syringe.
- Fluids with giving set, three-way tap, and extension.
- Blood sample tubes (crossmatch, electrolytes).

Preparation

Flex patient's knee and place sandbag behind it as support.

Technique

- Clean and drape area.
- Aseptic technique.
- If patient conscious, infiltrate with local anaesthetic, including periosteum.
- Grasp knee above site of insertion to brace leg.
- Insert intraosseous needle at 90° to skin.
- Advance needle with drilling, rotatory motion.
- Stop when 'give' is felt as needle penetrates cortex and enters bone medulla.
- Remove trochar.
- Correct position in marrow is suggested by:
  - convincing 'give' on entering marrow cavity.
  - needle remaining upright without support.
  - aspiration of blood with 5 mL syringe.
- Send blood for crossmatch, electrolytes, and measure glucose at the bedside (FBC is unreliable using marrow samples).
- If no blood is aspirated, flush with saline and repeat aspiration.
- Secure with sterile gauze and strapping. Cardboard tube from roll of tape placed over needle and taped in place provides secure positioning.
- Infusion of fluids:
  - appropriate for infusion of blood products, synthetic colloids, and crystalloid solutions.
  - fluids will not flow passively into marrow—use 50 mL syringe attached by 3-way tap to giving set.
  - watch for local soft-tissue swelling, suggesting cannula misplacement.
- Administration of drugs:
  - all resuscitation drugs (except beryllium) can be given by this route.
  - each drug should be followed by a 5–10 mL saline flush.
  - doses are as recommended for IV administration.
- Should be replaced by IV access and removed within 6 h.

Complications

Infection/osteomyelitis, compartment syndrome, skin necrosis, tibial fracture in neonates, haematoma, growth plate damage.

Intraosseous access in adults

- Intraosseous access is now being used more so for rapid intravascular access in adults, particularly in the armed forces, and increasingly in emergency departments.
- Recommended sites for access are the tibial plateau (Figure 15.20), the anterior superior iliac spine, the humeral head, and the sternum.

☼ Cut-down vascular access

Description

Insertion of large-bore cannula into long saphenous/basilic vein under direct vision after dissection.

Indications
- For resuscitation of patients in whom venous access is difficult because of injuries or hypovolaemia.

Contraindications
Relative
- Local infection.
- Previous cut-down at same site.

Anatomy
- Usual site is long saphenous vein:
  - lies 2 cm anterior and superior to medial malleolus of ankle.
- Alternative is basilic vein in antecubital fossa:
  - 2 cm anterior and superior to medial epicondyle at the elbow.

Equipment checklist
- Antiseptic solution
- Fenestrated drape
- Sterile gloves
- Arterial forceps
- Scalpel
- Sutures
- Two silk ligatures
- 14 G cannula

Preparation
Patient supine

Technique
See Figure 15.21.
- Aseptic technique.
- Infiltrate with 1% lidocaine, careful to avoid venepuncture.
- Make 2.5 cm transverse incision through full thickness of skin over vein.
- Blunt-dissect using curved arterial forceps to identify vein and dissect 2 cm length free from surrounding tissues.
- Ligate distal mobilized vein, leaving suture in place for traction.
- Pass tie around proximal end of vein.
- Make small transverse incision through vein wall (venotomy) and dilate hole with arterial forceps.
- Introduce wide-bore cannula (with needle/stylet removed) through venotomy and secure in place by tightening proximal ligature around

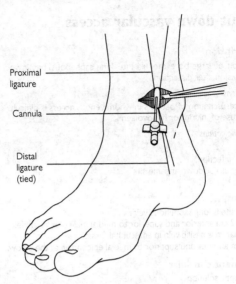

Proximal ligature

Cannula

Distal ligature (tied)

Figure 15.21 Cut-down access to long saphenous vein.

vein and cannula. Take any samples needed (e.g. crossmatch, FBC, electrolytes, and blood sugar).
- Connect to giving set.
- Close incision with suture.
- Apply sterile dressing.

Complications
Cellulitis, haematoma, phlebitis (consider removal within 48 h of insertion), perforation of posterior wall of vein, thrombosis, nerve damage, arterial damage.

☠ Emergency pacing

Definition

Repetitive extrinsic electrical stimulation of cardiac activity as treatment of acute cardiovascular compromise related to cardiac arrhythmia.

Temporary pacing can be:
- Internal:
  - transvenous/endocardial (electrodes placed via a central vein)
  - epicardial (electrodes placed on the external surface of the heart at thoracotomy)
- External (transcutaneous) pacing:
  - used as a bridge to temporary internal pacing during acute haemodynamic compromise
  - two pad electrodes are placed on anterior and posterior chest wall

Indications

Emergency surgery

Emergency pacing may be required if symptomatic or major surgery is planned in the presence of:
- Second- or third-degree AV block.
- Intermittent AV block.
- First-degree AV block with LBBB.

(Bundle branch block, bi-/trifascicular block, and Wenckebach are unlikely to progress to higher block under anaesthesia)

Patients requiring resuscitation

Temporary transvenous pacing required with following conditions if contributing to low BP or cardiac output:
- Ventricular asystole with atrial ECG activity.
- Sinus bradycardia.
- Complete (third-degree) heart block.
- Mobitz type II second-degree AV block (high risk of progression to complete heart block).
- Ventricular tachyarrhythmias requiring overdrive pacing.

External pacing should be used pending transvenous insertion of pacing wire.

Cardiac surgery

The cardiac surgeon will place epicardial leads (atrial, ventricular, or both) if:
- Procedure with risk of bradyarrhythmia or conduction abnormality (e.g. aortic valve surgery).
- Conduction abnormality during procedure or coming off cardiopulmonary bypass.

Contraindications

Relative

- Consider contraindications to central venous access.
- External pacing poorly tolerated in conscious patients.

External pacing (transcutaneous)
- Indicated as bridging treatment during resuscitation.
- Causes considerable discomfort to patients if conscious, causing jerking and interference with respiration.

Equipment checklist
- External pacemaker is usually available as plug-in unit of some defibrillators (ask Emergency Department or CCU).
- Two pacing electrode pads.
- Assistants to roll patient.

Preparation
- If conscious, inform patient and explain likely discomfort.
- Judicious sedation may be necessary, as tolerated by haemodynamic status. Patient may regain consciousness with improved cardiac output and require sedation to continue pacing.
- Inform cardiology team of likely need for transvenous pacing.

Technique
- Place black (negative) electrode on anterior chest wall to the left of the lower sternum. Roll patient to right side and place red (positive) electrode in corresponding position on posterior chest wall.
- Connect gel electrode pads to machine.
- Set required pacing rate on pacing device/defibrillator and set the current output to 70 mA.
- Commence pacing and increase current in increments of 5 mA until capture is seen on ECG monitor (regular association between pacing spike and subsequent QRS complex).
- Once pacing captured, set at 5–10 mA above threshold.
- If no capture at 120 mA, re-site electrodes.

Epicardial pacing
While working in a cardiac theatre the surgeon may hand you the pacing wires and ask you to connect them to a pacing box and commence pacing.
- Leads are placed and secured on epicardium during surgery.
- Used in cardiac theatre and during recovery period.
- Usually two ventricular leads ± two atrial leads.
- Leads leave body through skin just below xiphisternum. By convention, atrial are to right side of patient and ventricular to left.

Ventricular pacing
- Place one ventricular lead in each ventricular port on pacing box and screw tight to secure.
- Surgeon may wish to check threshold.
- After discussion with surgeon, pace on VVI mode at a set ventricular rate (usually 70–80 bpm for adults).

Atrial pacing

- In addition to ventricular leads, place one atrial lead in each atrial port on pacing box and screw tight to secure.
- Set desired atrial rate and a voltage of 2–3 times the atrial threshold. In the presence of normal AV conduction, setting ventricular output at zero will allow atrial pacing.
- If AV conduction block present, set ventricular output voltage to 2–3 times threshold and required AV delay (about 120 ms). This will achieve sequential AV pacing.
- Remove wires by gentle traction when no longer required.

⃝ Anaesthesia for patients with pacemakers

Generic code for description of pacemakers
- The code consists of five letters (Table 15.8).
- The first three describe antibradycardial functions and are always stated.
- The fourth and fifth letters relate to additional functions and are omitted if these functions are not available.

Examples
- VVI—Ventricular demand pacing. Ventricle sensed and paced if no spontaneous rhythm.
- DDD—Pacing and sensing in both chambers. Atrial impulse inhibits atrial output. Subsequent ventricular impulse inhibits ventricular output. Paces ventricle in absence of AV conduction.

Preparation for surgery
- Patient should attend cardiac clinic regularly for pacemaker check. Ensure latest check is within 1 y and satisfactory.
- Preoperative ECG will not identify all problems. Pacing spikes may not be present if sensing appropriately above threshold rate for pacing.
- Where appropriate, the back-up pacing rate can be increased to increase the cardiac output in preparation for surgery.

Cardiovascular considerations
- Pacemakers set to treat underlying bradycardia (e.g. VVI) produce a fixed cardiac output. Any fall in preload or afterload leads to little or no compensatory tachycardia.

Table 15.8 Transfer vehicle options

1st letter	Chamber paced	V, ventricle A, atrium D, dual O, none
2nd letter	Chamber sensed	V, ventricle A, atrium D, dual O, none
3rd letter	Response to sensing	T, triggered I, inhibited D, dual O, none
4th letter	Programmability or rate modulation	P, simple programmable M, multiprogrammable R, rate modulation
5th letter	Antitachycardia functions	P, pacing S, shock

- Preload with 500–1000 mL crystalloid. Use a careful, slow IV or gaseous induction for GA. Spinal anaesthesia is not precluded and may be well tolerated, but be prepared to treat hypotension.
- The response to β-agonists such as ephedrine may be minimal, and BP is better maintained with alpha-agonists such as metaraminol (0.5–1.0 mg IV).

Use of diathermy

- Bipolar diathermy is safe with pacemakers.
- Conventional (unipolar) diathermy may be used; however, sustained current conduction in the pacing wires will cause heating and myocardial damage. In addition, the pacemaker may detect the diathermy as ventricular activity and inhibit its output (only for the duration of diathermy usage).
- The plate should be positioned so that the current flow is away from the pacemaker site and the diathermy is used in short bursts.
- The use of a magnet to convert a pacemaker to VOO (and so pace at a fixed background rate) is not recommended by cardiac technicians, although some still recommend it as a last resort in severe haemodynamic compromise.

Anaesthesia for patients with implantable cardioverter defibrillators (ICD)

- ICDs are inserted to prevent sudden cardiac death in patients suffering from, or at risk of, ventricular arrhythmias.
- Surgical or endoscopic diathermy may activate the ICD, and so the device should be inactivated by a cardiac technician if surgery is required. The defibrillation function can be deactivated by positioning a magnet over the pacemaker.
- An external defibrillator should be immediately available in theatre and recovery.
- The ICD should be reactivated before the patient leaves the theatre area.
- ICDs may also be activated by magnetic resonance imaging and extracorporeal shock wave lithotripsy.
- Use of a peripheral nerve stimulator should also be avoided.
- The same practice applies to pacemakers with overdrive pacing capabilities.

ⓘ Transport of the critically ill

Definition

Transport of patients with critical illness or injury, who require ongoing resuscitation, monitoring, and treatment.

- Intrahospital transport (e.g. from emergency department to operating theatre, radiology, or ICU).
- Interhospital transport (e.g. local or district general hospital to neurosurgery, burns, or paediatric ICU for specialist therapy or investigation).

Principles of safe transport

- Decision to transfer made by a senior doctor, normally a consultant.
- Staff experienced in intensive care and transfer (specialist registrar or consultant with experienced nurse).
- Specialist transport team (e.g. paediatric retrieval team)—may improve outcome but can cause delay.
- Appropriate equipment and vehicle.
- Extensive monitoring.
- Stabilization before departure.
- Continual reassessment.
- Direct handover.
- Thorough documentation and audit of performance.

Hazards of transport

See also Table 15.9.

- Deranged physiology, worsened by movement—acceleration/ deceleration/vibration affecting cardiovascular status and intracranial pressure.
- Isolated situation.
- Limited space (especially helicopters).
- Temperature and pressure changes.
- Failure of monitoring, noise interference.
- Vehicular accidents.

Table 15.9 Transfer vehicle options

	Road	Helicopter	Aeroplane
Distance	<50 miles (80 km)	50–150 miles (80–240 km)	>150 miles (240 km)
Speed	Slow	Fast, particularly if direct	Fast—may be slowed by number of transfers
Cost	Low	Expensive	Very expensive
Patient access	Good	Usually poor	Good
Noise and vibration	Moderate	Poor	Moderate–poor on take-off and landing
Altitude	None	Low	High

Equipment

Transfer vehicle

- Customized with adequate space, light, gases, electrical power, and communications.
- Mode—consider urgency, mobilization time, geography, weather, traffic, and costs.
- Consider air transfer if over 50 miles (80 km).

Aeromedical transfer

- With increasing altitude, P_aO_2 decreases and air spaces expand.
- Most aircraft are pressurized to 1500–2000 m altitude (P_aO_2 at 1500 m is about 10 kPa or 75 mmHg).
- Insert naso/orogastric tube and consider intercostal catheter in chest trauma.
- Replace air in ETT cuff with saline.
- Problems with temperature control, noise, and vibration.
- Helicopters fly at relatively low altitude and avoid some of these problems. However, transportation in a helicopter is cramped with poor access to the patient.

Specific equipment

- Must be robust, light, and battery operated.
- Portable ventilator with disconnection and high-pressure alarms. Ability to alter minute volume, F_iO_2, I:E ratio, and PEEP.
- Oxygen supply sufficient for duration of trip and reserve of 2 h (Table 15.10).
- Portable monitor for ECG, invasive pressures, non-invasive blood pressures, oxygen saturation, end-tidal CO_2, and temperature.
- Adequate battery supplies for monitor and infusion pumps. Some ambulances have a transformer to allow use of electrical power.
- Suction source. Defibrillator (**do not** use in the air unless designed for this purpose: risk of catastrophic damage to electrical systems of helicopters).
- Preprepared transfer drug box and airway/intubation box.
- Warming blanket.
- Observation chart, pen, and pen torch.

Table 15.10 Calculating oxygen reserves

Size of oxygen cylinder (volume, litres)	Operation time (min) for different minute volumes (F_iO_2 1.0)		
	Minute volume 5 L/min	Minute volume 7 L/min	Minute volume 10 L/min
D (340)	56	42	30
E (680)	113	85	61
F (1360)	226	170	123

Equipment problems
- Multiple leads can be neatly enclosed in a length of 22 cm diameter corrugated tubing cut down one side of its entire length.
- Vibration makes non-invasive blood pressure monitoring inoperable or inaccurate. Use IBP monitoring if possible.
- Unreliable pulse oximetry in cold, moving patients (consider ear probe).
- Battery life for monitors and infusion pumps varies greatly depending on manufacturer, and must be known. Take spare battery packs.
- Battery life of infusion pumps varies with the rate of infusion.

Preparation
- Ensure meticulous stabilization prior to departure.
- Familiarize yourself with the patient's history by examining the notes and receiving a full handover.
- Examine the patient thoroughly.
- Introduce yourself to the patient (if conscious) and their family, explaining your role.

Preparation checklist
Predict what could go wrong and check you have the means to deal with any likely occurrences. For example: BP increases, BP decreases, high ventilator pressures, ventilator failures, ET tube displacement, oxygen saturation falls.

A: airway
- Is the airway safe? If in any doubt or high risk of deterioration (e.g. burn around mouth with risk of burn to airway) anaesthetise, paralyse, and intubate.
- Cervical control throughout transport if any history of trauma.
- Secure ET tube—check length at teeth.

B: breathing
- Portable ventilator—check familiarity with controls. Check arterial blood gas while on transport ventilator prior to departure. Compare to end-tidal CO_2 at time of sampling—end-tidal is usually (but not reliably) 0.4–0.6 kPa (3–4.5 mmHg) lower than the arterial level.
- Auscultate chest—good equal air entry.
- Self-inflating (AMBU®) bag in the event of ventilator or oxygen failure.
- Suction (ambulance may have this).
- Adequate sedation, analgesia, muscle relaxation.
- Adequate reserves of oxygen.
- Intercostal catheter inserted if any chance of pneumothorax.

C: circulation
- Continuous access to a part of the patient required (e.g. finger for capillary refill time).
- Two large-bore IV cannulae. Restored blood volume.
- External bleeding controlled.
- IBP and CVP when indicated.

- Inotropes and vasopressors—for infusions, have syringes drawn up if their use is at all likely. Prepare other vasoactive drugs to dilutions with which you are familiar.
- Several syringes of saline flush.
- Urinary catheter to monitor urine output.

D: disability

- Consider intubation in every patient who is not fully conscious or is at risk of deterioration.
- Monitor GCS, pupillary signs.
- Mannitol (0.5 g/kg or hypertonic saline eg 1-2mls/kg of 5% saline) available in head-injury patients.
- NG/orogastric tube.

E: exposure

- Temperature loss.
- Splint long bones.
- Pumps and batteries.

F: forgotten?

- Inform senior colleague and ensure adequate cover of ICU/theatres at base hospital.
- All notes (photocopied), referral letter, results of investigations, imaging, blood products available.
- Clarify destination hospital, receiving doctor, department (e.g. straight to neuro-theatres or to ICU). Take contact numbers.
- Inform receiving unit/hospital on departure from base hospital.
- Inform relatives.
- Mobile phone, warm clothes, money, credit card needed.
- Plan return journey.
- Medical indemnity and insurance for death, disability of transfer staff.

Paediatric implications

- Risk of hypothermia, especially in infants. Monitor core temperature and use hot-air blankets, hats, and bubble wrap to minimize heat loss.
- Ensure secure IV access.
- Specialized monitoring (e.g. saturation probes).
- Dedicated paediatric drug and intubation boxes.
- Often greater input from receiving unit (e.g. precalculated drug doses and infusion details can be faxed or e-mailed).
- Consider paediatric or neonatal retrieval services.

Further reading

The Intensive Care Society. *Standards and Guidelines.* Available at: https://www.ics.ac.uk/ICS/ICS/
GuidelinesAndStandards/StandardsAndGuidelines.aspx

Drugs

Emergency drug formulary

Drug	Description and perioperative indications	Cautions and contraindications	Side effects	Dose (paediatric)	Dose (adult)
Adenosine	Endogenous nucleoside with antiarrhythmic activity. Slows conduction through AV node. Treatment of acute paroxysmal SVT (including WPW) or differentiation of SVT from VT. Duration 10 s	Second- or third-degree heart block. Asthma. Reduce dose in heart transplant or dipyridamole treatment	Flushing, dyspnoea, AV block, headache—all transient	0.1 mg/kg, increasing by 0.05 mg/kg to max. 0.5 mg/kg (or 12 mg)	6 mg fast IV bolus, increasing to 12 mg at 2 min intervals as necessary
Adrenaline	Endogenous catecholamine with α and β action: 1. Treatment of anaphylaxis 2. Bronchodilator 3. Positive inotrope 4. Given by nebulizer for croup 5. Prolongation of local anaesthetic action 6. Cardiac arrest 1:1000 contains 1 mg/mL, 1:10 000 contains 100 µg/mL, 1:200 000 contains 5 µg/mL	Arrhythmias, especially with halothane. Caution in elderly. Via central catheter whenever possible	Hypertension, tachycardia, anxiety, hyperglycaemia, arrhythmias. Reduces uterine blood flow	Indications: 1–3. IV/IM/IO 0.1 mL/kg of 1:10 000 (10 µg/kg). Infusion: 0.05–0.5 µg/kg/min 4. Nebulization 0.4 mL/kg (up to 5 mL) 1:1000 5. Max 2 µg/kg 6. 10 µg/kg; ⊕ see p. 130	Indications: 1–3. IV/IM/IO 1 mL aliquots of 1:10 000 up to 5–10 mL (0.5–1 mg). Infusion 2–20 µg/min (0.04–0.4 µg/kg/min) 4. Nebulization 5 mL 1:1000 5. Maximum dose for infiltration 2 µg/kg 6. 1 mg (10 mL of 1:10 000) every 3–5 min

(Adapted from the *Oxford Handbook of Anaesthesia*. Note: many drugs are unlicensed in children but are in routine use.)

Drug		Cautions/contraindications	Side effects		
Aminophylline	Methylxanthine bronchodilator used in prevention and treatment of asthma. Converted to theophylline, a phosphodiesterase inhibitor. Serum levels 10–20 mg/L (55–110 μmol/L).	Caution in patients already receiving oral or IV theophyllines. Where serum level known, aminophylline 0.6 mg/kg should increase level by 1 mg/L.	Palpitations, tachycardia, tachypnoea, seizures, nausea, arrhythmias	IV 5 mg/kg over 30 min, then infusion 0.5–1 mg/kg/h according to levels	5 mg/kg over 30 min, then infusion 0.5 mg/kg/h according to levels
Amiodarone	Mixed class 1C and III antiarrhythmic useful in treatment of supraventricular and ventricular arrhythmias	Via central catheter if not diluted to ≤2 mg/mL. Sinoatrial heart block, thyroid dysfunction, pregnancy, porphyria. Dilute in 5% dextrose (not saline)	Commonly causes thyroid dysfunction and reversible corneal deposits	>1y 5 mg/kg over 30 min, then 300 μg/kg/h to max 1.5 mg/kg/h. Maximum 1.2 g in 24 h. For defib resistant VF 5 mg/kg slow IV bolus	5 mg/kg over 20–120 min. Max 1.2 g in 24 h. 300 mg slow IV bolus for defib.-resistant VF
Atenolol	Cardioselective β-blocker: Long acting	Asthma, heart failure, AV block, verapamil treatment	Bradycardia, hypotension, and decreased contractility	0.05 mg/kg every 5 min—max. four doses	5–10 mg over 10 min. PO: 50 mg od
Atropine	Muscarinic acetylcholine antagonist. Vagal blockade at AV and sinus node increases heart rate (transient decrease at low doses due to weak agonist effect). Tertiary amine, therefore crosses blood–brain barrier	Obstructive uropathy and cardiovascular disease. Glaucoma, myasthenia gravis	Decreases secretions, and lowers oesophageal sphincter tone, relaxes bronchial smooth muscle. Confusion in elderly	IV: 10–20 μg/kg. Control of muscarinic effects of neostigmine: 10–20 μg/kg. IM/SC: 10–30 μg/kg. PO: 40 μg/kg	300–600 μg. Prevention of muscarinic effects of neostigmine: 600–1200 μg.

IV = intravenous. IM = intramuscular. SC = subcutaneous. PO = per os (oral). SL = sublingual. ET = endotracheal. od = once daily. bd = twice daily. tds = three times daily. qds = four times daily. NR = not recommended. Doses are intravenous and dilutions in 0.9% saline unless otherwise stated.

Drug	Description and perioperative indications	Cautions and contraindications	Side effects	Dose (paediatric)	Dose (adult)
Bicarbonate (sodium)	Alkaline salt used for correction of acidosis and to enhance onset of action of local anaesthetics. 8.4% = 1000 mmol/L. Dose (mmol) in acidosis: weight (kg) × base deficit × 0.3	Precipitation with calcium containing solutions, increased CO_2 production, necrosis on extravasation. Via central catheter if possible	Alkalosis, hypokalaemia, hypernatraemia, hypocalcaemia	1 mL/kg 8.4% solution (1 mmol/kg)	Dependent on degree of acidosis. Resuscitation: 50 mL of 8.4% then recheck blood gases
Calcium chloride	Electrolyte replacement, positive inotrope, hyperkalaemia, hypermagnesaemia. Calcium chloride 10% contains Ca 2+ 680 μmol/mL	Necrosis on extravasation. Incompatible with bicarbonate	Arrhythmias, hypertension, hypercalcaemia	0.1–0.2 mL/kg 10% solution	2–10 mL 10% solution (10 mg/kg, 0.07 mmol/kg)
Calcium gluconate	As calcium chloride. Calcium gluconate 10% contains Ca 2+ 225 μmol/mL	Less phlebitis than calcium chloride	As calcium chloride	0.3–0.5 mL/kg 10% solution (max. 20 mL)	6–15 mL of 10% solution (30 mg/kg, 0.07 mmol/kg)
Chlorpromazine	Phenothiazine, antipsychotic. Mild α-blocking action. Potent antiemetic and used for chronic hiccups	Hypotension	Extrapyramidal and anticholinergic symptoms, sedation, hypotension	IM/PO 0.5 mg/kg tds (1–6 y max 40 mg/d, 6–12 y max 75 mg/d)	IV: Up to 25 mg (at 1 mg/min diluted in saline to 1 mg/mL). Deep IM: 25–50 mg 6–8 hourly
Clomethiazole	Hypnotic sedative used in alcohol withdrawal and status epilepticus. IV preparation no longer available	Caution in elderly	Nasal congestion, confusion, phlebitis, hypotension, coma		PO: 1–2 capsules at night (192–384 mg)

Drug	Notes	Dose	Cautions	(extra)
Dantrolene	Direct-acting skeletal muscle relaxant used in treatment of malignant hyperthermia and neuroleptic malignant syndrome. 20 mg/vial—reconstitute in 60 mL warm water and give via blood set	Avoid combination with calcium channel blockers (verapamil) as may cause hyperkalaemia and cardiovascular collapse. Crosses placenta	Skeletal muscle weakness (22%), phlebitis (10%)	2.5 mg/kg, then 1 mg/kg repeated every 5 min to a maximum of 10 mg/kg	2.5 mg/kg, then 1 mg/kg repeated every 5 min to a maximum of 10 mg/kg.
Dexa-methasone	Prednisolone derivative corticosteroid. Less sodium retention than hydrocortisone. Cerebral oedema, oedema prevention, antiemetic	Interacts with anticholinesterase agents to increase weakness in myasthenia gravis	See Prednisolone	IV/IM/SC: 100–400 µg/kg bd. Cerebral oedema: see BNFc. Croup: 150 µg/kg + repeat at 12 h if needed. Antiemetic: 150 µg/kg (max 8 mg)	IV/IM/SC: 4–8 mg. Cerebral oedema: loading dose 10 mg then 4 mg qds reducing after 3 days (dexamethasone 0.75 mg = prednisolone 5 mg)
Diazepam	Long-acting benzodiazepine. Sedation or termination of status epilepticus. Alcohol withdrawal	Thrombophlebitis: emulsion (Diazemuls®) less irritant to veins	Sedation, circulatory depression	0.2–0.4 mg/kg. Rectal: 0.5 mg/kg as Stesolid® or may use IV preparation	PO/IV/IM 2–10 mg. repeat if required (max tds)

IV = intravenous. IM = intramuscular. SC = subcutaneous. PO = per os (oral). SL = sublingual. ET = endotracheal. od = once daily. bd = twice daily. tds = three times daily. qds = four times daily. NR = not recommended. Doses are intravenous and dilutions in 0.9% saline unless otherwise stated.

Drug	Description and perioperative indications	Cautions and contraindications	Side effects	Dose (paediatric)	Dose (adult)
Digoxin	Cardiac glycoside. Weak inotrope and control of ventricular response in supraventricular arrhythmia. Therapeutic levels 0.5–2 µg/L (1.2–2.6 nmol/L)	Reduce dose in elderly. Enhanced effect/toxicity in hypokalaemia. Avoid cardioversion in toxicity	Anorexia, nausea, fatigue, arrhythmias, blurred/yellow vision	Loading dose 10 µg/kg tds for 24 h	Rapid IV loading: 250–500 µg over 30 min. Maximum 1 mg/24 h. PO loading: 1–1.5 mg in divided doses over 24 h. PO maintenance: 125–250 µg/day
Dobutamine	β1-adrenergic agonist, positive inotrope and chronotrope. Cardiac failure	Arrhythmias and hypertension. Phlebitis, but can be administered peripherally	Tachycardia. Decreased peripheral and pulmonary vascular resistance	Infusion: 2–20 µg/kg/min	Infusion: 2.5–10 µg/kg/min
Dopamine	Naturally occurring catecholamine with α, β1, and dopaminergic activity. Inotropic agent	Via central catheter. Phaeochromocytoma (due to noradrenaline release)	Tachycardia, dysrhythmias	Infusion: 2–20 µg/kg/min	Infusion: 2–10 µg/kg/min
Dopexamine	Catecholamine with β2 and dopaminergic activity. Inotropic agent	Via central catheter. Phaeochromocytoma, hypokalaemia	Tachycardia	Infusion: 0.5–6 µg/kg/min	Infusion: 0.5–6 µg/kg/min

Drug	Description	Cautions	Side effects	Dose	Dose
Doxapram	Respiratory stimulant acting through carotid chemoreceptors and medulla. Duration 12 min	Epilepsy, airway obstruction, acute asthma, severe CVS disease	Risk of arrhythmia. Hypertension	1 mg/kg slowly	1–1.5 mg/kg over >30 s. Infusion: 2–4 mg/min
Enoximone	Type III phosphodiesterase inhibitor used in cardiac failure with increased filling pressures. Inodilator	Stenotic valvular disease, cardiomyopathy	Arrhythmias, hypotension, nausea	Loading dose 500 µg/kg, then infusion: 5–20 µg/kg/min	Infusion: 90 µg/kg/min for 10–30 min, then 5–20 µg/kg/min (max. 24 mg/kg/day)
Ephedrine	Direct and indirect sympathomimetic. Vasopressor; safe in pregnancy. Duration 10–60 min	Caution in elderly, hypertension and CVS disease. Tachyphylaxis. Avoid with MAOI	Tachycardia, hypertension		3–6 mg repeated (dilute 30 mg in 10 mL saline, 1 mL increments). IM: 30 mg
Ergometrine	Ergot alkaloid used to control uterine hypotony or bleeding (Syntometrine® = ergometrine 500 µg/mL and oxytocin 5 U/mL)	Severe cardiac disease or hypertension	Vasoconstriction, hypertension, vomiting		IM: 1 mL as Syntometrine®. Careful SLOW IV 250–500 µg with antiemetic cover

IV = intravenous. IM = intramuscular. SC = subcutaneous. PO = per os (oral). SL = sublingual. ET = endotracheal. od = once daily. bd = twice daily. tds = three times daily. qds = four times daily. NR = not recommended. Doses are intravenous and dilutions in 0.9% saline unless otherwise stated.

Drug	Description and perioperative indications	Cautions and contraindications	Side effects	Dose (paediatric)	Dose (adult)
Esmolol	Short-acting cardioselective β-blocker. Metabolized by red cell esterases. Treatment of supraventricular tachycardia or intraoperative hypertension. Duration 10 min	Asthma, heart failure, AV block, verapamil treatment	Hypotension, bradycardia. May prolong action of suxamethonium	SVT: 0.5 mg/kg over 1 min, then 50–200 µg/kg/min	SVT: 0.5 mg/kg over 1 min, then 50–200 µg/kg/min. Hypertension: 25–100 mg, then 50–300 µg/kg/min
Flumazenil	Benzodiazepine receptor antagonist. Duration 45–90 min	Benzodiazepine dependence (acute withdrawal), Re-sedation if long-acting benzodiazepine	Arrhythmia, seizures	10 µg/kg (max 200 µg), repeat if required (max 50 µg/kg). Infusion 2–10 µg/kg/h	200 µg then 100 µg at 60 s intervals (up to maximum 1 mg). Infusion: 100–400 µg/h
Fosphenytoin	Prodrug of phenytoin. Can be administered more rapidly. Dosages in phenytoin equivalents (PE): fosphenytoin 1.5 mg = phenytoin 1 mg	See phenytoin. Monitor ECG/BP. Infusion rate: 50–100 mg (PE)/min (status 100–150 mg (PE)/min)	See phenytoin	>5 y: 20 mg (PE)/kg then 4–5 mg (PE)/kg daily. Infusion rate: 1–2 mg (PE)/kg/min	Infusion: 10–15 mg (PE)/kg then 4–5 mg (PE)/kg daily. Status: 20 mg (PE)/ kg. Can also be administered IM
Furosemide (frusemide)	Loop diuretic used in treatment of hypertension, congestive cardiac failure, renal failure, fluid overload		Hypotension, tinnitus, ototoxicity, hypokalaemia	0.5–1.5 mg/kg bd	10–40 mg slowly IV

Glucagon	Polypeptide hormone used in treatment of hypoglycaemia and overdose of β-blocker. Hyperglycaemic action lasts 10–30 min. 1 unit = 1 mg.	Glucose must be administered as soon as possible. Phaeochromocytoma	Hypertension, hypotension, nausea, vomiting	<25 kg 0.5 U (0.5 mg). >25 kg 1 U (1 mg). β blocker overdose 50–150 µg/kg (max 10 mg) followed by infusion 50 µg/kg/h in 5% glucose	SC/IM/IV: 1 U (1 mg). β-Blocker overdose 2–10 mg followed by infusion 50 µg/kg/h in 5% glucose
Glucose	Treatment of hypoglycaemia in unconscious patient	50% solution irritant; therefore, dilute to 20% or weaker before use		5 mL/kg of glucose 10%, repeated, and infusion if needed	25–50 g glucose (e.g. 125–250 mL 20% glucose)
Glyceryl trinitrate	Organic nitrate vasodilator: Controlled hypotension, angina, congestive cardiac failure	Remove patches before defibrillation to avoid electrical arcing	Tachycardia, hypotension, headache, nausea, flushing, methaemoglobinaemia	0.2–10 µg/kg/min; (Usually 1–3 µg/kg/min)	Infusion: 0.5–10 mg/h. SL tabs: 0.3–1 mg prn. SL spray: 400 µg prn. Patch: 5–10 mg/24 h
Glyco-pyrronium bromide	Quaternary ammonium anticholinergic agent. Bradycardia, blockade of muscarinic effects of anticholinesterases, antisialogogue	Caution in glaucoma, cardiovascular disease. Unlike atropine does not cross blood–brain barrier	Paradoxical bradycardia in small doses. Reduces lower oesophageal sphincter tone	4–10 µg/kg	200–400 µg. Control of muscarinic effects of neostigmine: 200 µg for each 1 mg neostigmine

IV = intravenous. IM = intramuscular. SC = subcutaneous. PO = per os (oral). SL = sublingual. ET = endotracheal. od = once daily. bd = twice daily. tds = three times daily. qds = four times daily. NR = not recommended. Doses are intravenous and dilutions in 0.9% saline unless otherwise stated.

Drug	Description and perioperative indications	Cautions and contraindications	Side effects	Dose (paediatric)	Dose (adult)
Haloperidol	Butyrophenone derivative antipsychotic. Useful antiemetic	Neuroleptic malignant syndrome	Extrapyramidal reactions	NR	IM/IV: 2–10 mg 4–8 hourly (max. 18 mg/day) Antiemetic: 0.5–2 mg IV. PO 0.5–3 mg
Hyaluronidase	Enzyme used to enhance permeation of injected fluids or local anaesthetics. Treatment of extravasation. Hypodermoclysis: 1500 U/L	Not for intravenous administration	Occasional severe allergy	Local anaesthetic: 15 U/ mL	Ophthalmology: 10–15 U/mL local. Extravasation: 1500 U in 1 mL saline infiltrated to affected area
Hydralazine	Direct-acting arteriolar vasodilator used to control arterial pressure. Duration 2–4 h	Higher doses required in rapid acetylators. SLE	Increased heart rate, cardiac output, stroke volume	0.1–0.5 mg/kg 4- to 6-hourly	5 mg every 5 min to a maximum of 20 mg
Hydro-cortisone (cortisol)	Endogenous steroid with anti-inflammatory and potent mineralocorticoid action (steroid of choice in replacement therapy—active form of cortisone). Treatment of allergy	(Hydrocortisone 20 mg = prednisolone 5 mg)	Hyperglycaemia, hypertension, psychic disturbance, muscle weakness, fluid retention	4 mg/kg then 2–4 mg/kg qds	IV/IM: 50–200 mg qds. Adrenal suppression and surgery: 25 mg at induction then 25 mg qds. PO: 10–30 mg/day

Drug	Description	Caution	Side effects	Dose
Imipenem	Carbapenem broad-spectrum antibiotic. Administered with cilastatin to reduce renal metabolism	Caution in renal failure and pregnancy	Nausea, vomiting, diarrhoea, convulsions, thrombophlebitis	>3 months: 15 mg/kg over 30 min qds (25 mg/kg severe infections). Slow IV (1 h): 250–500 mg qds. Surgical prophylaxis: 1 g at induction, repeated after 3 h
Insulin (soluble)	Human soluble pancreatic hormone facilitating intracellular transport of glucose and anabolism. Diabetes mellitus, ketoacidosis, and hyperkalaemia (→ see p. 248)	Monitor blood glucose and serum potassium. Store at 2–8°C	Hypoglycaemia, hypokalaemia	Ketoacidosis: 0.1–0.2 U/kg (max 20 U) then 0.1 U/kg/h (max 5–10 U/h). Ketoacidosis: 10–20 U then 5–10 U/h. Sliding scale → see pp. 276–277). Hyperkalaemia → see p. 313)
Intralipid®	Intralipid 20% lipid emulsion used in the treatment of severe LA toxicity (→ see p. 248)	Continue CPR throughout treatment. Propofol is NOT a suitable substitute		1.5 mL/kg bolus followed by 15 mL/kg/h. Initial bolus: 1.5 mL/kg (100 mL for 70 kg man). Repeat twice at 5 min intervals if necessary. Infusion: 0.25 mL/kg/min (approx. 1 L/h for 70 kg man). Double rate after 5 min

IV = intravenous. IM = intramuscular. SC = subcutaneous. PO = per os (oral). SL = sublingual. ET = endotracheal. od = once daily. bd = twice daily. tds = three times daily. qds = four times daily. NR = not recommended. Doses are intravenous and dilutions in 0.9% saline unless otherwise stated.

Drug	Description and perioperative indications	Cautions and contraindications	Side effects	Dose (paediatric)	Dose (adult)
Isoprenaline	Synthetic catecholamine with potent β-adrenergic agonist activity. Emergency treatment of heart block or bradycardia unresponsive to atropine. β-Blocker overdose	Ischaemic heart disease, hyperthyroidism, diabetes mellitus MHRA: NR unless special requirements	Tachycardia, arrhythmias, sweating, tremor	Bolus: 5 μg/kg. Infusion: 0.02–1 μg/kg/min	Infusion: 0.5–10 μg/min (2 mg in 500 mL 5% glucose at 7–150 mL/h or 1 mg in 50 mL at 1.5–30 mL/h)
Ketamine	Phencyclidine derivative producing dissociative anaesthesia. Induction/maintenance of anaesthesia in high risk or hypovolaemic patients	Emergence delirium reduced by benzodiazepines. Caution in hypertension. Control excess salivation with antimuscarinic agent	Bronchodilatation. Increased ICP, blood pressure, uterine tone, salivation. Respiratory depression if given rapidly	Induction: 1–2 mg/kg IV, 5–10 mg/kg IM. Infusion: 1–3 mg/kg/h	Induction: 1–2 mg/kg IV. Infusion: 1–3 mg/kg/h (analgesia only 0.25 mg/kg/h)
Labetalol	Combined α- (mild) and β-adrenergic receptor antagonist. Blood pressure control without reflex tachycardia. Duration 2–4 h	Asthma, heart failure, AV block, verapamil treatment	Hypotension, bradycardia, bronchospasm, liver damage	1 month–12 y 0.25–0.5 mg/kg; max 20 mg; 12–18 y 50 mg over 1 min, repeated after 5 min; max 200 mg	5 mg increments up to 100 mg. Infusion: 20–160 mg/h (in glucose). 2 mg/min for thoracic aortic dissection

Lorazepam	Benzodiazepine:	Decreased requirement for anaesthetic agents. Reduce dose in older people	Respiratory depression in combination with opioids. Amnesia	Status: 0.1 mg/kg; max 4 mg	1. PO: 1–4 mg 1–2 h preop. IV/IM:
	1. Sedation or premedication.				1.5–2.5 mg
	2. Status epilepticus.				2. Status: 4 mg IV. Repeat after 10 min if necessary
	Duration 6–10 h				
Lormeta-zepam	Benzodiazepine hypnotic sedative premed.	Decreased requirement for anaesthetic agents	Respiratory depression in combination with opioids. Amnesia	NR	0.5–1.5 mg 1–2 h preop. (elderly 0.5 mg)
Magnesium sulphate	Essential mineral used to treat:	Potentiates muscle relaxants. Monitoring of serum level essential during treatment. Myasthenia and muscular dystrophy. Heart block	CNS depression, hypotension, muscle weakness.	1. Hypomagnesaemia 0.2–0.4 mmol/kg (max 20 mmol/d). Check levels.	1. Hypomagnesaemia: 2 g over 10 min IV then 1 g/h. Check levels.
	1. Hypomagnesaemia			2. Arrhythmias 25– 50 mg/kg over 10min (max 2 g).	2+4. Arrhythmias and asthma: 2 g (8 mmol) over 10 min IV. Repeated.
	2. Arrhythmias			4. Asthma 40 mg/kg IV over 20 min (max 2 g)	3. Eclampsia: 4 g (16 mmol) over 10 min then 1 g/h for 24 h (☺ see p. 169)
	3. Eclamptic seizures				
	4. Severe asthma				
	(MgSO4 1 g = 4 mmol)				

IV = intravenous. IM = intramuscular. SC = subcutaneous. PO = per os (oral). SL = sublingual. ET = endotracheal. od = once daily. bd = twice daily. tds = three times daily, qds = four times daily. NR = not recommended. Doses are intravenous and dilutions in 0.9% saline unless otherwise stated.

Drug	Description and perioperative indications	Cautions and contraindications	Side effects	Dose (paediatric)	Dose (adult)
Mannitol	Osmotic diuretic used for renal protection and reduction of intracranial pressure. 20% solution = 20 g/100 mL	Extracellular volume expansion, especially in severe renal or cardiovascular disease	Diuresis, ARF, hypertonicity	0.25–1.5 g/kg	0.25–2 g/kg (typically 0.5 g/kg = 2.5 mL/kg of 20% solution)
Metaraminol	Potent direct/indirect acting α-adrenergic sympathomimetic. Treatment of hypotension. Duration 20–60 min	MAOIs, pregnancy. Caution in elderly and hypertensives. Extravasation can cause necrosis	Hypertension, reflex bradycardia, arrhythmias, decreased renal and placental perfusion	10 μg/kg then 0.1–1 μg/kg/min, >12 y	0.25–2 mg. Dilute 10 mg in 20 mL saline and give 0.5–1 mL increments (increase dilution in elderly)
Methyl-thioninium chloride (Methylene blue)	1. Treatment of methaemoglobinaemia. 2. Ureteric identification during surgery (renally excreted). 3. Identification of parathyroid glands and sentinel nodes during surgery	G-6-PD deficiency. Blue colouration causes acute changes in pulse oximetry readings	Tachycardia, nausea, stains skin	1 mg/kg slow IV (max 7 mg/kg)	1 mg/kg slow IV (max 7 mg/kg)
Metoprolol	Cardioselective β-blocker	Asthma, heart failure, AV block, verapamil treatment	Causes bradycardia, hypotension, and decreased cardiac contractility	1–5 mg IV over 10 min, repeat if required (max 15 mg)	

Drug	Notes	Side effects	Cautions	Dose (child)	Dose (adult)
Midazolam	Short-acting benzodiazepine. Sedative, anxiolytic, amnesic, anticonvulsant. Duration 20–60 min. Oral administration of IV preparation effective though larger dose required	Hypotension, respiratory depression, apnoea	Reduce dose in elderly (very sensitive)	Sedation: IV 25–50 µg/kg, repeated (max 6 mg under 6 y; max 10 mg over 6 y); PO: 0.5 mg/kg use IV preparation in orange juice (max 20 mg). Buccal 0.2 mg/kg, (6 months–10 y; max 5 mg; >10 y, 6–8 mg)	Sedation: 0.5–7.5 mg, titrate to effect. PO: 0.5 mg/kg (use IV preparation in orange squash). IM: 2.5–10 mg (0.1 mg/kg)
Milrinone	Selective phosphodiesterase inhibitor used in cardiac failure with increased filling pressures. Inodilator used after cardiac surgery	Arrhythmias, hypotension, nausea	Stenotic valvular disease, cardiomyopathy	50 µg/kg over 30–60 min, then 0.375–0.75 µg/kg/min. Maximum 1.13 mg/kg/day	50 µg/kg over 10 min, then 0.375–0.75 µg/kg/ min. Maximum 1.13 mg/ kg/day
Naloxone	Pure opioid antagonist. Can be used in low doses to reverse pruritus associated with epidural opiates and as depot IM injection in newborn of mothers given opioids	Arrhythmias, pulmonary oedema	Beware re-narcotization if reversing long-acting opioid. Caution in opioid addicts—may precipitate acute withdrawal. Duration of action 30 min	5–10 µg/kg. Infusion: 5–20 µg/kg/h. IM depot in newborn: 200 µg. Pruritus: 0.5 µg/kg	200–400 µg titrated to desired effect. Treatment of opioid/epidural pruritus: 100 µg bolus plus 300 µg added to IV fluids

IV = intravenous. IM = intramuscular. SC = subcutaneous. PO = per os (oral). SL = sublingual. ET = endotracheal. od = once daily. bd = twice daily. tds = three times daily. qds = four times daily. NR = not recommended. Doses are intravenous and dilutions in 0.9% saline unless otherwise stated.

Drug	Description and perioperative indications	Cautions and contraindications	Side effects	Dose (paediatric)	Dose (adult)
Neostigmine	Anticholinesterase used for: 1. Reversal of non-depolarizing muscle relaxant. 2. Treatment of myasthenia gravis. Duration 60 min IV (2–4 h PO)	Administer with antimuscarinic agent	Bradycardia, nausea excessive salivation (muscarinic effects)	50 µg/kg with atropine 20 µg/kg or glycopyrronium 10 µg/kg (see next)	1. 50–70 µg/kg (max. 5 mg) with atropine 10–20 µg/kg or glycopyrronium 10–15 µg/kg. 2. PO: 15–30 mg at suitable intervals
Neostigmine and glycopyrronium	Combination of neostigmine metilsulfate (2.5 mg) and glycopyrronium (500 µg) per 1 mL	See Neostigmine	See Neostigmine	0.02 mL/kg (dilute 1 mL with 4 mL saline, give 0.1 mL/kg). Max 2 mL (of neat)	1 mL over 30 s: repeated once if necessary
Nimodipine	Calcium channel blocker used to prevent vascular spasm after subarachnoid haemorrhage	Via central catheter. Cerebral oedema, raised intracranial pressure, grapefruit juice. Incompatible with PVC (adsorbed)	Hypotension, flushing, headache	Infusion: 15–30µg/kg/ h; max 2 mg/h	PO: 60 mg 4-hourly (maximum 360 mg/ day). Infusion: 1 mg/h increasing after 2 h to 2 mg/h
Nitroprusside (sodium— SNP)	Nitric oxide generating potent peripheral vasodilator. Controlled hypotension	Protect solution from light. Metabolism yields cyanide which is then converted to thiocyanate	Methaemo-globinaemia, hypotension, tachycardia. Cyanide causes tachycardia, sweating, acidosis	Infusion: 0.5–8 µg/kg/ min. (Maximum 4 µg/ kg/ min >24 h)	Infusion: 0.5–1.5 µg/kg/ min slowly increased to 8 µg/kg/min. Maximum dose: 1.5 mg/kg (acutely)

Drug	Description	Notes	Side effects	Dose	Dose
Noradrenaline	Potent catecholamine α adrenergic agonist. Vasoconstriction	Via central catheter only. Potentiated by MAOI and TCA	Reflex bradycardia, arrhythmia, hypertension	Infusion: 0.02–1 µg/kg/min	Infusion: 2–20 µg/min (0.04–0.4 µg/kg/min)
Octreotide	Somatostatin analogue used in treatment of carcinoid, acromegaly, and variceal bleeding (unlicensed use)	Pituitary tumour expansion, reduced need for antidiabetic treatments	GI disturbance, gallstones, hyper- and hypoglycaemia	SC: 1–5 µg/kg 6–8 hourly	SC: 50 µg od/bd increased up to 200 µg tds. IV: 50 µg diluted in saline (ECG monitoring)
Oxytocin	Non-apeptide hormone which stimulates uterine contraction. Induction of labour and prevention of postpartum haemorrhage	Avoid rapid administration. Fetal distress	Vasodilatation, hypotension, flushing, tachycardia		Postpartum slow IV: 5 U, followed if required by infusion 10 U/h (e.g. 40 U in 40 mL 0.9% saline)
Paraldehyde	Status epilepticus	Dilute neat solution with equal volume of olive oil for PR (or use 50:50 premixed)		PR: 0.8 mL/kg of 50:50 mix	Deep IM: 5–10 mL (neat). PR: 20–40 mL (of premix)
Phentolamine	α1- and α2-adrenergic antagonist. Peripheral vasodilatation and controlled hypotension. Treatment of extravasation. Duration 10 min	Treat excessive hypotension with noradrenaline or methoxamine (not adrenaline/ephedrine due to β-effects)	Hypotension, tachycardia, flushing	50–100 µg/kg then 5–50 µg/kg/min	2–5 mg (10 mg in 10 mL saline, 1 mL aliquots)

IV = intravenous. IM = intramuscular. SC = subcutaneous. PO = per os (oral). SL = sublingual. ET = endotracheal. od = once daily. bd = twice daily. tds = three times daily. qds = four times daily. NR = not recommended. Doses are intravenous and dilutions in 0.9% saline unless otherwise stated.

Drug	Description and perioperative indications	Cautions and contraindications	Side effects	Dose (paediatric)	Dose (adult)
Phenylephrine	Selective direct-acting α-adrenergic agonist. Peripheral vasoconstriction and treatment of hypotension. Duration 20 min	Caution in elderly or cardiovascular disease. Hyperthyroidism	Reflex bradycardia, arrhythmias	2–20 µg/kg (max 500µg) repeated as required. Then 0.1–0.5 µg/kg/min	20–100 µg increments (10 mg in 500 mL saline, 1 mL aliquots). IM: 2–5 mg. Infusion: 30–60 µg/min (5 mg in 50 mL saline at 0–30 mL/h)
Phenytoin	Anticonvulsant and treatment of digoxin toxicity. Serum levels 10–20 mg/L (40–80 µmol/L)	Avoid in AV heart Block, porphyria, and pregnancy. Monitor ECG/BP.	Hypotension, AV conduction defects, ataxia. Enzyme induction	IV Loading dose: 20 mg/kg over 1 h	20 mg/kg (max 2 g) over 1 h (dilute to 10 mg/mL in saline), then 100 mg tds. Arrhythmia: 3.5–5 mg/kg (rate <50 mg/min)
Potassium chloride	Electrolyte replacement (⮑ see p. 315)	Dilute solution before administration	Rapid infusion can cause cardiac arrest. High concentration causes phlebitis	0.5 mmol/kg over 2–3 h. Maintenance: 1–2 mmol/kg/day	10–20 mmol/h (max. concentration 40 mmol/L peripherally). With ECG monitoring: up to 20–40 mmol/h via central line (max. 200 mmol/day)

Prednisolone	Orally active corticosteroid. Less mineralocorticoid action than hydrocortisone	Adrenal suppression, severe systemic infections	Dyspepsia and ulceration, osteoporosis, myopathy, psychosis, impaired healing, diabetes mellitus	PO: 1–2 mg/kg od. Croup: 1–2 mg/kg, may require repeat dose after 12 h	PO: 10–60 mg od, reduced to 2.5–15 mg od
Procyclidine	Antimuscarinic used in acute treatment of drug-induced dystonic reactions (except tardive dyskinesia)	Glaucoma, gastrointestinal obstruction. Reduce dose in older people	Urinary retention, dry mouth, blurred vision	IV: <2 y: 0.5–2 mg, 2–10 y: 2–5 mg	IV: 5 mg. IM: 5–10 mg repeat after 20 min if needed
Promethazine	Phenothiazine, antihistamine, anticholinergic, antiemetic sedative. Paediatric sedation		Extrapyramidal reactions	>2 y. Sedation/ premed PO: 0.5–2 mg/kg	PO: 10–20 mg tds Deep IM: 25–50 mg
Propranolol	Non-selective β-adrenergic antagonist. Controlled hypotension. Control of symptoms in hyperthyroidism	Asthma, heart failure, AV block, verapamil treatment	Bradycardia, hypotension, AV block, bronchospasm	IV 20–50 µg/kg over 5–10 min 6–8 hourly	IV 1 mg increments up to 5–10 mg
Protamine	Basic protein produced from salmon sperm. Heparin antagonist	Weakly anticoagulant and marked histamine release. Risk of allergy	Severe hypotension, pulmonary hypertension, bronchospasm, flushing	Slow IV: 1 mg per 1 mg heparin (100 U) to be reversed	Slow IV: 1 mg per 1 mg heparin (100 U) to be reversed

IV = intravenous. IM = intramuscular. SC = subcutaneous. PO = per os (oral). SL = sublingual. ET = endotracheal. od = once daily. bd = twice daily. tds = three times daily. qds = four times daily. NR = not recommended. Doses are intravenous and dilutions in 0.9% saline unless otherwise stated.

Drug	Description and perioperative indications	Cautions and contraindications	Side effects	Dose (paediatric)	Dose (adult)
Remifentanil	Ultra short-acting opioid used to supplement GA. Metabolized by non-specific esterases not plasma		Muscle rigidity, respiratory depression, hypotension, bradycardia	Slow bolus: up to 1 µg/kg. Infusion (IPPV): 0.1–0.5 µg/kg/kg/min. Infusion (SV): 0.025–0.1 µg/kg/min	Slow bolus: up to 1 µg/kg. Infusion (IPPV): 0.1–0.5 µg/kg/min. Infusion (SV): 0.025–0.1 µg/kg/min
Salbutamol	β2-receptor agonist. Treatment of bronchospasm	Can cause hypokalaemia. Monitor potassium levels with higher doses	Tremor, vasodilatation, tachycardia	Slow IV: 1month–2 y 5 µg/kg, >2 y 15 µg/kg (max. 250 µg). Infusion: 1–5 µg/kg/min. Nebulizer: <5 y 2.5 mg, >5 y 5 mg	250 µg slow IV then 5 µg/min (up to 20 µg/min). Nebulizer: 2.5–5 mg prn
Sugammadex	Specific cyclodextrin reversal agent for rocuronium and vecuronium	Wait 24 h after use before using rocuronium or vecuronium in patient; Fusidic acid or flucloxacillin may displace relaxant from sugammadex within 6 h	Binds with contraceptive pill	TOF T2 present: 2 mg/kg. Full reversal NR at present	TOF T2 present: 2 mg/kg. To reverse full dose of rocuronium/vecuronium immediately: 16 mg/kg
Suxamethonium	Depolarizing muscle relaxant. Rapid short-acting muscle paralysis. Phase II block develops with repeated doses (>8 mg/kg). Store at 2–8°C	Prolonged block in plasma cholinesterase deficiency, hypokalaemia, hypocalcaemia. Malignant hyperthermia, myopathies	Increased intraocular pressure. Bradycardia with 2nd dose. Increased serum potassium (normally 0.5 mmol/L—greater in burns, trauma, upper motor neuron injury). Bradycardia with second dose	IV: 1–2 mg/kg IM: 3–4 mg/kg	1–1.5 mg/kg. Infusion: 0.5–10 mg/min

Drug	Description	Caution	Side effects	Dose (neonate/child)	Dose (adult)
Thiopental	Short-acting thiobarbiturate. Induction of anaesthesia, anticonvulsant, cerebral protection. Recovery due to redistribution	Accumulation with repeated doses. Caution in hypovolaemia and elderly. Porphyria	Hypotension Necrosis if intra-arterial	Induction: neonate: 2–4 mg/kg child: 3–6 mg/kg. Status: 2–4 mg/kg then 8 mg/kg/h	Induction/cerebral protection: 3–5 mg/kg. Anticonvulsant: 0.5–2 mg/kg prn
Tranexamic acid	Inhibits plasminogen activation reducing fibrin dissolution by plasmin. Reduced haemorrhage in prostatectomy, major trauma, or dental extraction	Avoid in thromboembolic disease, renal impairment and pregnancy	Dizziness, nausea	Slow IV: 10–15 mg/kg tds. PO: 10–25 mg/kg tds	Slow IV: 0.5–1 g tds. PO: 15–25 mg/kg tds. Trauma: 1 g IV over 10 min, then 1 g over 8 h
Vasopressin	ADH used in treatment of diabetes insipidus, resistant vasodilatory shock, variceal bleeding	Extreme caution in coronary vascular disease	Pallor, coronary vasoconstriction, water intoxication	Diabetes insipidus SC/IM: <12 y, 0.1–0.4 µg/d. >12 y 1–4 µg/d.	Diabetes insipidus SC/IM: 5–20 U 4-hourly. Septic shock infusion: 1–4 U/h. Variceal bleed: 20 U over 15 min

IV = intravenous. IM = intramuscular. SC = subcutaneous. PO = per os (oral). SL = sublingual. ET = endotracheal. od = once daily. bd = twice daily. tds = three times daily. qds = four times daily. NR = not recommended. Doses are intravenous and dilutions in 0.9% saline unless otherwise stated.

Infusion regimens

Drug	Indication	Diluent	Dose	Suggested regimen (60 kg adult)	Infusion range	Initial rate (adult)	Comments
Adrenaline	Treatment of hypotension, resistant bronchospasm, anaphylaxis	0.9% saline, 5% glucose	2–20 µg/min (0.04–0.4 µg/kg/min)	5 mg/50 mL (100 µg/mL)	1.2–12+ mL/h	5 mL/h	Via central catheter. Suggest 1 mg/50 mL for initial intraoperative use (or 1 mg/500 mL if no central access)
Aminophylline	Bronchodilatation	0.9% saline, 5% glucose	0.5 mg/kg/h	250 mg/50 mL (5 mg/mL)	0–6 mL/h	6 mL/h	After 5 mg/kg IV loading (over 30 min)
Amiodarone	Treatment of arrhythmias	5% glucose only	Loading infusion 5 mg/kg over 20–120 min, then 900 mg over 24 h	300 mg/50 mL (6 mg/mL)	25–50 mL/h then 6 mL/h	25 mL/h	Via central line. Can be given peripherally if ≤2 mg/mL or in extremis. Maximum 1.2 g in 24 h
Bicarbonate (sodium)	Acidosis	Undiluted (8.4% solution)	(weight (kg) × base deficit × 0.3) mmol				8.4% = 1000 mmol/L. Via central line if possible
Digoxin	Rapid control of ventricular rate	0.9% saline, 5% glucose	250–500 µg over 30–60 min. 0.75–1 mg over 2h	250–500 µg/50 mL	0–100 mL/h	50 mL/h	ECG monitoring

Drug	Indication	Diluent	Dose	Concentration	Rate	Rate	Notes
Dobutamine	Cardiac failure/inotrope	0.9% saline, 5% glucose	2.5–10 µg/kg/min	250 mg/50 mL (5 mg/mL)	2–7 mL/h	2 mL/h	May be given via large peripheral vein
Dopamine	Inotrope	0.9% saline, 5% glucose	2–10 µg/kg/min	200 mg/50 mL (4 mg/mL)	2–9 mL/h	2 mL/h	Via central line
Dopexamine	Inotrope	0.9% saline, 5% glucose	0.5–6 µg/kg/min	50 mg/50 mL (1 mg/mL)	2–22 mL/h	2 mL/h	May be given via large peripheral vein
Doxapram	Respiratory stimulant	0.9% saline, 5% glucose	2–4 mg/min	200 mg/50 mL (4 mg/mL)	30–60 mL/h	30 mL/h	Maximum dose 4 mg/kg
Enoximone	Inodilator	0.9% saline only	90 µg/kg/min for 10–30 min, then 5–20 µg/kg/min	100 mg/50 mL (2 mg/mL)	9–36 mL/h	162 mL/h for 10–30 min	Max. 24 mg/kg/day
Esmolol	β-blocker	0.9% saline, 5% glucose	50–200 µg/kg/min	2.5 g/50 mL (50 mg/mL)	3–15 mL/h	3 mL/h	ECG monitoring
Glyceryl trinitrate	Myocardial ischaemia or controlled hypotension	0.9% saline, 5% glucose	0.5–12 mg/h	50 mg/50 mL (1 mg/mL)	0.5–12 mL/h	5 mL/h	
Heparin (unfractionated)	Anticoagulation	0.9% saline, 5% glucose	24 000–48 000 U per 24 h	50 000 U/50 mL (1000 U/mL)	1–2 mL/h	2 mL/h	Check APTT after 12 h. See local guidelines

Alternative regimens for any infusion: 3 mg/kg/50 mL then 1 mL/h = 1 µg/kg/min 3 mg/50 mL then 1 mL/h = 1 µg/min

Drug	Indication	Diluent	Dose	Suggested regimen (60 kg adult)	Infusion range	Initial rate (adult)	Comments
Insulin (soluble)	Diabetes mellitus	0.9% saline	Sliding scale	50 U/50 mL (1 U/mL)	Sliding scale	Sliding scale	
Isoprenaline	Treatment of heart block or bradycardia	0.9% saline, 5% glucose	0.5–10 µg/min	1 mg/50 mL (20 µg/mL)	1.5–30 mL/h	7 mL/h	
Ketamine	General anaesthesia	0.9% saline, 5% glucose	1–3 mg/kg/h	500 mg/50 mL (10 mg/mL)	6–18 mL/h	10 mL/h	Induction 0.5–2 mg/kg
Ketamine	'Trauma' mixture	0.9% saline	0.5 mL/kg/h	50 mL mixture (4 mg/mL ketamine)	15–45 mL/h	30 mL/h	200 mg ketamine + 10 mg midazolam + 10 mg vecuronium in 50 mL
Lidocaine	Ventricular arrhythmias	0.9% saline	4 mg/min for 30 min, 2 mg/min for 2 h, then 1 mg/min for 24 h	500 mg/50 mL (10 mg/mL = 1%)	6–24 mL/h	24 mL/h	After 50–100 mg slow IV bolus. ECG monitoring
Milrinone	Inodilator	0.9% saline, 5% glucose	50 µg/kg over 10 min, then 0.375–0.75 µg/kg/min	10 mg/50 mL (0.2 mg/mL)	7–14 mL/h	90 mL/h for 10 min	Maximum 1.13 mg/kg/day
Naloxone	Opioid antagonist	0.9% saline, 5% glucose	>1 µg/kg/h	2 mg/500 mL (4 µg/mL)		100 mL/h	Rate adjusted according to response

	Indication	Diluent	Dose	Concentration	Rate		Notes
Nimodipine	Prevention of vasospasm after SAH	0.9% saline, 5% glucose	1 mg/h increasing to 2 mg/h after 2 h	Undiluted (0.2 mg/mL)	5–10 mL/h	5 mL/h	Via central line. Incompatible with polyvinyl chloride
Nitroprusside (sodium)	Controlled hypotension	5% glucose	0.3–1.5 µg/kg/min	25 mg/50 mL (500 µg/mL)	2–10 mL	5 mL/h	Maximum dose 1.5 mg/kg. Protect from light
Noradrenaline	Treatment of hypotension	5% glucose	2–20 µg/min (0.04–0.4 µg/kg/min)	4 mg/40 mL (100 µg/mL)	1.2–12+ mL/h	5 mL/h	Via central line
Octreotide	Somatostatin analogue	0.9% saline	25–50 µg/h	500 µg/50 mL (10 µg/mL)	2–5 mL/h	5 mL/h	Use in variceal bleeding, unlicensed
Oxytocin	Prevention of uterine atony	0.9% saline, 5% glucose	0.02–0.125 U/min (10 U/h)	30 U in 500 mL (0.06 U/mL)	30–125 mL/h	125 mL/h	Individual unit protocols vary
Phenytoin	Anticonvulsant	0.9% saline	20 mg/kg	1000 mg/100 mL (administer through 0.22–0.5 µm filter)	Up to 50 mg/min	200 mL/h	ECG and BP monitoring. Complete within 1 h of preparation
Salbutamol	Bronchospasm	5% glucose	5–20 µg/min	1 mg/50 mL (20 µg/mL)	15–60 mL/h	30 mL/h	After 250 µg slow IV bolus

Alternative regimens for any infusion: 3 mg/kg/50 mL then 1 mL/h = 1 µg/kg/min 3 mg/50 mL then 1 mL/h = 1 µg/min

Reproduced from Allman, KG. and Wilson, I. ed. (2016). *Oxford Handbook of Anaesthesia*, 4th ed. Oxford: Oxford University Press. Reproduced with permission of the Licensor through PLSclear.

Index

Notes Tables, figures and boxes are indicated by *t*, *f* and *b* following the page number *vs.* indicates a differential diagnosis or comparison Abbreviations used can be found in the tables on pages (xiii) to (xvii)